CEDAR MILL
COMMUNITY LIBRARY
12505 NW CORNELL RD.
PORTLAND, OR 97229
503-644-0043

WITHDRAWN
CEDAR MILL LIBRARY

D0957634

Herbal Goddess

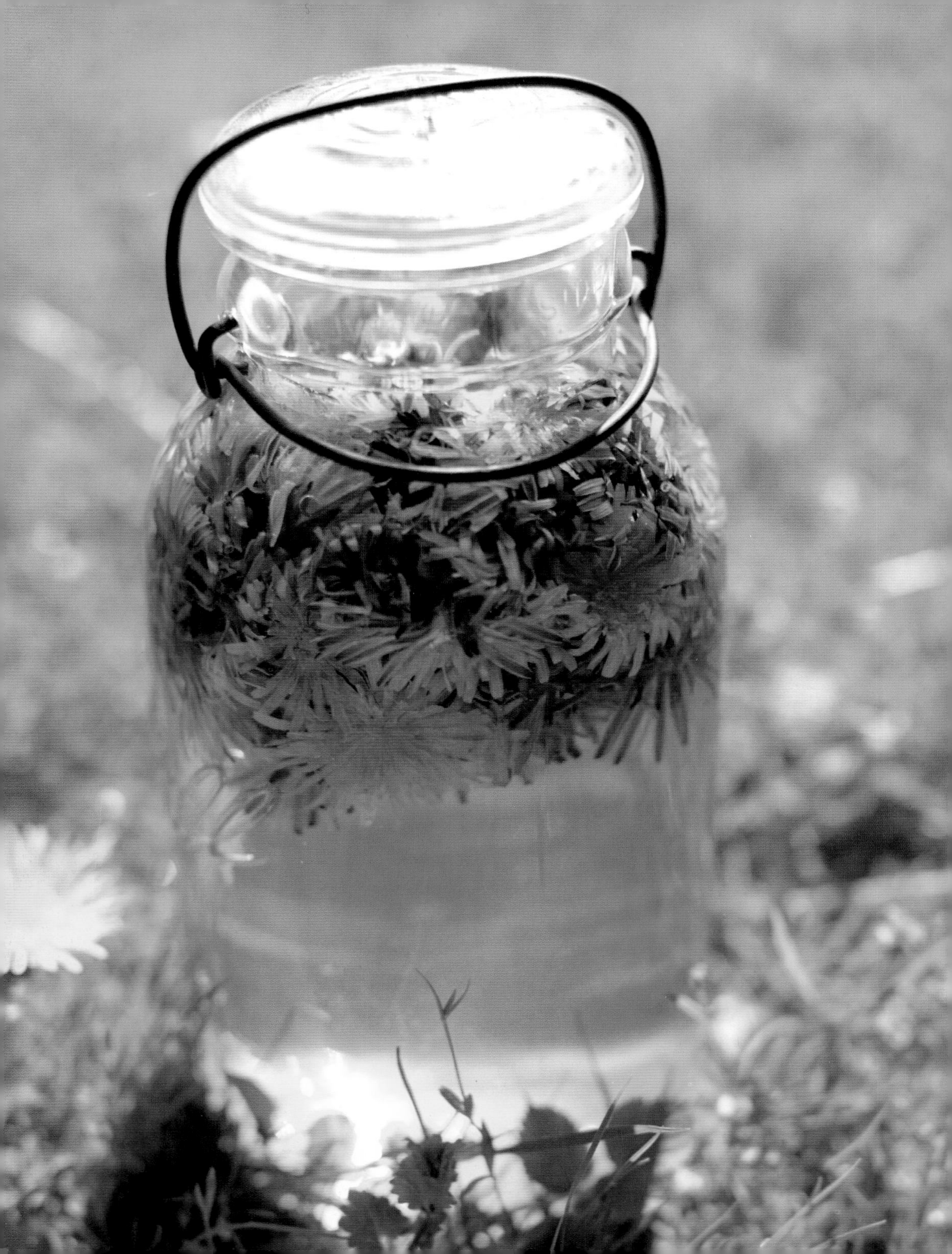

Herbal Goddess

discover the amazing spirit of 12 healing herbs with teas, potions, salves, food, yoga, and more

Amy Jirsa

photographs by
Winnie Au

Storey Publishing

The mission of Storey Publishing is to serve our customers by publishing practical information that encourages personal independence in harmony with the environment.

EDITED BY Sarah Guare and Deborah Balmuth
ART DIRECTION AND BOOK DESIGN BY Carolyn Eckert
TEXT PRODUCTION BY Jennifer Jepson Smith
INDEXED BY Samantha Miller

COVER AND INTERIOR PHOTOGRAPHY BY © Winnie Au, except for those credited on page 256.
PHOTOGRAPHY STYLING BY Sally Staub

© 2015 by Amy Jirsa

The publisher would like to thank Ward's Nursery (wardsnursery.com) for supplying plants and pots for the photo shoot.

All rights reserved. No part of this book may be reproduced without written permission from the publisher, except by a reviewer who may quote brief passages or reproduce illustrations in a review with appropriate credits; nor may any part of this book be reproduced, stored in a retrieval system, or transmitted in any form or by any means — electronic, mechanical, photocopying, recording, or other — without written permission from the publisher.

The information in this book is true and complete to the best of our knowledge. All recommendations are made without guarantee on the part of the author or Storey Publishing. The author and publisher disclaim any liability in connection with the use of this information.

Storey books are available for special premium and promotional uses and for customized editions. For further information, please call 1-800-793-9396.

STOREY PUBLISHING
210 MASS MoCA Way
North Adams, MA 01247
www.storey.com

Printed in China by R.R. Donnelley
10 9 8 7 6 5 4 3 2 1

Library of Congress Cataloging-in-Publication Data

Jirsa, Amy, author.
Herbal goddess / by Amy Jirsa.
pages cm
Includes index.
ISBN 978-1-61212-412-4 (pbk. : alk. paper)
ISBN 978-1-61212-413-1 (ebook) 1. Herbs—Theraputic use. 2. Materia medica, Vegetable. I. Title.
RM666.H33J57 2015
615.3'21—dc23

2014033793

Acknowledgments

Writers know how many people it truly takes to publish a book — from its inception to the inspiration to put words on the page to the actual publication of the physical book; I could fill pages with the names of people who deserve my undying gratitude, but, for all of our sakes, I'll keep it short.

To Sean: endless gratitude for your unwavering support, help, unconditional love, and constant grounding. To Sarah Gaffney: thank you for always being my first and last reader, kindred spirit, fellow poet, and soul sister. To my family: thank you for sharing your love, your recipes, and your love for all things green and growing. To Mom, Em, and Curt: thank you, thank you, thank you. For everything.

To herbalists like Deb Soule who brought herbs back into the forefront of health and culture and who are still out there growing, writing, advocating, and making it happen: thank you.

To Ward's Nursery in Great Barrington, Massachusetts: thank you for supplying the gorgeous plants for the photo shoot.

And, finally, huge thanks to Deb, Jennifer, Sarah, Carolyn, and the entire Storey Publishing family. I have found a home with you — you guys rock!

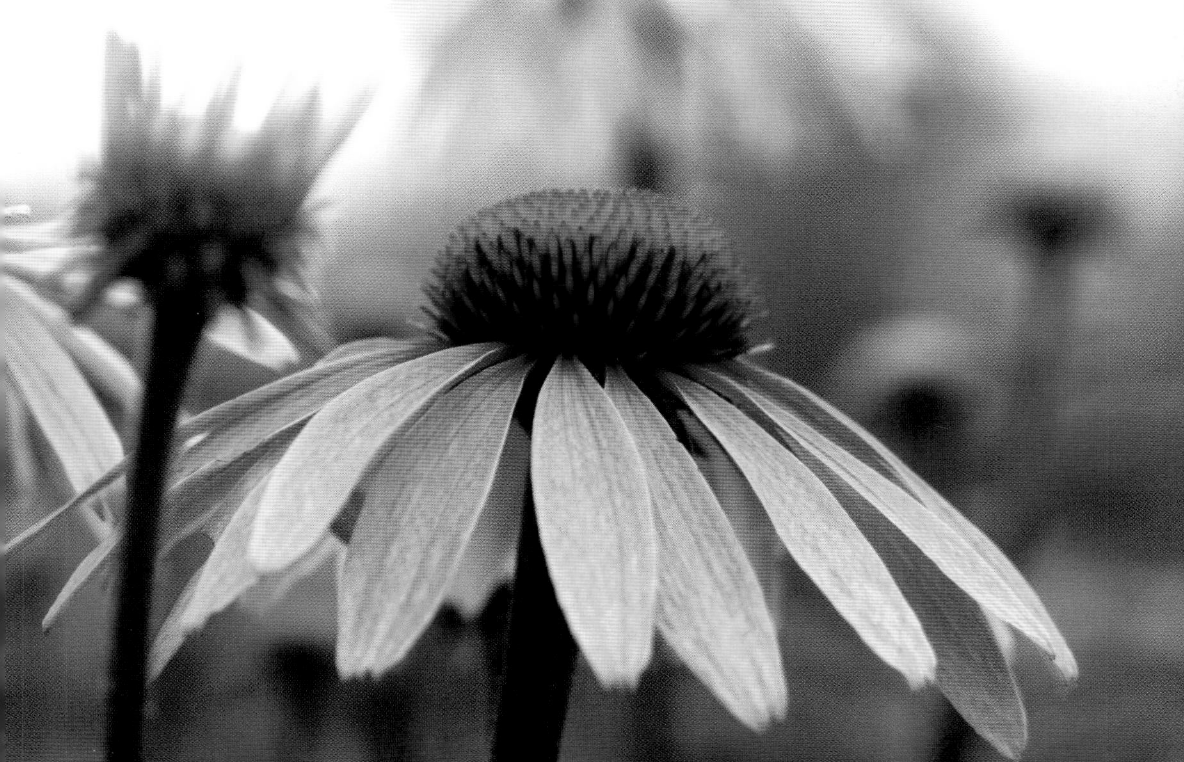

contents

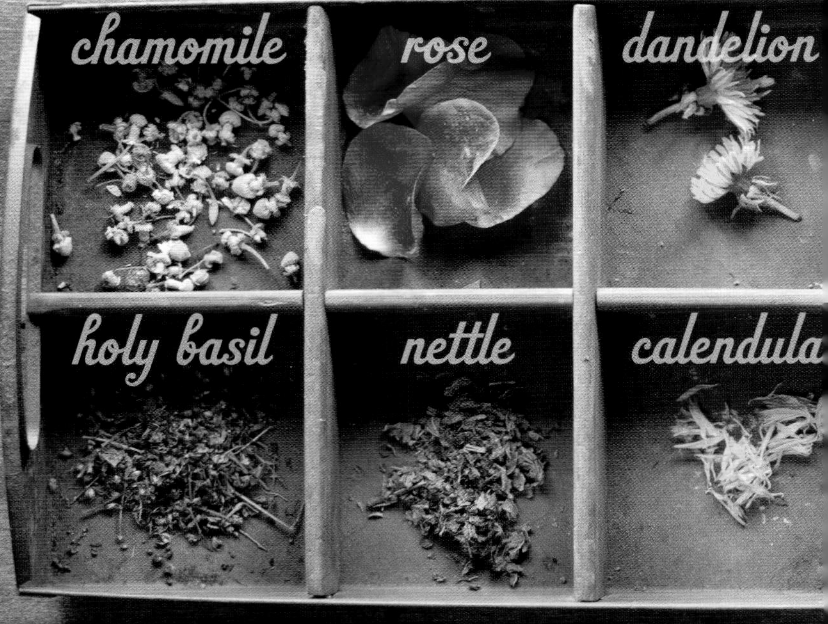

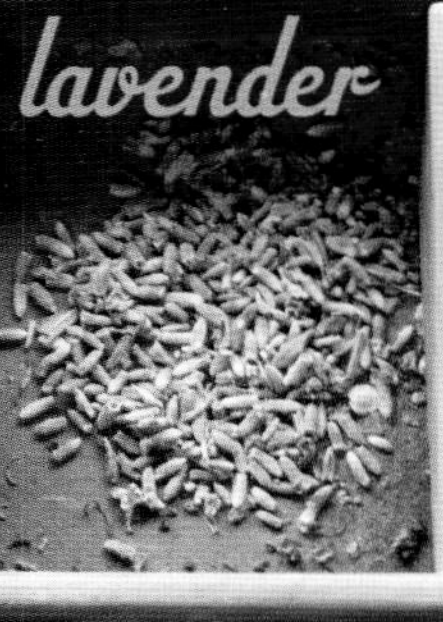
lavender

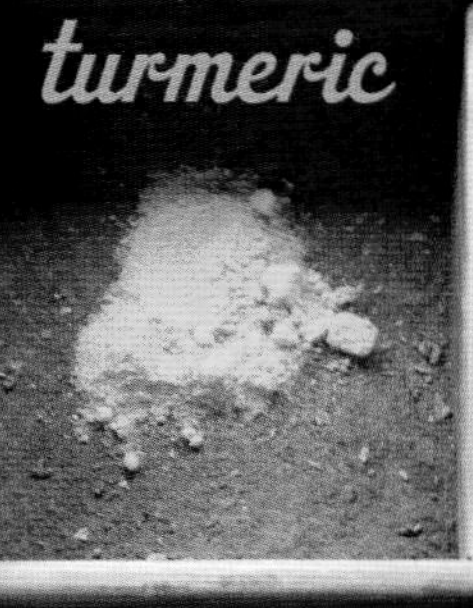
turmeric

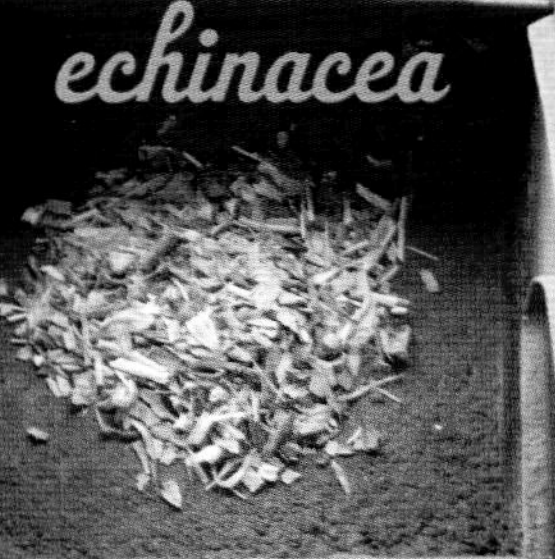
echinacea

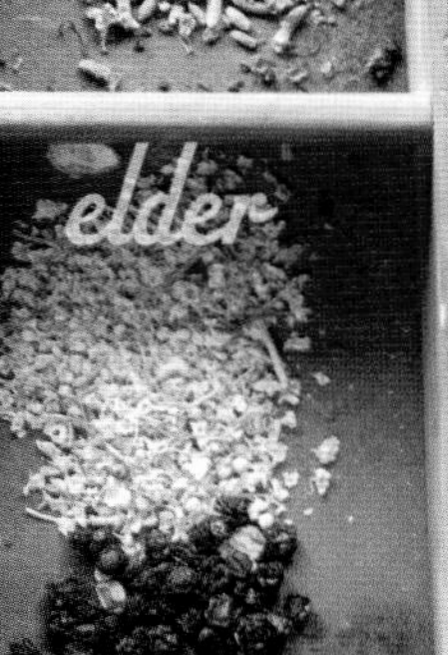
elder

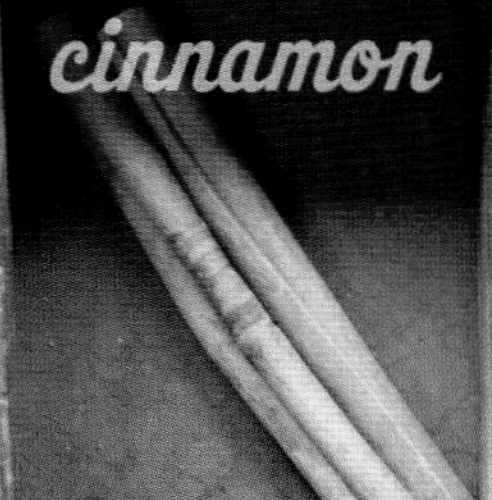
cinnamon

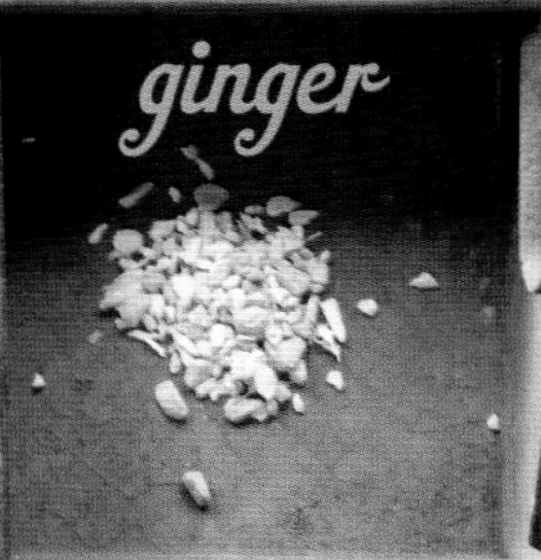
ginger

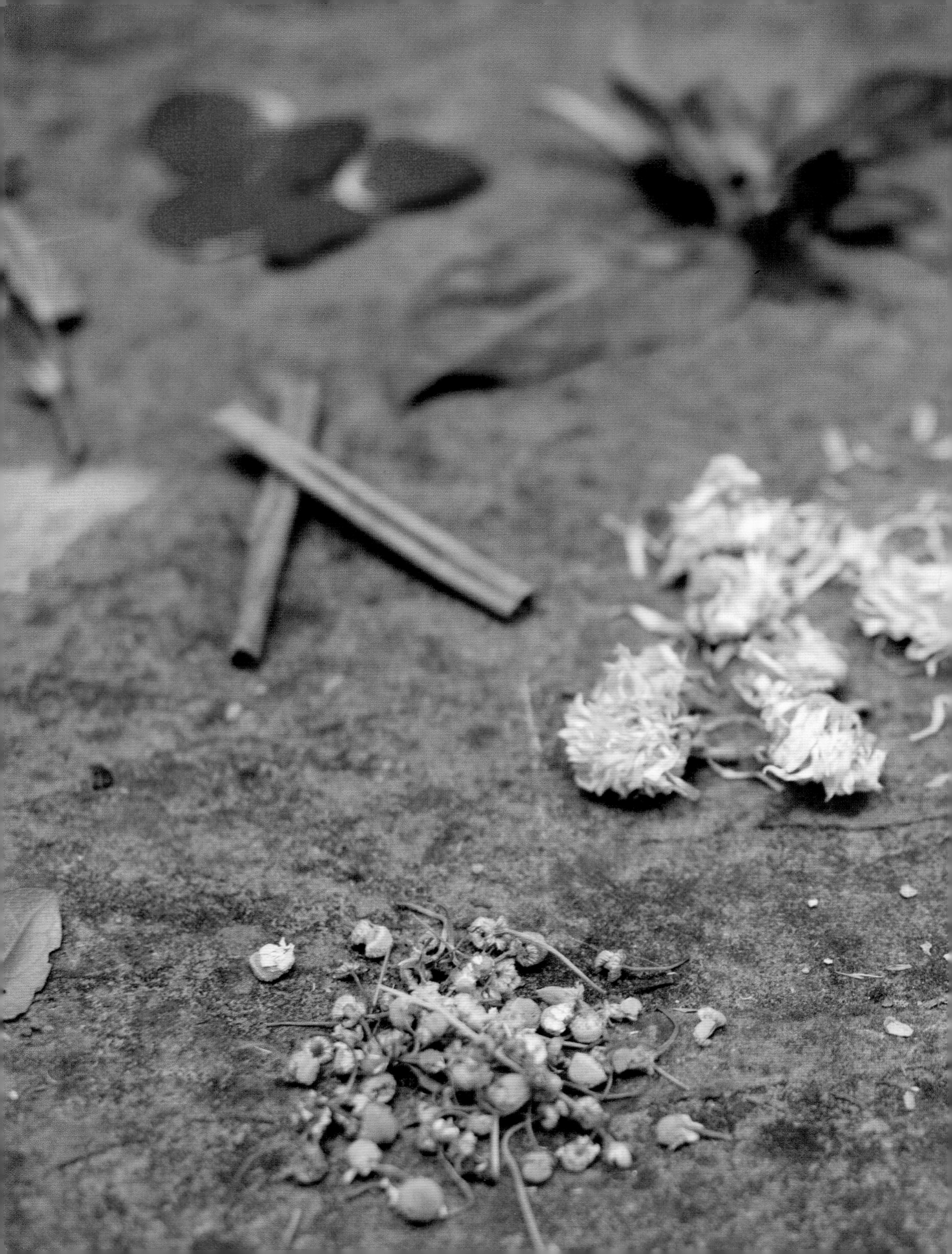

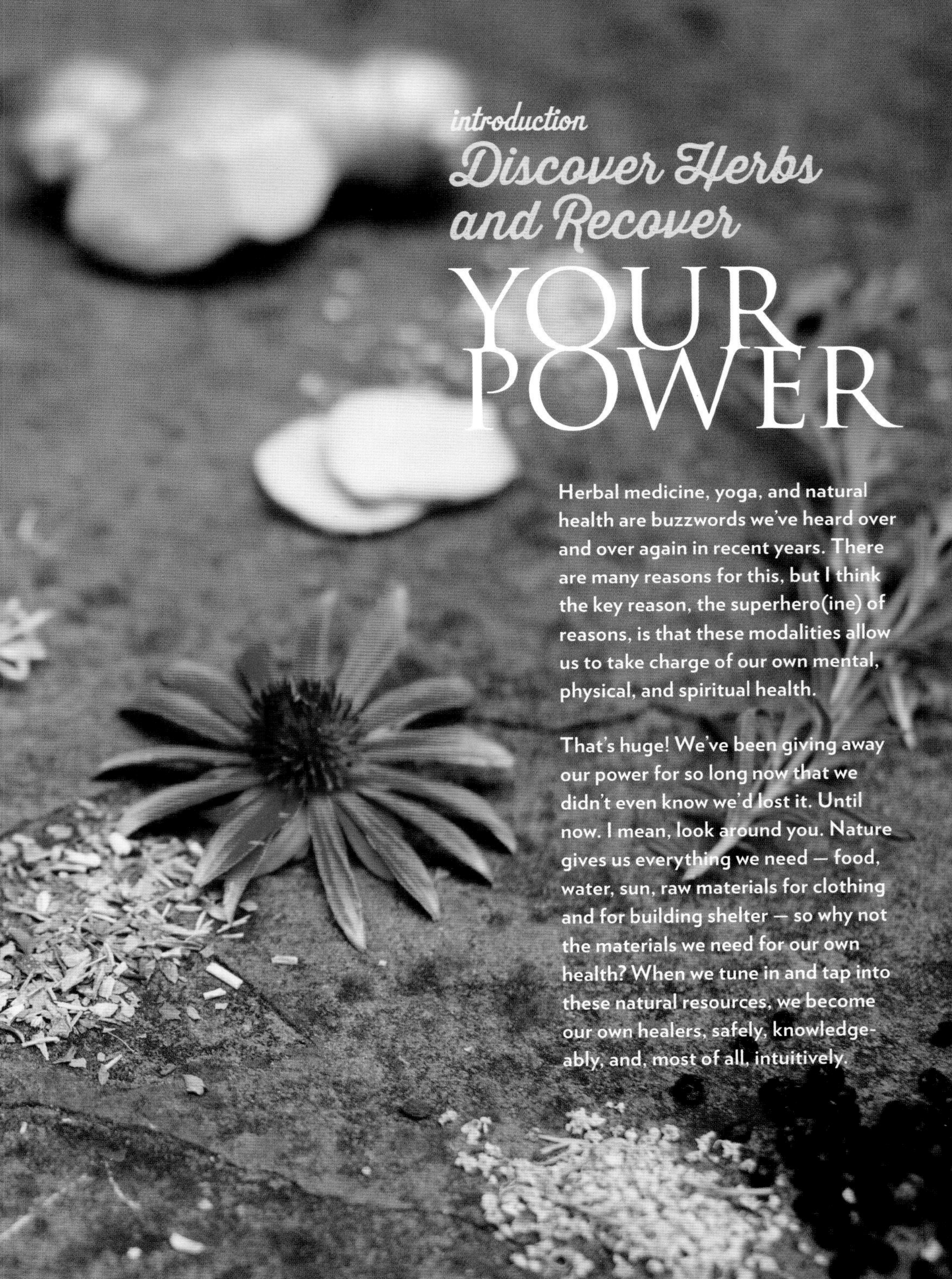

introduction

Discover Herbs and Recover YOUR POWER

Herbal medicine, yoga, and natural health are buzzwords we've heard over and over again in recent years. There are many reasons for this, but I think the key reason, the superhero(ine) of reasons, is that these modalities allow us to take charge of our own mental, physical, and spiritual health.

That's huge! We've been giving away our power for so long now that we didn't even know we'd lost it. Until now. I mean, look around you. Nature gives us everything we need — food, water, sun, raw materials for clothing and for building shelter — so why not the materials we need for our own health? When we tune in and tap into these natural resources, we become our own healers, safely, knowledge-ably, and, most of all, intuitively.

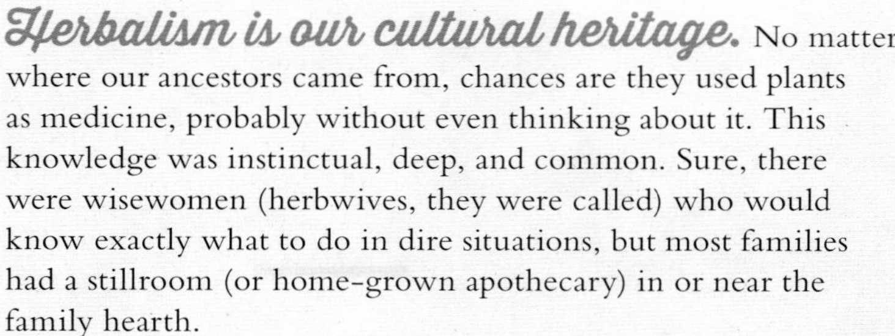

Herbalism is our cultural heritage. No matter where our ancestors came from, chances are they used plants as medicine, probably without even thinking about it. This knowledge was instinctual, deep, and common. Sure, there were wisewomen (herbwives, they were called) who would know exactly what to do in dire situations, but most families had a stillroom (or home-grown apothecary) in or near the family hearth.

Yes, we might have lost some of that knowledge along the way, but the instincts are still there. It's still in our genes or collective subconscious. We reach for peppermint when we want to freshen our breath or cool down, for instance; chamomile when we want to relax; and tea when we want to wake up. Yup — black, green, oolong, and rooibos teas are all herbs. In fact, you might be rather surprised to see so many "non-traditional" herbs in this little volume.

Technically, an herb is any plant that produces seeds, has a non-woody stem, and dies down after flowering. But to an herbalist, any plant that has medicinal, culinary, or aromatic mojo is considered an herb. Trust me — every plant I've included is an herb by that definition. There's major mojo here.

I know that, taken as a whole, learning about herbs seems like a lot of work. The sheer amount of information out there — on websites, in books, and in periodicals — can be overwhelming. And when you think of every possible medicinal plant out there? Ye gads! It is a lot. It's too much for most professional herbalists, even. That's why I've limited this book to 12 herbs.

You may be wondering, "How on earth can one herbalist decide on just 12 herbs?" Well, that choice came down partially to intuition; I've worked with many herbs over the years and these 12 continue to stand out to me as some of the most versatile and easiest to work with and source. These are my favorite go-to herbs, the ones that offer a range of solutions for healthy living from the outside to the inside, from the mind to the body to the spirit. These are the herbs my apothecary is never without. With these 12 herbs, I feel confident that I can take care of (almost) anything that might crop up in day-to-day living. Plus, there's a good variety here — some are beautiful, aromatic, and surprising (like the rose); some are familiar and, perhaps, already in your pantry (like chamomile). So that's it: just 12. Easy. Fun. Intuitive.

Sure, there are scads more than 12 herbs out there (enough to dedicate your life to their exploration, let's put it that way). But I'll tell you a secret: Most herbalists are intimately familiar with a handful of herbs (say, 30 or so) and we spend a long time getting to know each herb that we work with. So here's my suggestion: Try focusing on one herb at a time, and spend an entire month getting to know each one. It's the best way to become really familiar with how each herb affects you.

Think of the close relationships in your life. Think of the time it takes to really get to know someone — how much care and attention that kind of cultivation requires. You don't take that time with everyone you run into, but you know when it's worth it. It's the same thing with herbs. They, too, will become more familiar with time and attention. This is your moment of introduction. And if you're already acquainted, this is your time to go deeper. This is late-night-chardonnay-drinking sisterhood time.

To that end, I've supplied you with not only lots of specific recipes, but also some general formulas throughout the appendixes. These master recipes will allow you to blend, create, and invent your very own herbal preparations, from teas and tinctures to salves and cosmetics; from herbal oils and vinegars to flower essences. Here you'll learn the ins and outs of herbal crafting as you become inspired to build your own personalized herbal apothecary. You'll take your health into your own hands, secure in the knowledge that you are intimately familiar with every ingredient going into every remedy.

And speaking of your health and your hands — you'll notice yoga poses scattered throughout this book, each herb's spirit inspiring a yogic posture of its own. I included these because, to me, yoga is as close to connecting to plant spirits as our bodies can get. This isn't a book about yoga, so I'm assuming some basic familiarity with these poses; there

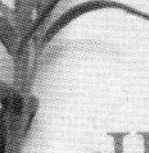

are lots of reference guides out there if you'd like to explore yoga more fully. Just flow with it; if it inspires you, fantastic!

And on that note, feel free to read this book in any order. You'll find, I think, that this guide becomes a starting place for your herbal exploration — that learning about these herbs will springboard learning about other herbs, and your studies will continue organically, with you creating the course and the curriculum. I'm giving you the basics so that you can become your own master teacher and Herbal Goddess down the road.

To my mind, you're an Herbal Goddess when you find that moment of inspiration, of inspired action that spurs you to experiment in your own way and to do your own exploring. To be an Herbal Goddess means to create your own craft of wellness, your own traditions, your own heritage while tapping into those of your sisters — both here-and-now and long gone. Because that knowledge is never really lost, is it? We may have strayed from the path of natural healing in recent decades, but herbs have a mysterious aspect to them — an ancient energy and wisdom. Just like any source of inspiration, this energy speaks to us.

Herbs have long been a part of spiritual and magical traditions, and those traditions are intricately woven into their healing properties and history. In honor of that sister-herbalist-goddess lineage, you'll find lots of magical applications for your herbs here as well.

Whether this is all new to you or provides a deeper exploration of herbs that you're already familiar with, you will find room to play here. There are always new avenues to take, even when heading for familiar homes.

At any rate, read at your leisure, have fun, and explore.

Be bold, be creative, and be healthy.

Oh, and be sure to goddess it up, you divine creatures, you!

HERBAL PREPARATION BASICS

Versatility is such a highly prized quality these days. It's a high compliment to be called a versatile actor, artist, parent, or student. Well, the herb world is no different.

Plants have been used for medicinal purposes for as long as we've been walking the earth. It just makes sense that different preparations will offer different results, and that how you prepare your herbal remedy depends on the situation, the herb used, and the body part effected. Here is a bit of what you'll encounter on the following pages.

TERMS TO KNOW

Dried herbs. We probably all know what dried herbs look like, right? We use them in tea and see them in the bulk section of the grocery store, classified as culinary or medicinal (or both!). Drying herbs is really the easiest way to preserve a harvest, and since dried herbs are available year-round, they're the most convenient for medicine-making purposes.

Fresh herbs. Have a garden? Fresh herbs are the most potent form of the herb because they contain the most water, nutrients, and fiber possible. Lots of fresh herbs can be eaten as is, or brewed in tea or steeped in vinegar. I prefer to use fresh herbs as much as possible and save dried herbs for such long-term preservations as tinctures and salves.

Compress. A compress is basically a length of cloth that has been soaked in a very strong, very warm, herbal infusion (or tea) and then applied to an injured or affected area of the skin.

Decoction. A decoction is like a tea made from the woody parts of herb (think bark, stems, and roots). Since you won't extract all the medicinal goodness from these hardier plant parts by steeping them in hot water alone, they are simmered in water for 10 minutes, strained, and then taken as you would take a cup of tea.

Essential oil. An essential oil is steam-distilled aromatic oil from the leaves and flowers of herbs. This undiluted and very potent oil preserves the volatile oils (the stuff that makes plants smell awesome) as perfectly as possible.

Herbal oil. An herbal oil is simply oil infused with herb matter. It can be used for culinary, medicinal, or skincare purposes.

Herbal vinegar. Just like herbal oil, herbal vinegar is made by steeping herbal matter in a vinegar of choice. It

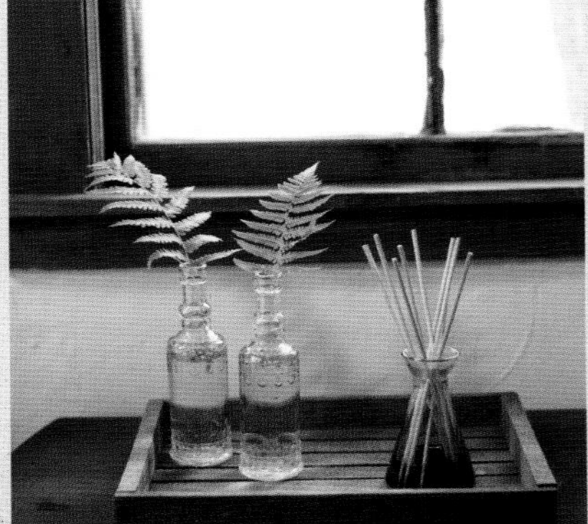

can be used in the kitchen, on the skin, or in beverages for medicinal purposes.

Poultice. Think herbal mash. A poultice is an herb that's been chewed up or bruised using warm water in order to break its cellular structure and release its healing qualities (it works best with fresh herbs, but you can reconstitute dried herbs as well). This mash is then applied directly to an affected area of the skin and covered with a warm, damp cloth.

Salve. A salve is an herbal oil that is heated and mixed with wax in order to form a balm-like application (think body butter or lip balm).

Tea. Herbal teas are technically called infusions (the word "tea" is reserved for the caffeinated varieties; but, eh, semantics). For the purposes of this book, a tea is a quantity of dried or fresh herb steeped in hot to boiling water for a prescribed period of time.

Tincture. A tincture is a liquid extract of the medicinal qualities of an herb. Alcohol, vinegar, glycerin, and water are all common menstruums (liquids used for extraction purposes). This is my favorite way to prepare herbs, since it really preserves the important constituents, has a long shelf life, and is super-easy to take.

STILLROOM STAPLES

You know how cookbooks have a little section on "pantry staples"? Well, the stillroom is the herbalist's pantry. Gather a small cache of these essentials and you'll be ready for any herbal project or inspiration, from a cup of tea to a full-body herbal clay treatment.

Beeswax. Beeswax is what we add to herbal oils in order to make salves (think lip balm). Vegan alternatives include candelilla wax, which is made from boiling the leaves and stems of the candelilla shrub.

Carrier oils. Since essential oils are so potent, they're often too strong to put directly onto the skin. Carrier oils are mild, unscented or lightly-scented oils — such as almond, apricot, or coconut — used to "carry" essential oils.

Charcoal disks. When you want to use loose, dried herbs as incense, you need a heat source they can smolder on. Enter the charcoal disk. Simply place the small disk in a heat-proof dish and hold a match to it. Once it begins to spark, it should self-light. This can take a few tries. Once lit, take a pinch of dried herb and drop it onto the disk. The herb will dampen the flame, and the disk will continue to smolder, releasing the aromatic smoke from your herb.

Cosmetic clays. Clay is loaded with minerals, and your skin is an amazing, absorptive organ. When you pair the two together, you get a formula for good health. The cleansing, detoxifying, and drawing power of clay is unparalleled.

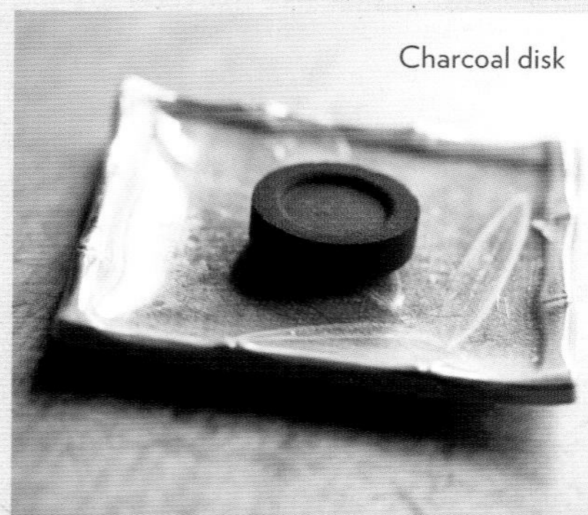
Charcoal disk

There are many varieties of clay. My favorites are French green clay, bentonite clay, and white cosmetic clay, but no matter which clay you choose, all are stellar for cleansing, exfoliating, boosting circulation, and deodorizing.

French green clay (also called sea clay) is a powerful drawer of oils and is perfect for acne-troubled or oily skin. The green color comes from decomposed plant matter, which is loaded with nutrients and minerals. Green clay brings fresh blood and circulation to damaged skin cells and tightens pores. You can even use it as a spot treatment for acne. Right before bed, dab a little moistened green clay on any trouble spots/outbreaks and wake to a clearer complexion.

Bentonite clay is one of the most powerful healers out there. When mixed with water, it becomes electrically charged and swells into a gentle, healing sponge. Because it carries a negative charge, it will pull impurities, such as heavy metals and toxins, out of the skin. Since this is a powerful healer, I don't use it in everyday masks and cosmetic applications. Instead, I save it for healing after a long illness, heavy metal or radiation exposure, or a long course of pharmaceutical drugs.

White cosmetic clay (sometimes called china clay or kaolin clay) is the gentlest and most versatile clay. This is perfect for daily use, even if you have sensitive, dry, or mature skin, since it doesn't draw oil from the skin.

Cocoa butter. Cocoa butter is pressed from the seeds of the cacao tree (yup — same tree that gives us life-sustaining chocolate) and is used as a moisturizer either on its own or in salve or lotion recipes. This is my absolute favorite moisturizer. It is rich, creamy, thick, and scented ever-so-slightly of chocolate.

Glycerin. Glycerin is a by-product of the vegetable oil-making process. It's a naturally occurring solvent, which is perfect for drawing medicinal qualities of herbs into tinctures for children and others who want to avoid alcohol and don't like the taste of vinegar (glycerin is naturally sweet).

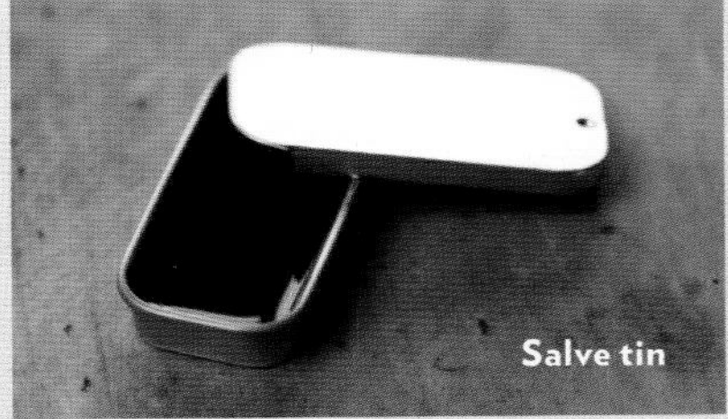
Salve tin

Salve tins. I always have a variety of small tins lying around. Many of these I reuse from store-bought products, but I also seem to have friends who will just give me their old tins because they know I'll reuse them. I find it best to have a variety of sizes; the most common are ½ ounce, 1 ounce, 2 ounce, and 4 ounce.

Shea butter. Derived from the karite tree, shea butter is an amazing, softening, water-resistant skin moisturizer. You can use it on its own or in lotion or salve recipes.

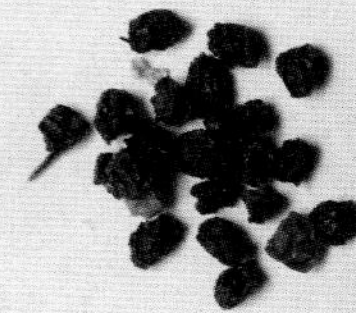

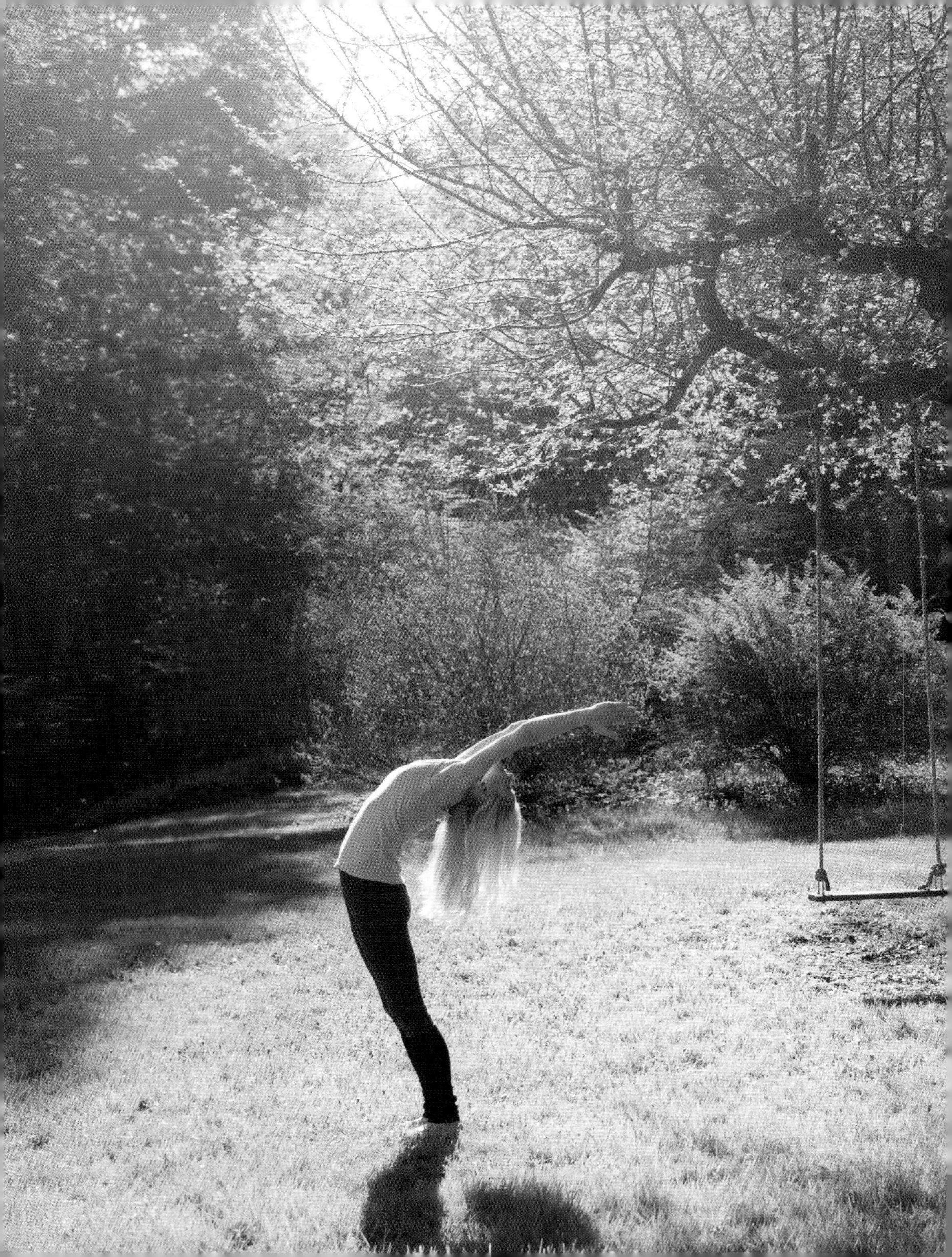

1

Discovering the Sunny Side of CHAMOMILE

Who could use a little sunshine, a little happiness, in their day? Hey, who couldn't, right? Well, you're in luck, because here we're exploring sunny, daisy-like, little chamomile (*Matricaria recutita* and *Chamaemelum nobilis*) — right at the beginning. Who knows why you picked up this book. Maybe you were looking to learn more about herbs (yay!), or maybe you've just come off a holiday/long winter binge, or maybe you're just looking for a little renewal. Anyway, the *why* doesn't really matter in the long run.

Most of us (including yours truly) put so much faith and hope into some shiny promise of renewal that we inevitably fail; our expectations are so high that we doom ourselves never to live up to them. Couple that with the letdown that follows this so-called failure, and you become overwhelmed.

So let's take it down a notch. Let's narrow our focus and choose one thing we can do for ourselves each day to improve our health, our well-being, and our focus. That's what this book is for, and what better place to start than with chamomile, the tiny, joyful cousin of the sunflower? In this first chapter let's hand our hearts and our minds over to the sun — the source of life, health, and happiness; chamomile is the perfect herb for the job.

You've probably tasted chamomile tea before. Maybe you even prefer it to other hot tea or coffee-like beverages. No surprise there; chamomile tea is the second most popular tea in the world (after black tea). And, for that reason, it's taken for granted. I mean, it's not a sexy tea, is it? It's a stay-at-home, before-bed, warm-and-cozy tea, isn't it? Oh-ho! I beg to differ.

Okay, so maybe chamomile will never have the sex appeal of the rose (see chapter 2) or the rock-star status of echinacea (see chapter 9). But chamomile can be your best friend — maybe even one of those friends who becomes more than "just friends" once you get to know them better. (And then again, maybe that's just taking the metaphor a bit too far . . . .) Trust me, this is a truly versatile herb and, once you've familiarized yourself with it over the coming weeks, you'll find it is an invaluable addition to your herbal survival kit.

Here's the skinny: Chamomile boasts anti-inflammatory, antibiotic, anti-spasmodic, calming, diuretic, and tonic properties. See? You'll use chamomile for everything. But the best news? It's completely safe for adults and children alike. One note, though — as chamomile is a member of the ragweed family, if you suffer from severe ragweed allergies, start slowly with this herb to see how it treats you. (This should be the practice when introducing any and all herbs, by the way.)

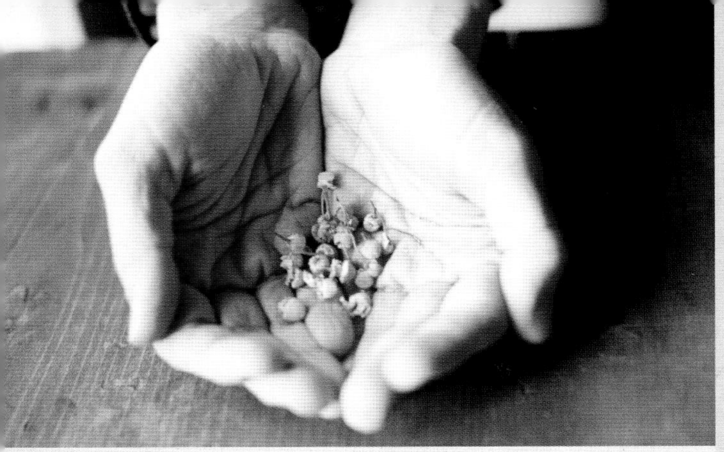

As a member of the happy-go-lucky daisy family, chamomile is recognizable by its yellow center and 10 or more petals surrounding it. This tiny flower grows on a very thin stalk, which can reach up to 2 feet tall. The leaves are delicate, divided, and rather feathery. The scent is sweetly intoxicating, uplifting, and mildly bitter. Like all herbs, chamomile is a wild-growing plant, but due to invasive farming, city sprawl, and widespread development of natural landscapes, it's pretty rare to find it anywhere but in cultivated gardens.

DRYING BLOSSOMS

If you can get your hands on fresh chamomile blossoms, you can use them in tea or as an addition to an aromatic and soothing bath. If you want to preserve them for use throughout the year or in other medicinal forms such as salves or tinctures (see appendixes), spread your blossoms on a screen and let them dry indoors, away from direct sunlight. Keep these dried blossoms stored in an airtight container for up to a year. Oh, and speaking from experience here, make sure you put your herbs away as soon as they've dried; otherwise you've got a whole lot of dusty, wasted effort (not to mention wasted medicinals and, most likely, a less-than-happy plant spirit).

CHAMOMILE

Matricaria recutita and *Chamaemelum nobilis*

Parts used: Flowers
How to harvest: After a little nod of gratitude, snip flower heads from the stalk mid-morning after the dew has dried
Effects on body: Boosts digestive fire, eases intestinal maladies and pain, strengthens metabolism, and cleanses blood
Effects on mind and spirit: Calming, cooling, pacifying; eases anxiety and irritability
Safety first: Go slowly if you have a ragweed allergy; though rare, it could cause a reaction

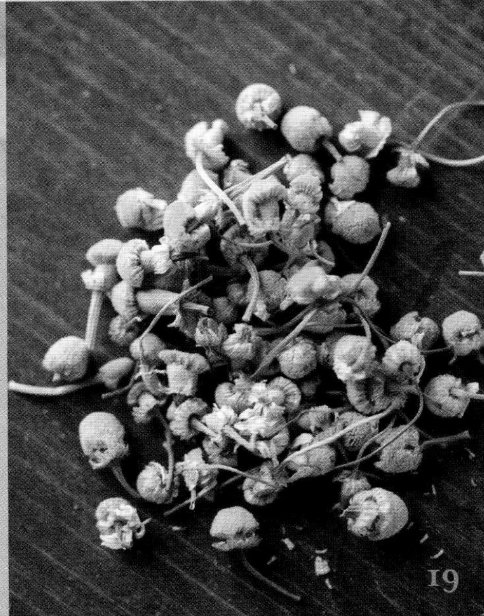

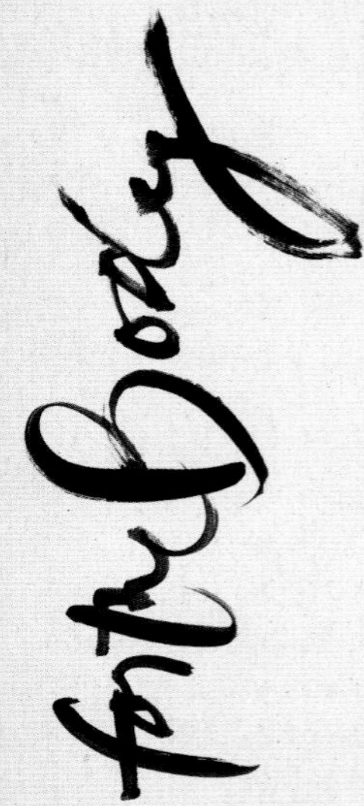

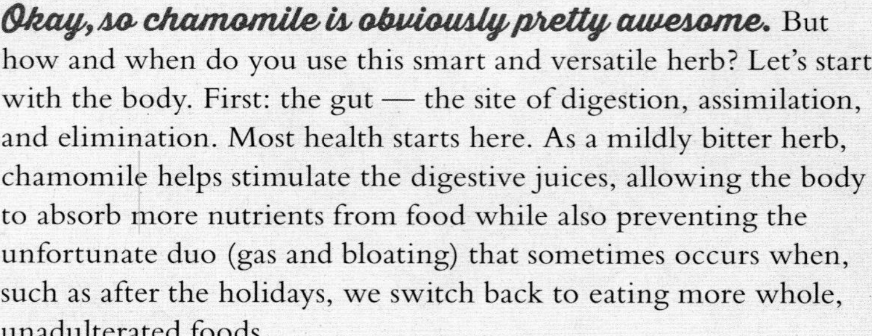

Okay, so chamomile is obviously pretty awesome. But how and when do you use this smart and versatile herb? Let's start with the body. First: the gut — the site of digestion, assimilation, and elimination. Most health starts here. As a mildly bitter herb, chamomile helps stimulate the digestive juices, allowing the body to absorb more nutrients from food while also preventing the unfortunate duo (gas and bloating) that sometimes occurs when, such as after the holidays, we switch back to eating more whole, unadulterated foods.

Chamomile also strengthens the metabolism by aiding the kidneys in cleansing the blood. That scent you associate with chamomile? That's the volatile oil, which stimulates the liver and kidneys, encouraging their purging of toxins. Let's face it, after your third week of, say, eggnog and gingerbread for breakfast, this is support your body could certainly use (see tea recipes on page 25).

After any fabulous period of indulgence, not only are there toxins to purge, but there are storehouses of nutrients to restock. Sugar, caffeine, and excess fat and dairy can deplete our body's energy and nutrients. Chamomile is a monster source of niacin, magnesium, and essential fatty acids. Inevitably, at least at first, you're going to miss the extravagance, but stockpiling your body with nutrients will help cut down on the cravings that so often haunt us when we try to change our body's routine.

Adding chamomile to your daily diet can increase plant-based compounds (called polyphenols) in your system, which, in turn, increase antibacterial activity in your body. The analgesic (pain-relieving) and anti-inflammatory actions of chamomile help soothe sinus pain, headaches, sore throats, and swollen lymph glands.

Exercise, too, will help ward off illnesses and hurry you through this detox process. Yup, you guessed it: Chamomile is a good support for the workout regimen which typically accompanies most attempts to get back on the healthy train. As an anti-spasmodic, chamomile can help reduce muscle cramps and inflammation. If you suffer from nerve pain, such as sciatica or lumbago, chamomile can be used internally or externally.

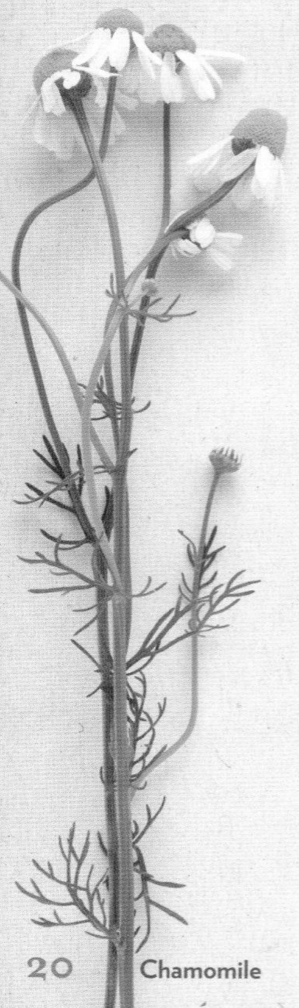

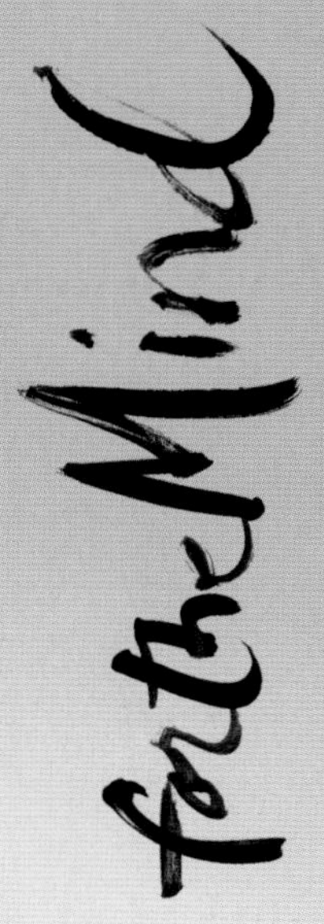

So far, we've just touched on depression and blues; sometimes, getting up and getting going is no easy task. It's no wonder that anxiety and depression often trail us around, whether we're making major changes or not. But allow chamomile to do its work here, too; as a nervine and mild sedative, chamomile will soothe all (okay, *most*) of your worries. The volatile oils of chamomile (especially from fresh, not dried, flowers) are especially soothing, in particular for those with a tendency toward whining (both child and adult varieties).

You can also use chamomile in flower essence form (an oh-so-groovy magical potion that capitalizes on a flower's unique vibration; see box on page 22). All you need to do is put a few drops in a glass of water or directly under the tongue. Are you easily upset, irritable, or holding emotional tension? Well, chamomile's got a vibration for that. What about easing addictions, anger, anxiety, depression, insomnia, nervousness, and chronic stress or tension (especially when it's felt in the stomach)? Yup — that, too. What about the kiddos? Is this safe for them? You bet — this flower essence is especially soothing and effective for the 12-and-under population.

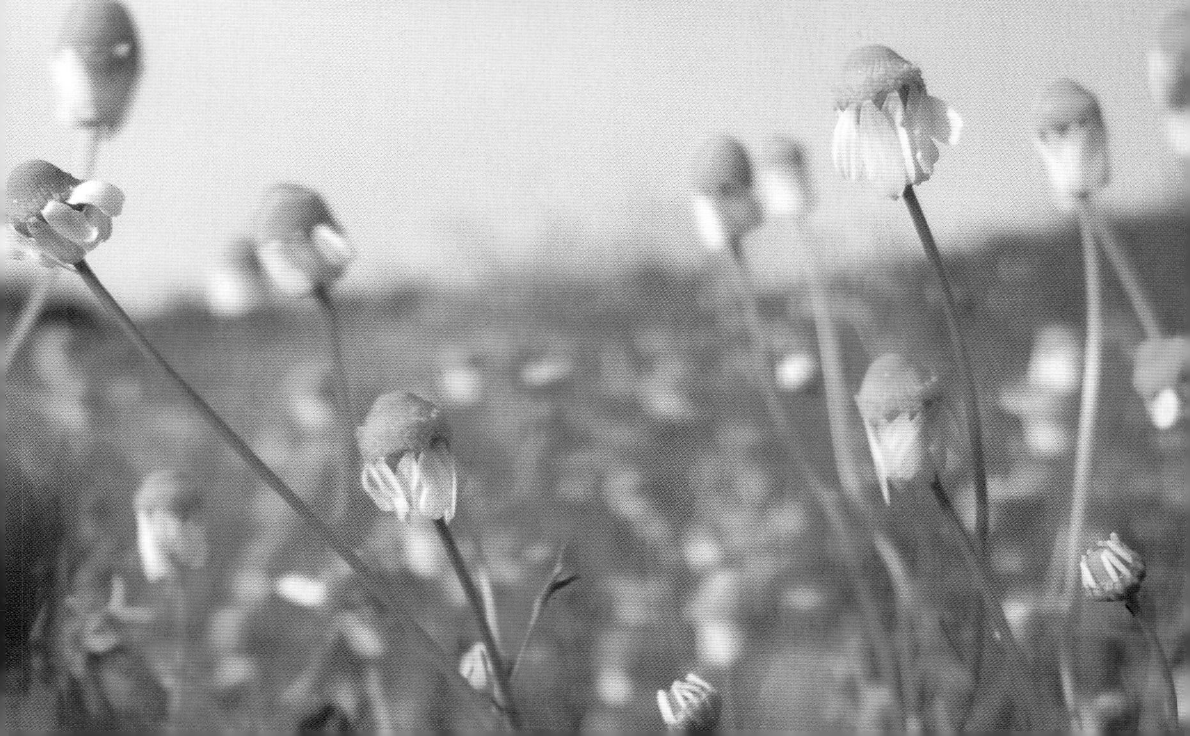

FLOWER ESSENCE VS. ESSENTIAL OIL

When we talk about herbs "for the mind," we're going to be referring primarily to flower essences, which are different than essential oils. Now, I know that these two plant-derived healing modalities can be a bit confusing at first, so let's break it down.

Essential oils are the distilled volatile oils or the "essence" — the compounds that make up the scent — of a particular plant. Essential oils work by way of your sense of smell (aromatherapy).

Flower essences, on the other hand, work from the assumption that every living thing has a vibration. Think back to basic science. Remember atoms and molecules? Remember how they're always moving, and that even a seemingly solid object is just a bunch of moving parts? It's the same thing with us, with plants, and with flowers. So, flower essences capture a flower's vibration and harness it for better health. Flower essences are made by infusing the fresh flowers of a plant in spring water and leaving them to steep in the sun. The idea is that the vibrations of the flowers change the molecular structure of the water. Basically, this "charged" water helps to stimulate our own self-healing vibrations.

How do you get your hands on this miracle brew? Well, you can easily purchase ready-made essences, or create your own, which is truly a grounding, mystical, and fun process — talk about getting to know your plants (see Appendix I for flower essence instructions).

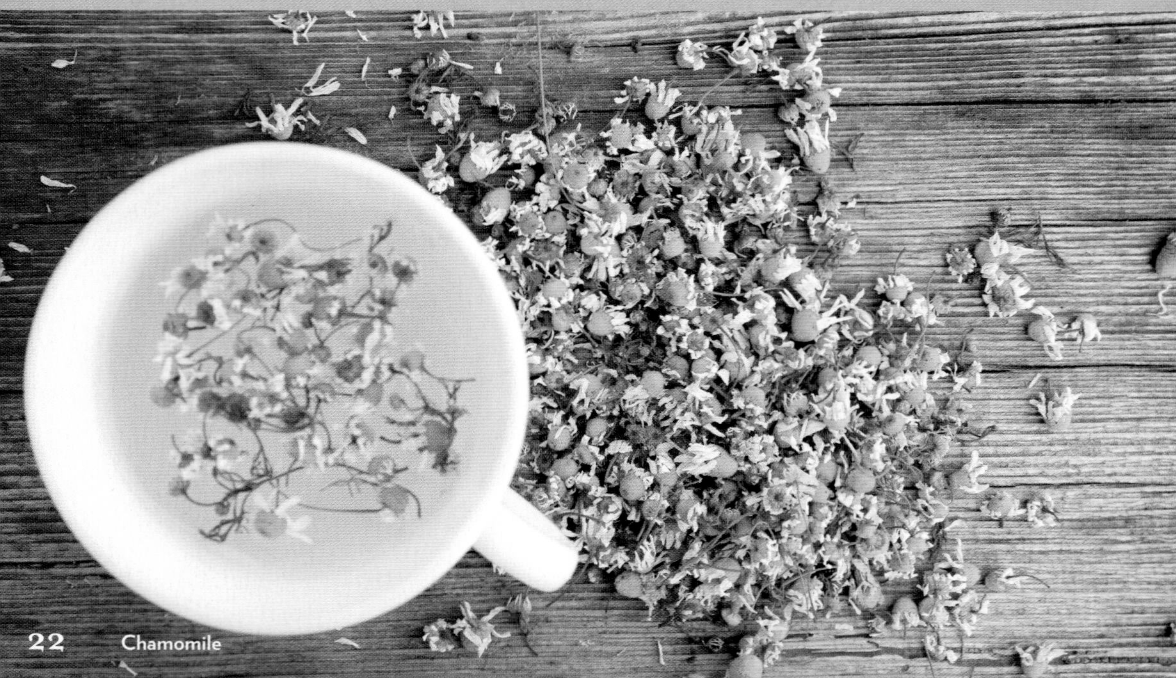

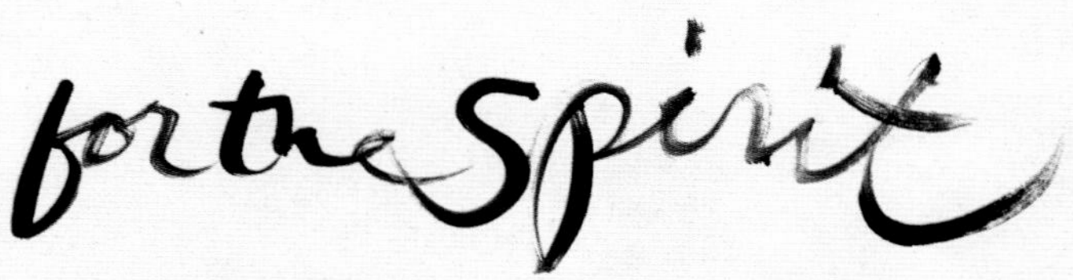

All magical herbs have a gender, planet, and element attached to them. Why? Well, it's kind of a long story (isn't that always the truth with good stories?). Essentially, these attachments were a classification tool.

The gender of a plant was based on how its vibration felt, presumably a judgment made by someone with a lot more sensitivity than yours truly. Basically, think of gender as describing warming or cooling energy. "Masculine" energy is warming and "feminine" energy is cooling.

Traditionally, certain planets were associated with different outcomes in magic (the sun for protection and the moon for fertility, for example). So, when herbs were found to bring about certain outcomes, they were assigned to a particular planet for classification purposes.

You can think of the elements in the same way as the planets. The four elements (earth, air, fire, and water) consist of everything one needs to create and sustain life. The earth element is linked to prosperity and fertility, air to wisdom and intelligence, and so on. So, long story short (too late for that, maybe . . .), it's all about classification and cross-reference.

As is par for the course in all ancient wisdom, no one (it seems) really agrees upon anything. For chamomile, I've found various magical attachments and have decided that the practitioner will just have to decide for herself which feels true, thank you very much. For example, I've found that chamomile's gender is either masculine or feminine, depending on the source behind the research. The planet is the sun and/or Venus, and the element is water (everyone pretty much agrees on this). Chamomile offers help in the areas of protection, prosperity, wealth, fame, riches, sleep, love (this might explain the Venus connection), purification, and achieving goals. So, how can you get your magic on? Drinking and bathing in chamomile and using the flower essence are definitely a few ways to cover your bases. See others below.

CHAMOMILE MAGIC

TO KEEP YOU ON YOUR PATH

You can place a pinch of the dried herb in a sachet and keep this in your purse or pocket or wear it around your neck. Its presence will help remind you of your goals every time you see or feel it. If you have charcoal disks lying around, you can place one on a heat-proof surface, light it, and sprinkle some chamomile flowers on the disk, allowing the incense to smolder. Meditate (or just lie down and relax) while inhaling the fragrance.

FOR PROTECTION

To invoke protection, you can sprinkle chamomile around the outside of your house to ward off ill luck, unwelcome visitors, or negative energy. Walking in a clockwise direction, sprinkle the chamomile with either hand (I use my left hand, since it's closest to the heart, but do what works for you), visualizing the kind of energy you want to dwell with you in your home. While away from home, wear chamomile in a sachet or tuck a pouch of the herb in your car to extend the protection as you travel.

A NOTE ON MAGIC

Do you have to be well versed in magical dealings to use herbs toward a specific end? I don't think so. I think a lot of magic is about your intention and then about amplifying that intention. Figure out what you need and then use the herb to amplify that need and blast it into the magical universe.

TEAS

Digestive support. Try this little number: Steep a cup of chamomile tea (2 teaspoons dried flowers per 1 cup just-boiled water) for 10 to 15 minutes. Since the volatile (essential) oils of chamomile are so important to this digestive kick, be sure to cover your tea as it steeps. Drink about 20 minutes before you eat. A warning, though: This tea will be a wee bit bitter; try sweetening it with stevia or honey and adding non-dairy milk (the proteins in regular milk interfere with the medicinal effects of the herb).

Basic tea for workouts, anxiety, and insomnia. Brew 2 teaspoons in a cup of water and let steep for only 3 to 5 minutes, in order to avoid bitterness. Add honey or maple syrup for a little sugar-and-nutrient boost.

For rejuvenating and rehydrating after your workout, drink the tea chilled. For anxiety relief, have a cup as soon as anxiety begins. Inhale the steam from the tea for a few moments before drinking — the volatile oils released in the steam will do wonders for anxiety. For guaranteed (inner and outer) beauty sleep, try a cup of chamomile tea an hour or so before bed.

Chamomile for cranky, colicky children. If you have little ones around, chamomile is a wonderful herb for cranky, colicky, or teething infants and children. For better sleep, make the following tea. A chamomile infusion can also be rubbed on the gums of teething infants.

Gently warm 1 cup milk (dairy or non-dairy) on the stove, being careful not to scald it. Turn off the heat and add 1 teaspoon dried chamomile flowers. Let steep, covered, for 5 minutes. Sweeten with honey (if the child is older than 2) if you like.

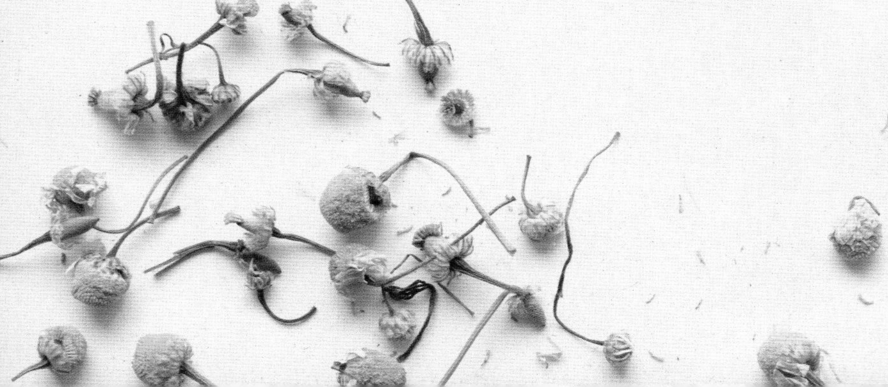

CHAMOMILE AROMATHERAPY

For anxiety. Feeling stressed before a big project or presentation? Sniff from a little vial of chamomile essential oil to soothe mental tension, helping you focus on the present rather than worrying and projecting into the future. (A side note: from personal experience, I can tell you that it's probably best to do this in a bathroom cubicle or somewhere else equally private, or else learn to ignore questions and curious looks . . .)

For insomnia. Try a warm bath with a few cups of strongly brewed chamomile tea or a few drops of chamomile essential oil added to the water. The heat of the bath will help relieve tension, while the aromatherapeutic effects of the chamomile will soothe the senses.

Alternatively, make an aromatherapy diffuser to place next to the tub or in the bedroom. Blend essential oils with a carrier oil and then add porous diffuser reeds. The reeds wick the liquid, and the scent evaporates into the air.

For headaches. If tension causes you to suffer regularly from headaches, try steeping a strong chamomile infusion laced with a few drops of chamomile essential oil. Dip a washcloth in the infusion and drape the cloth over your forehead (use cooled or heated water, depending on what sounds best to you at the moment). Relax in a dark room. If you don't have time for this treatment, try uncapping a bottle of chamomile essential oil and inhaling its fragrance as you close your eyes; you can also try massaging a drop or two into the temples and at the base of the skull.

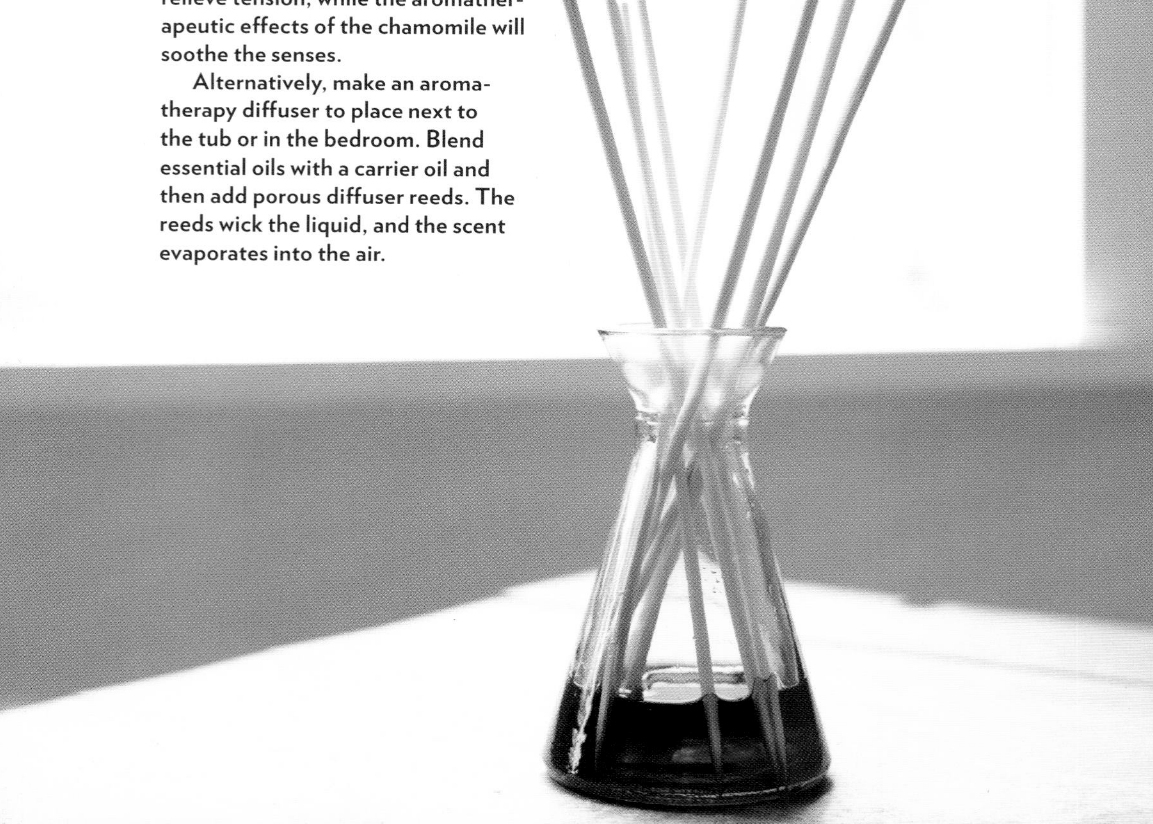

BODY CARE

recipes

Cold and Flu Steam

For the inevitable cold or flu that always seems to follow a period of detox, try an herbal steam featuring chamomile.

3 drops essential chamomile oil or 6 tablespoons dried chamomile flowers

1. Add the oil to a steaming pot of water, or if making tea, add the dried flowers to a quart of hot water.
2. Place a towel, tent-like, over your head and breathe in the steam for 10 minutes. Make sure the water isn't boiling; we want healing, not burning, happening here. As an anti-inflammatory and antimicrobial, chamomile will heal the lungs and sinuses, while the heat drains the mucus from the body (as a bonus, you'll end up with gorgeous, glowing, detoxed skin as well).

Chamomile Lip Balm/Stress Reliever

This is a general lip balm recipe, but I like to boost the essential oil component and then rub it on my temples or pulse points when I'm feeling stressed or anxious. Also, with the high-scent factor, just rubbing the balm on my lips easily allows the scent to travel to my aromatherapy machine (aka my nose) .

2 tablespoons beeswax

2 tablespoons shea butter

2 tablespoons almond oil

2 vitamin E capsules (this acts as a preservative)

20 drops chamomile essential oil

6 ½-ounce tins (see Resources)

1. Sterilize your tins and any wooden spoons or measuring cups you'll be using in boiling water for 10 minutes. If using plastic spoons and measuring cups, run them through the hottest cycle in your dishwasher.
2. Melt the wax and shea butter in a double boiler (or in a heat-safe bowl perched above a pan of simmering water). Add the almond oil. When

Recipe continues on next page

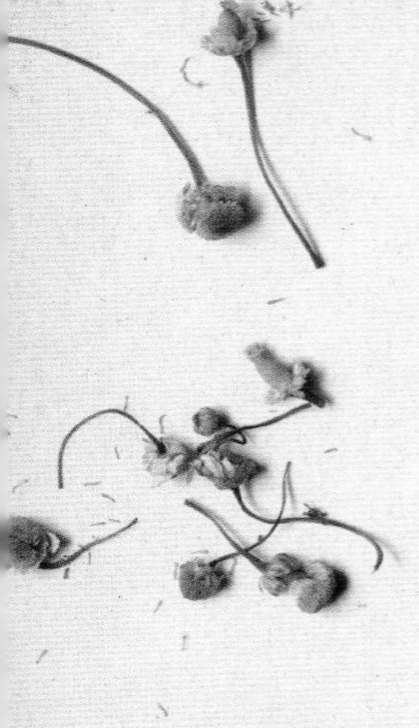

all the ingredients have melted, remove from heat.

3. Puncture the vitamin E capsules with a sterilized pin, and add the contents to the mixture, along with the chamomile essential oil. Mix gently.

4. Carefully pour the mixture into the tins. Leave off the lids and let the balm cool, undisturbed. This will take a few hours. Decorate and/or label the tins as desired. Keep or give away!

Makes 3 ounces

Chamomile Herb Sachets

These sachets can be tucked into drawers, tossed into the dryer, slipped into a pocket and sniffed (surreptitiously) when anxious, or tucked beneath your pillow at night to ensure a sound sleep. If making your own bags, consider stamping them with fabric-safe ink or choosing fabric that reflects your personality.

Handmade bags (in the size of your choice) of cotton or muslin, or pre-made cotton tea bags

Coarsely ground chamomile flowers

Chamomile essential oil

Stuff each bag with dried flowers and add a few drops of essential oil to boost the aromatherapeutic power.

Chamomile Body Wash

Herb-infused soaps are a wonderful addition to your daily shower — especially if you don't have time for an aromatherapeutic bath every day.

5 drops chamomile essential oil

1 teaspoon jojoba or almond oil

1 16-ounce bottle castile soap

3 drops tea tree oil (optional)

3 drops peppermint essential oil (optional)

3 drops citrus essential oil (optional)

1. Add the chamomile essential oil and jojoba or almond oil to the bottle of castile soap. For an invigorating wash, add the tea tree and peppermint oil; for a soothing wash, add the citrus oil. Shake it, shake it, shake it up.

2. Stick that bottle in the shower and use it daily. If you wish to dilute the castile soap, which can dry out your skin on its own, you may wish to put the soap in a foaming pump bottle. Fill the bottle one-third full of soap and two-thirds full of water. Screw on the pump top and *voilà*! Foaming soap, gentle (and fun!) enough to use every day.

Makes 16 ounces

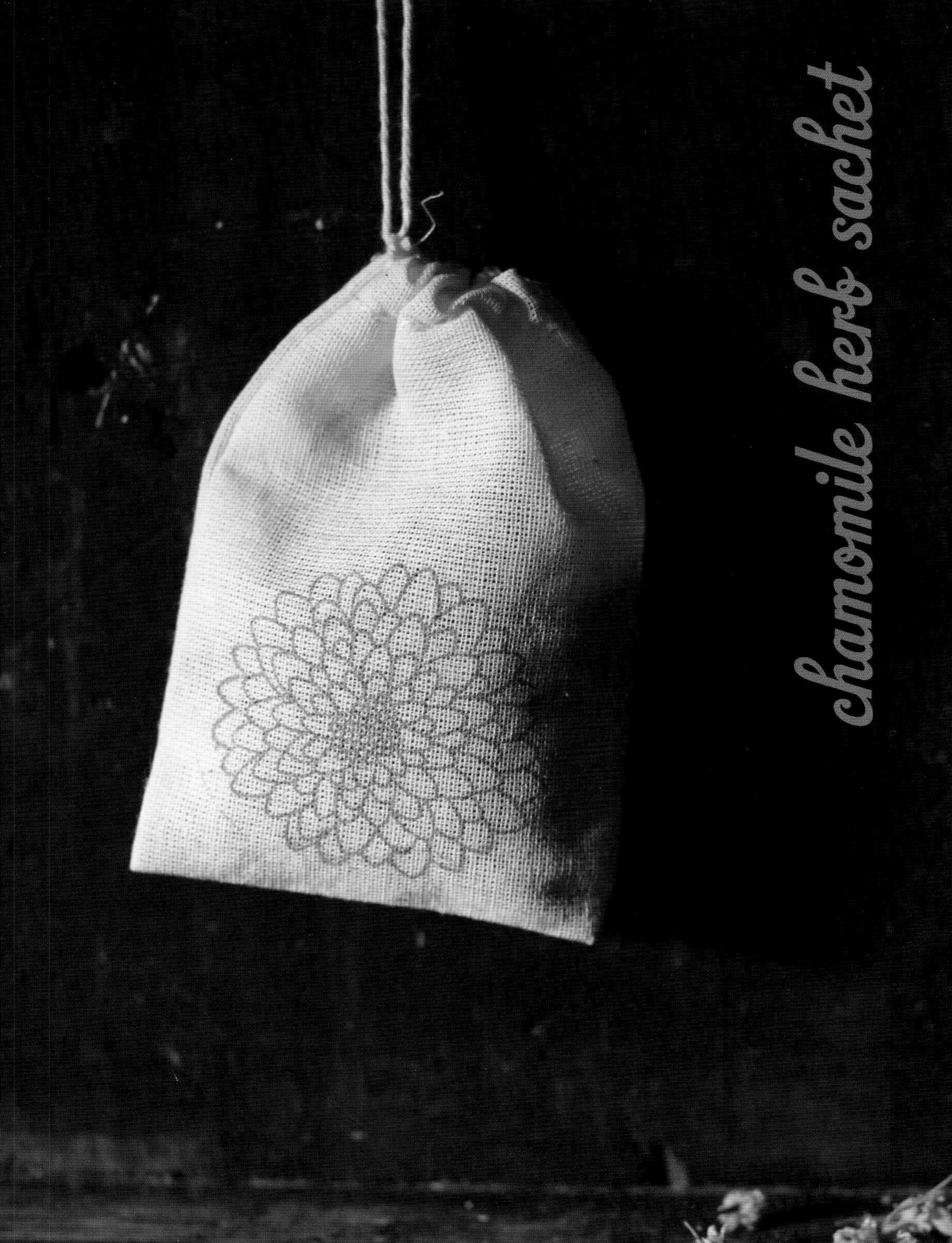
chamomile herb sachet

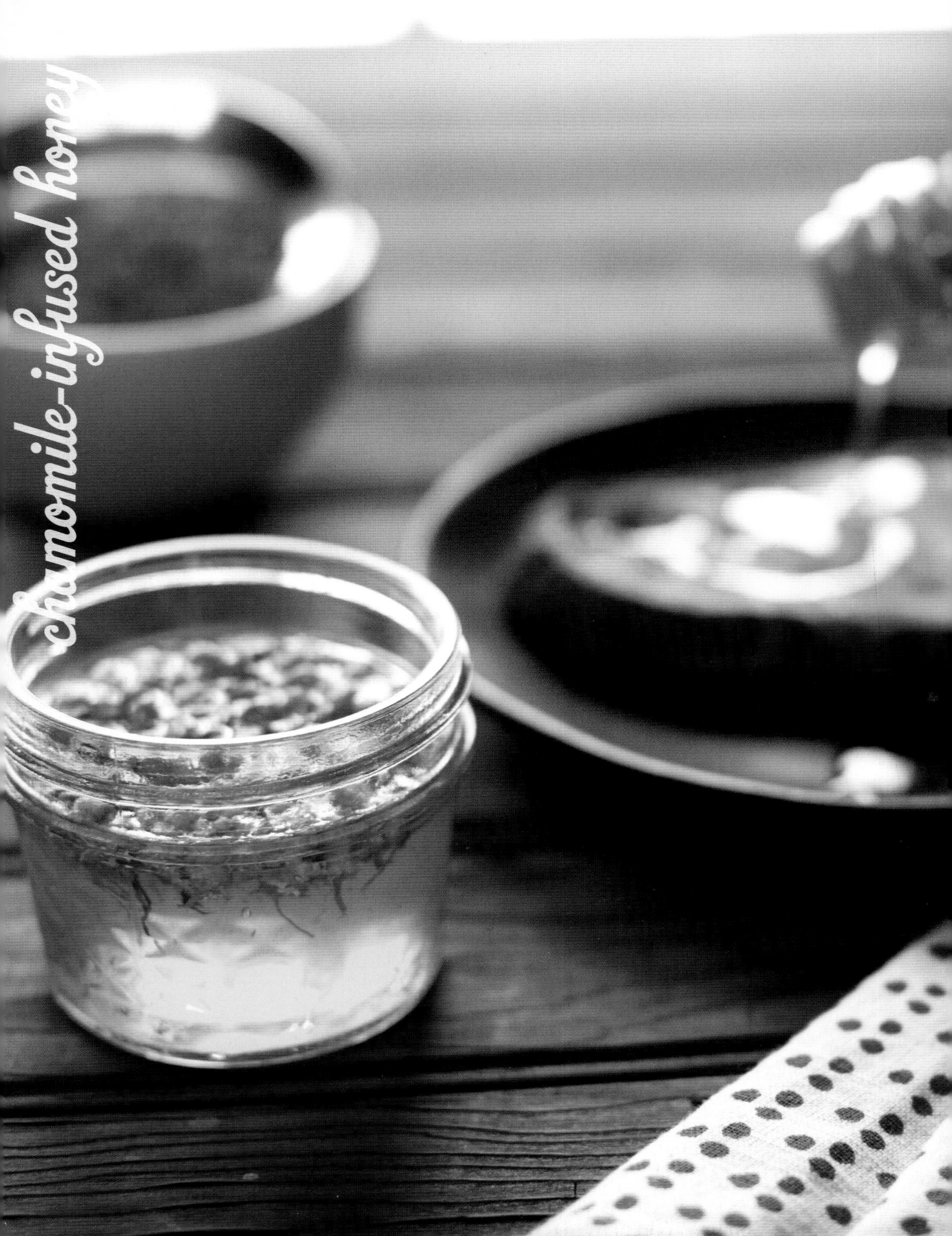
chamomile-infused honey

FOOD

Butterscotch Chamomile Clusters

This recipe comes down from my great-aunt, and, since I'm a sucker for butterscotch, I've kept it around, making little additions here and there. Chamomile is a surprisingly good mesh with the sweetness of the 'scotch.

- **2 cups butterscotch chips**
- **2 tablespoons nut butter of choice**
- **4 cups organic brown rice crisps cereal**
- **1 batch chamomile-infused sugar (recipe follows)**

1. Put the chips and nut butter in a double boiler (or heat-proof glass bowl over simmering water) and place it over low heat. Stir constantly until melted, then remove from heat (this should take 5 minutes or so once your water gets simmering).
2. Add the rice cereal and stir carefully until coated. Drop by tablespoons onto parchment paper and let harden a few minutes.
3. Roll the batter into balls between palms and then roll them in chamomile sugar. Set them aside until firm.

Makes about 3 dozen clusters

Chamomile-Infused Honey (Standard Method)

Infused honeys are just a fabulous, fabulous invention. I'm sure they were first derived to preserve the herbal harvest, as well as present a good (and palatable) delivery method for all kinds of herbal goodness. Now there are endless ways to use these sweet infusions, from baked treats to tea to ice creams to cough medicines. If you grow your own chamomile, gather flowers in the morning, after the dew has dried.

- **2 cups honey (I prefer raw, organic, local honey)**
- **3–5 tablespoons fresh chamomile blossoms or 2–4 tablespoons dried flowers**

1. Sterilize a 1-pint mason jar by boiling it in water for 10 minutes and allowing it to air-dry. Alternatively, run it through your dishwasher on the hottest setting.
2. Put the chamomile blossoms in the jar and cover them with honey. If you don't want the mess of straining the honey after the steeping period, you can put the herbs in a reusable tea bag.
3. Set the jar in a sunny windowsill for 1 week. Gaze at it lovingly (there's

Recipe continues on next page

nothing more beautiful than flowers suspended in honey on a sunny windowsill).

4. Taste the honey. If the flavor is strong enough, strain the herbs and discard (or compost or use in one of the above recipes). If it's not strong enough for you, then either add more herbs or let the honey steep for another week.

Makes about 2 cups

Chamomile-Infused Honey (Fast Method)

If you just can't wait two weeks for your herb-infused honey, try this. Use this honey to treat coughs (take a tablespoon every few hours or add to hot water, lemon, and brandy — brandy is optional), to add flavor to teas, for baking, or for spreading on your breakfast toast, oatmeal, or muffins.

- **2 cups honey**
- **2 cups fresh chamomile blossoms or 1 cup dried**

1. Pour the honey into a double boiler or a heat-proof bowl set over a pan of simmering water at low heat. Add the chamomile blossoms directly to the honey, or place them in small muslin sachet bags if you don't want to strain the honey. Heat the mixture to 180°F/80°C (use a candy thermometer) and keep it there for 10 to 12 minutes.
2. Strain the mixture (or discard the muslin bag) into a glass jar.

Chamomile-Infused Sugar

Use the sugar, herb flecks and all, in any recipe. You can also get creative — try lavender, rose, rosemary, ginger, vanilla, or any combination of herbs to flavor your sugars.

- **⅓ cup dried chamomile flowers**
- **2 cups organic sugar (white or brown)**

Add the flowers to the bottom of a clean 1-quart mason jar (there will be space in the jar — no worries; you want room for shaking). Cover with the sugar and shake. Let this stand for at least 2 weeks in a cool, dry place. Shake the jar and contents daily.

Makes about 2 cups

Chamomile Energy Bars

These guys are so fabulous for long car trips, airplane rides, hikes, camping, and school lunches — plus they're endlessly versatile. My mom used to switch it up and pack different varieties for us every week.

- **3 cups oatmeal**
- **3 tablespoons veggie oil**
- **½ cup bran cereal**
- **½ cup chopped nuts of your choice**
- **⅓ cup chamomile-infused honey (recipes, pages 31 and 32)**
- **½ cup dried cherries or dried fruit of choice**
- **½ cup candied, dried ginger (optional; if you skip this, add ½ cup dried fruit of choice)**

1. Preheat the oven to 375°F/190°C.
2. Put the oatmeal, oil, cereal, nuts, and honey in a large bowl and mix well. Spread the mixture on an ungreased baking sheet (I like to line it with parchment paper — makes life much easier) and bake for 20 minutes.
3. Sprinkle dried ginger on top, gently pressing them into the bars. When cool, cut into squares.

Makes 15 good-size bars

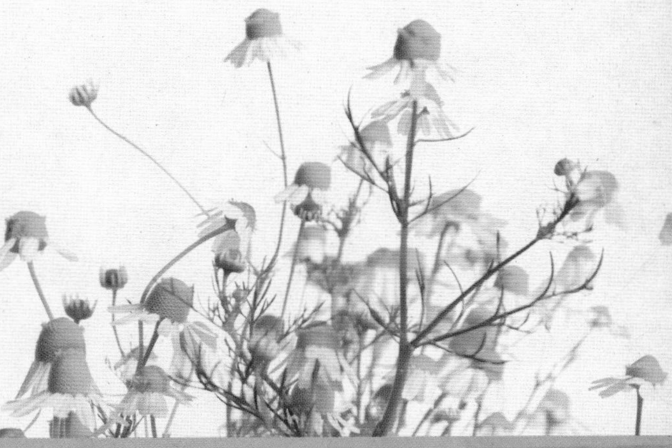

CHAMOMILE BLOND-ING

Got blond? Or want to get blond? Chamomile can be added to your hair care regimen. In the winter months, highlights can fade. Bring a little of that chamomile sunshine into your hair by brewing a strong infusion of chamomile (6 tablespoons per quart of water). Keep this mixture in the refrigerator and use as a hair toner after you shampoo and condition — no need to rinse. The chamomile will bring out the natural blond and gold tones in your hair and subtly lighten dark hair.

CHAMOMILE YOGA

Since chamomile is uplifting, associated with the sun, and specially formulated to get us out of our doldrums, I thought I would offer up a sunny posture that cannot help bringing some joy into your day: Standing Salute.

Beginning in Mountain Pose (*Tadasana*). Feel all four corners of your feet on the ground. Engage your knees and quadriceps (the muscles that run along the front of your thighs). Tuck your pelvis slightly so that you have a nice, long spine. Pull your navel in toward your spine a bit, for support. Lift through your heart so that you can breathe easily. Make sure your shoulder blades are sliding down your back, shoulders relaxed. Tuck your chin slightly so that your neck isn't strained.

Moving into Standing Salute. Bring your palms together at heart center (and if you can do this before a sunny window, even better). Inhale and sweep your arms out to the sides and then overhead. You can leave your hands shoulder-width apart here, fingers spread, or clasp them in what I call Charlie's Angels Mudra (clasp the hands together, making a gun out of your first finger and thumb).

On your next inhale, lean back slightly — don't lose your balance. Go just far enough for a small, but invigorating, backbend. Exhale and return to standing, with arms still stretched toward the ceiling (or, in other words, the sun!) for Standing Salute.

Finishing. One more inhale and stretch your arms up; exhale and sweep them around and down, then gather them together again at heart's center. Do this as many times as you like. First thing in the morning, as the sun is rising, always sets the tone of the day for me.

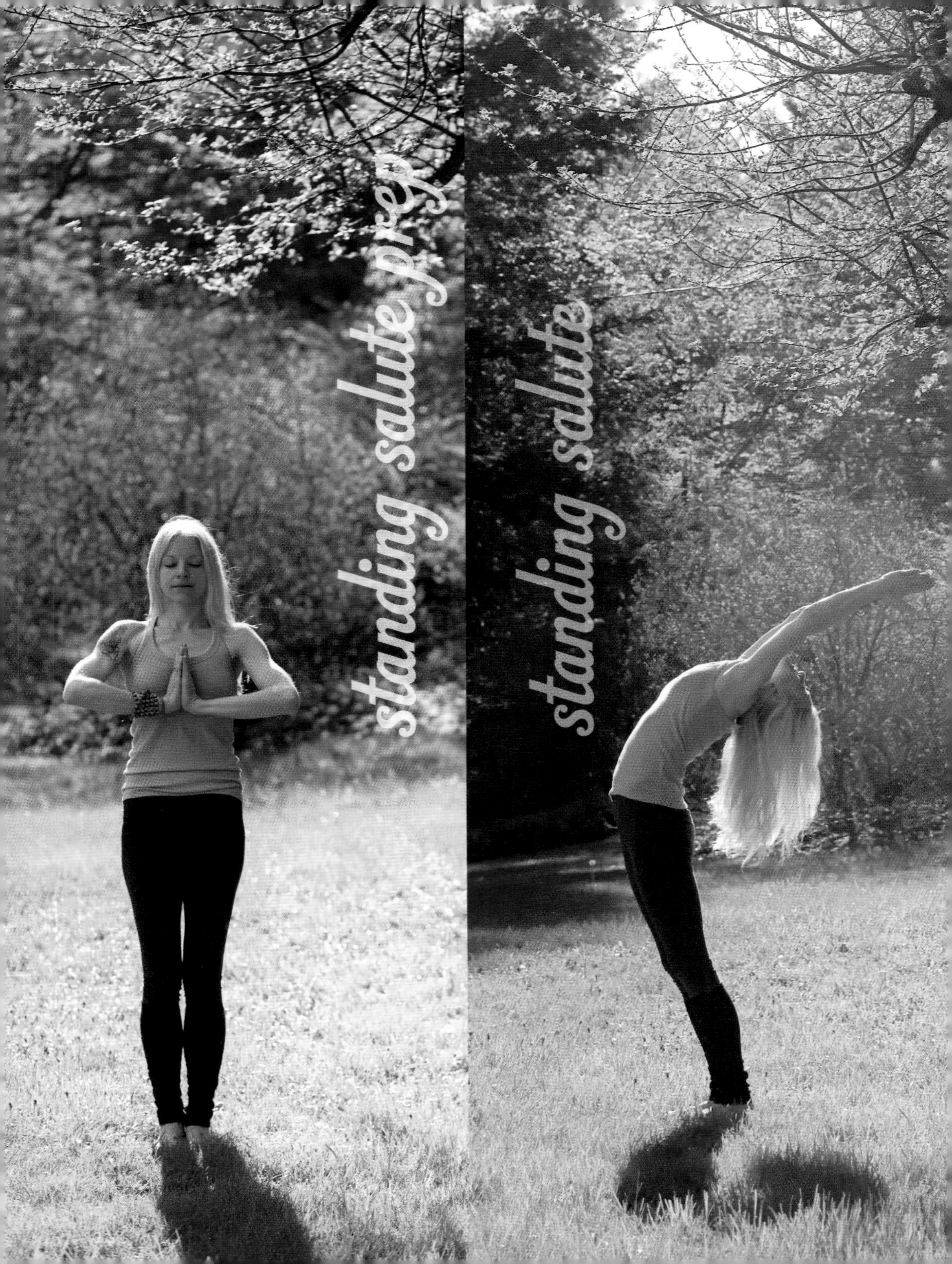
standing salute prep
standing salute

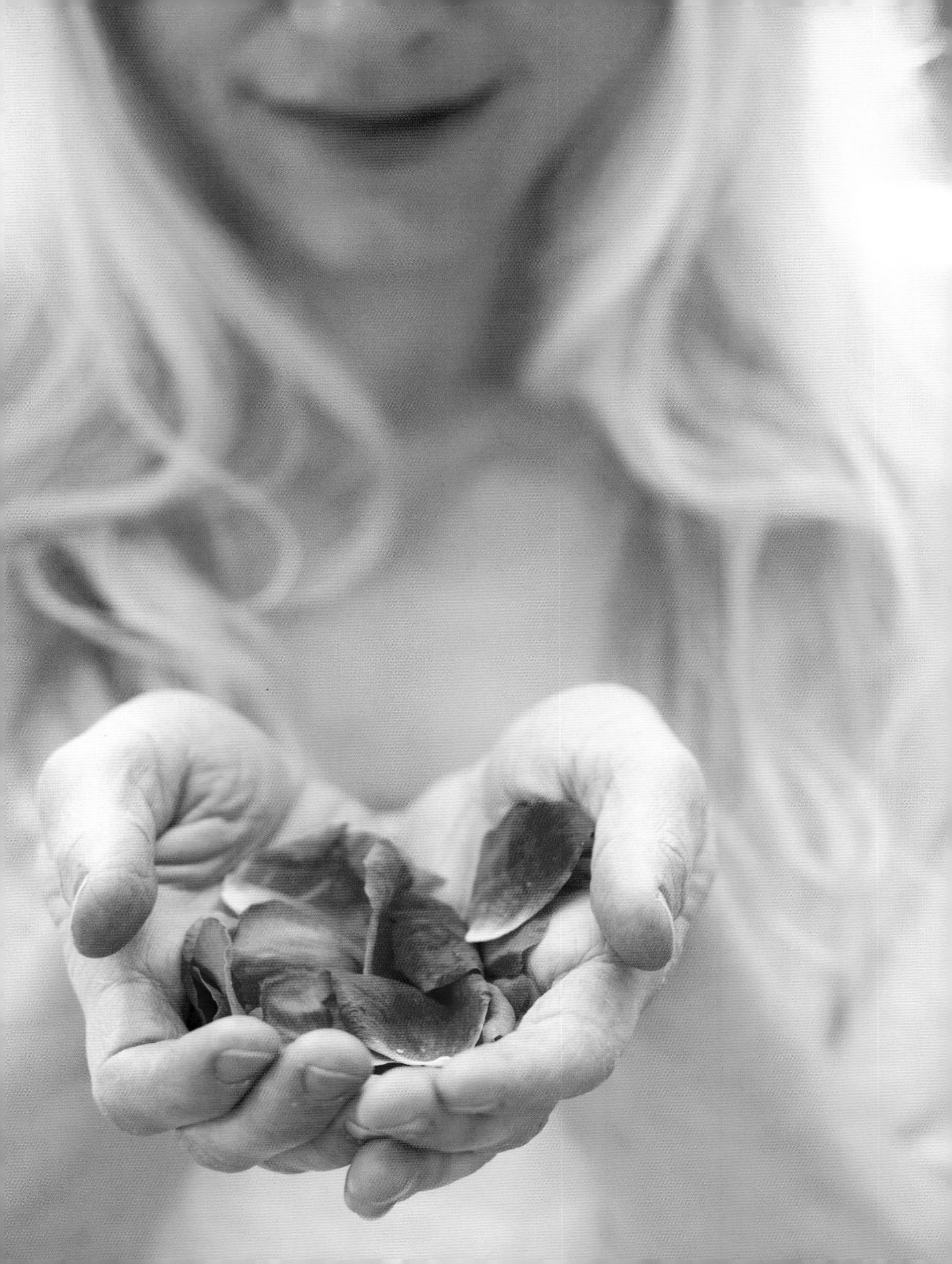

2

Rediscovering the MOST ROMANTIC BLOOM

Ah, roses; ah, love. Enter a beautiful medicinal with the most romantic history (and associations). No matter where you fall on the love it/hate it rose-love symbolism spectrum, you have to admit that there's nothing like the jolt from the sight and smell of a rose (a species of the *Rosa* genus). Casting love and its myriad consequences aside, roses (as herbs) are soothing and therapeutic to the body, mind, and spirit.

Now, we're not talking the seriously sexy, long-stemmed, perfectly velvet-red roses you find for a zillion dollars a dozen in any florist's Valentine window display. We're talking the untamed, undomesticated, uncultivated, wily, wanton, and wild rose (my favorite varietal is *Rosa rugosa*, or the rugosa rose). As you develop your relationship with these medicinal herbs, you'll find that, just like people, you get better results when you just let them live the way they want to live.

You can grow wild roses in your herbal plot. You just want to stay away from the hybrids, which are cultivated for scent and/or beauty, because their medicinal value has been more or less sacrificed in favor of brighter colors and deeper scents. And although beauty is subjective (the one lesson we all come away with in regard to love . . .), I must say that I much prefer the rowdy charm of the wild roses. If you're interested in sowing some wild roses, take some time to plot a medicinal rose garden. Choose the wild varietals such as *Rosa rugosa* (the rugosa, Japanese, or beach rose), *Rosa rubiginosa* (the eglantine or sweet briar rose), or *Rosa canina* (the dog rose).

If you have roses nearby, you can harvest the flower petals throughout the summer. You can also cut blossoms from the plant on a sunny day, after the dew has evaporated. Be sure to leave some flowers untouched, allowing them to ripen into rosehips. You can gather the fruit after the first frost in the fall; waiting this long allows the rosehip's sweetness to develop. You can use the petals and hips fresh or dried; if dried, keep them in an airtight container for up to a year.

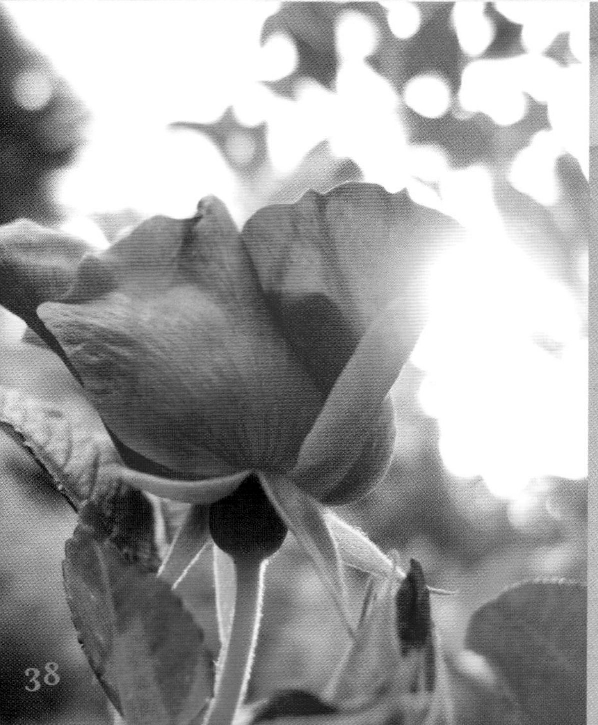

ROSE

Species of the *Rosa* genus

Parts used: Flower petals and rosehips
How to harvest: Cut flower heads on a sunny morning after the dew has dried; harvest rosehips after the first frost
Effects on body: Anti-inflammatory, antiseptic, tonic for the heart and circulatory system
Effects on mind and spirit: Uplifting, cheering, calming, heart-opening
Safety first: Avoid taking if you are pregnant. Be sure to harvest your roses far from roadsides, and never harvest flowers that have been subject to chemical fertilizers or pesticides.

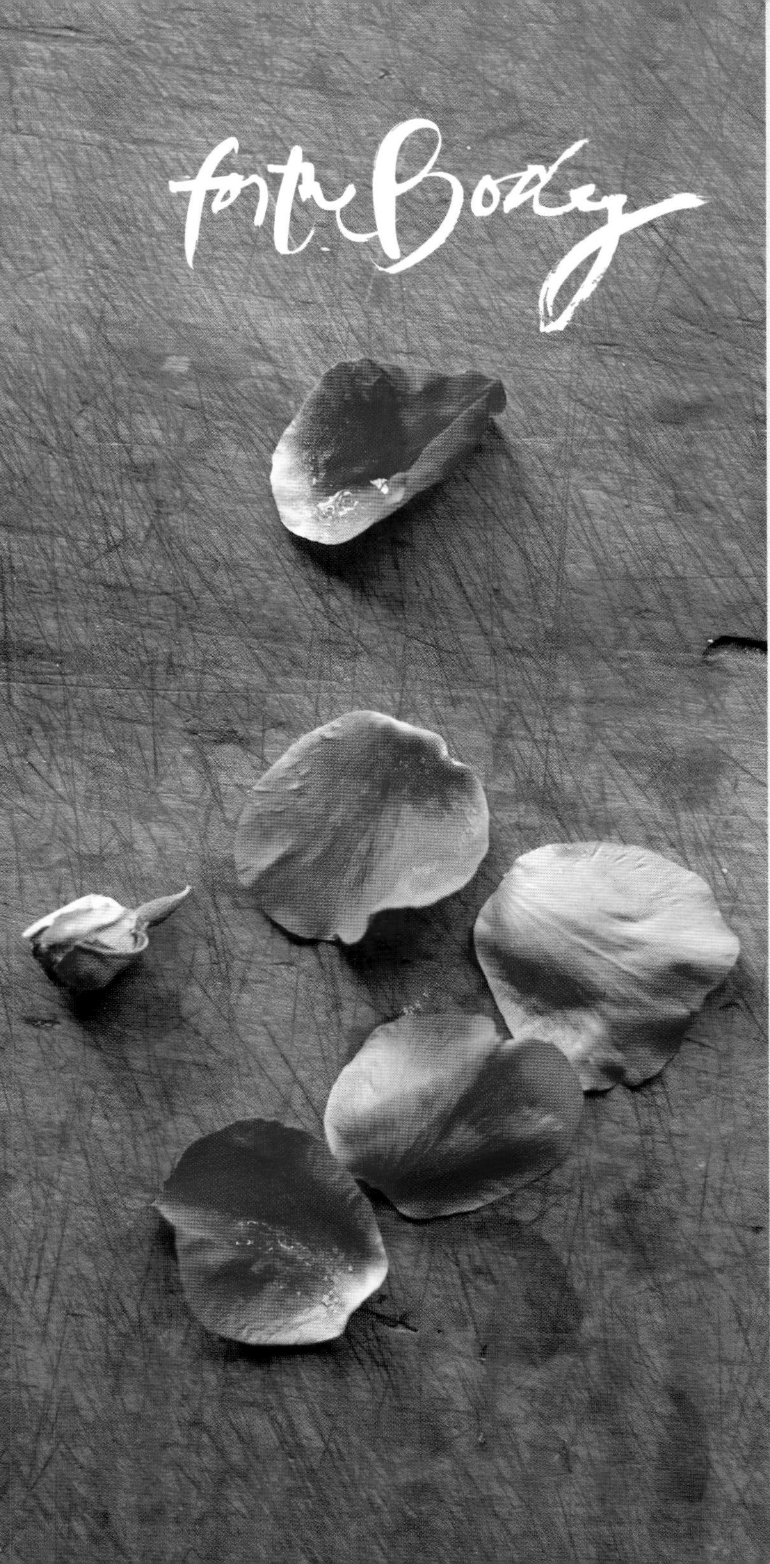

In herbal medicine, we use the petals and fruit (rosehips) of the rose. Rose petals are mildly sedative, antiseptic, anti-inflammatory, and anti-parasitic. They're also mild laxatives, a good supportive tonic for the heart, and great for lowering cholesterol (romantic, right?).

The antiseptic nature of rose petals makes them a wonderful treatment for wounds, bruises, rashes, and incisions. Taken internally, their anti-inflammatory properties make them a wonderful treatment for sore throats or ulcers. They can stimulate the liver and increase appetite and circulation.

Got flu? Rose can also lower your body temperature and help bring down a fever or cool you off in the summer. As an anti-spasmodic, it helps relieve spasms in the respiratory system (asthma and coughs), in the intestinal tract (cramping, constipation), and in the muscles (cramps and sports injuries). Adding its antiviral qualities, you've got an entire winter's medicine chest in one herb.

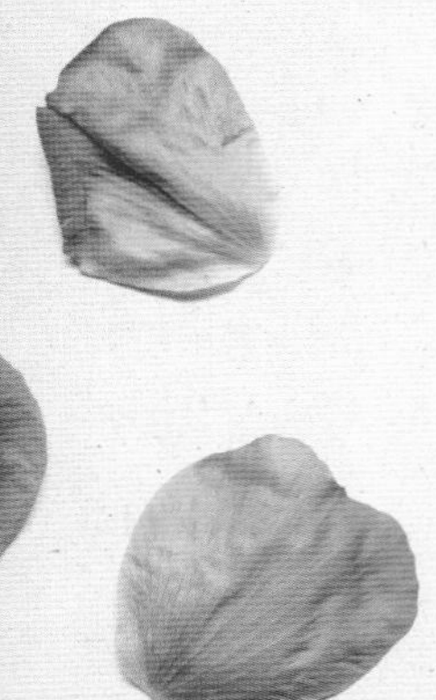

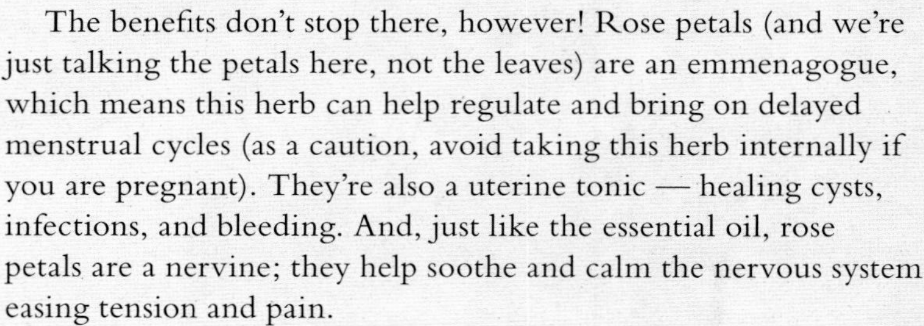

The benefits don't stop there, however! Rose petals (and we're just talking the petals here, not the leaves) are an emmenagogue, which means this herb can help regulate and bring on delayed menstrual cycles (as a caution, avoid taking this herb internally if you are pregnant). They're also a uterine tonic — healing cysts, infections, and bleeding. And, just like the essential oil, rose petals are a nervine; they help soothe and calm the nervous system, easing tension and pain.

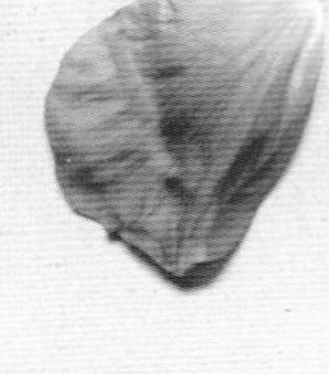

Okay, so that's just the flower. (What?! There's more?!) Once the flower has run its course, we're left with rosehips, or the fruit of the rose. Rosehips are wonderful little packages that are delicious in teas or even substituted for your favorite fruit in recipes for preserves. High in vitamin C, especially, but also containing vitamins A, B_3, D, and E, rosehips are an effective nutritive — especially helpful during the long cold and flu season. Rosehips are also a strong antioxidant, protecting you from the ravaging effects of the free radicals that are a part of any urban lifestyle.

Rosehips also contain iron, which is therapeutic for anemia as well as for easing pain and discomfort during one's monthly cycle. Their flavonoid content makes rosehips strong antioxidants that protect the body from free radicals (read: anti-aging tonic for inner and outer beauty). Their anti-inflammatory nature helps soothe all kinds of pain, including arthritis, gout, and sore muscles.

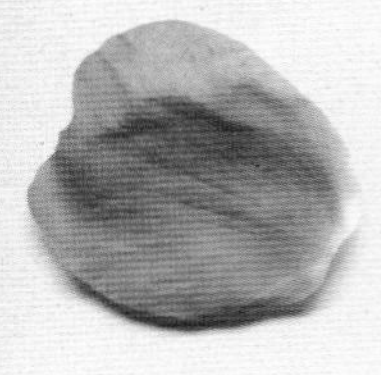

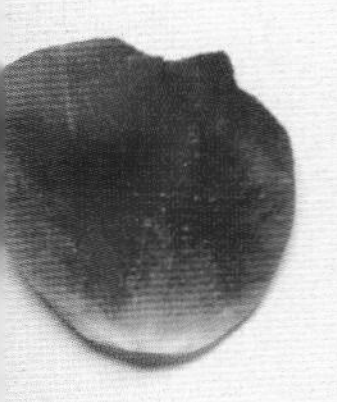

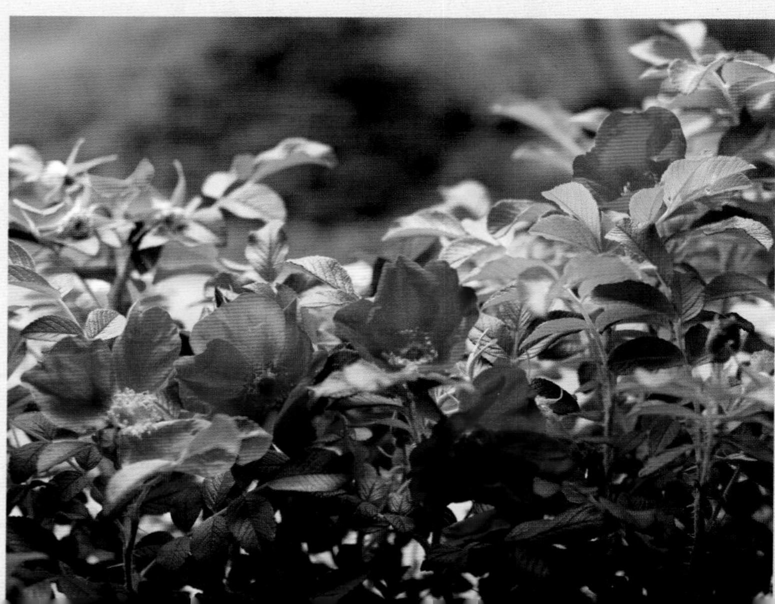

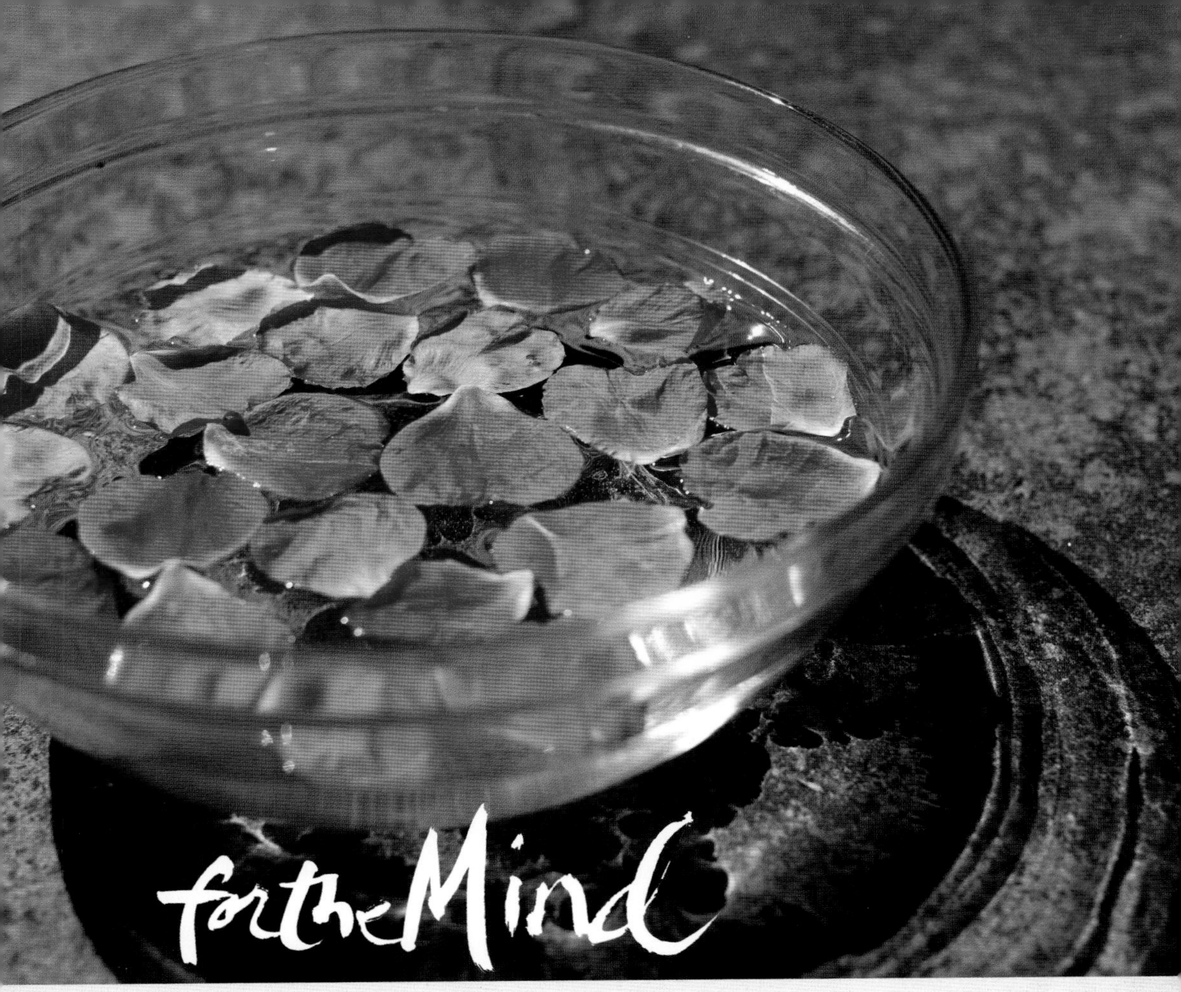

for the Mind

The smell of rose essential oil is soothing to the senses, inviting calm and focus. While it increases concentration, it can also bring on pleasant dreams if you scent your pillow with a few drops of oil at night.

For those who believe they are incapable of love (and we've all been there), rose flower essence (see box on essences on page 22) helps to open up the heart to that emotion. The essence also helps foster a feeling of community and belonging when you're feeling lost or alone. Experiencing a lot of responsibility in a difficult situation? Rose essence helps caregivers, nurses, hospice patients, social workers, and parents find patience, compassion, and understanding and overcome the fear of death. The flower essence also deepens and instills grace in those who take it, fostering an ability to experience life openly and objectively, instead of subjectively (through the emotions).

Already found your soul mate? Worried about stagnation in the relationship (aren't we all, at one point or another)? Rose essence helps long-standing couples re-ignite love and rekindle passion in their relationships.

What about the most essential relationship — the one between your "mundane" self and your divine, higher self? Deepen your relationship to the divine (whatever that is for you) with this essence. One way this works is by dissolving judgments and putting an end to long prejudices (realized or subconscious). Alternatively, it can also help you to find the strength and understanding needed to move on from a relationship, be it a personal or a professional one, when it is no longer working for you (bonus: this essence helps you do so with grace, poise, and no regrets).

Lastly, but certainly not the least of its benefits: rose creates a sense of compassion and empathy for all living creatures. When you take this flower essence, the veil is withdrawn and you awaken to the secret that all beings unite and relate.

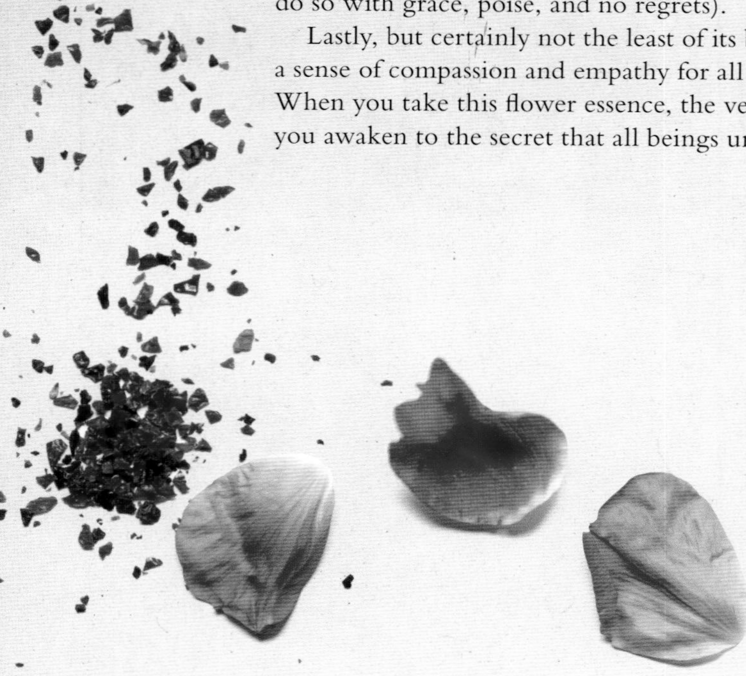

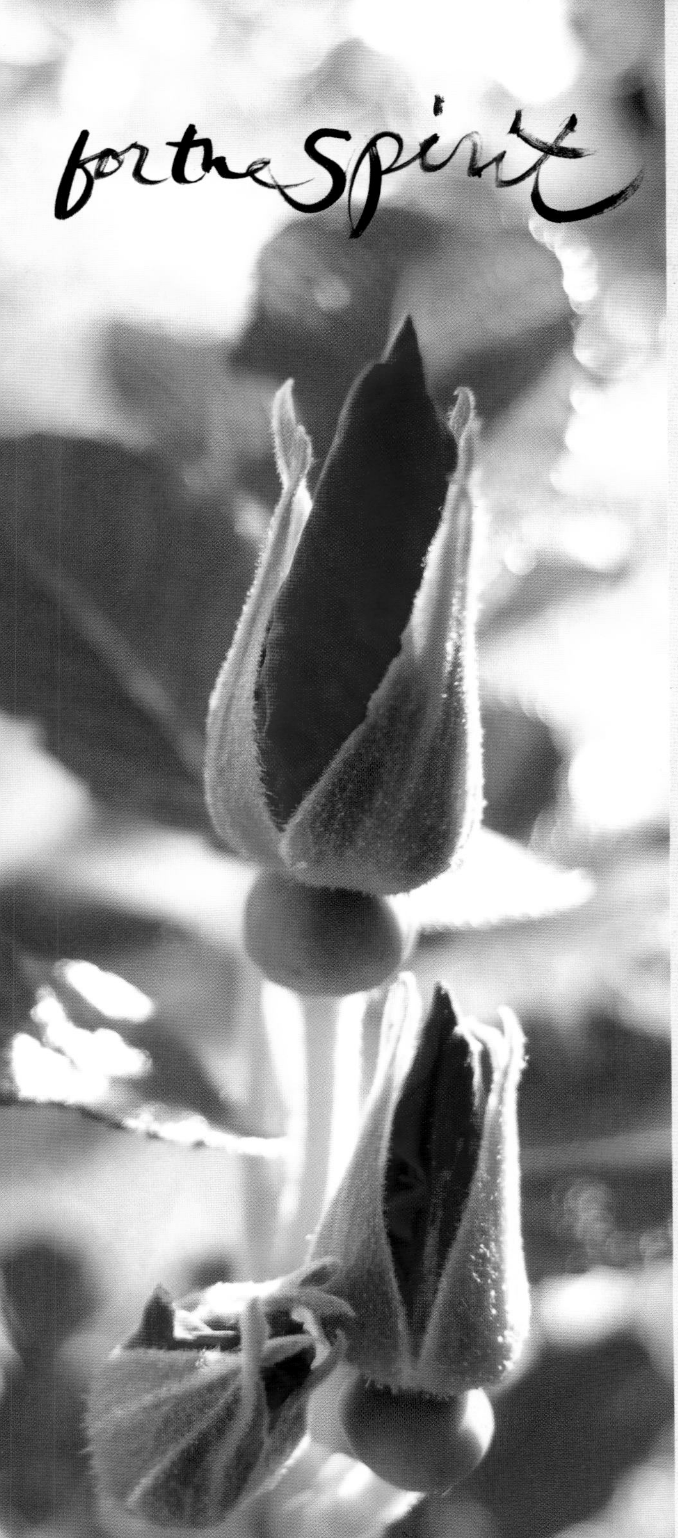

As with all things in nature, mind, body, and spirit tend to overlap. You can easily see how fostering universal compassion — a key benefit of the rose flower essence — crosses over into the spiritual realm (indeed, it helps *open* you to the spiritual realm by ramping up sensitivity and dispelling fear). And, surely, you already know some of the common magical qualities of the rose. A rose invites romance, expresses sympathy, and conveys love and friendship simply with the gift of its presence; the rose signifies the bond between people, from passion to devotion to condolence and commiseration. Either way, roses say more than words ever could; this, my friends, is the definition of true magic.

As for magical associations, the gender of the rose is feminine (no surprise there), the elements are fire and water (we are talking passion, after all), and the planets are Mars and Venus (masculine and feminine, don't ya know?). The rose possesses the power to aid in healing, love, luck, protection, and psychic powers.

Roses are a talisman for good luck in romance. Sometimes objects are magical because they've been used for so long for one particular purpose, and sometimes they've been used for one particular purpose because their magic is that strong. Roses? I think it's a little bit of both.

ROSE MAGIC

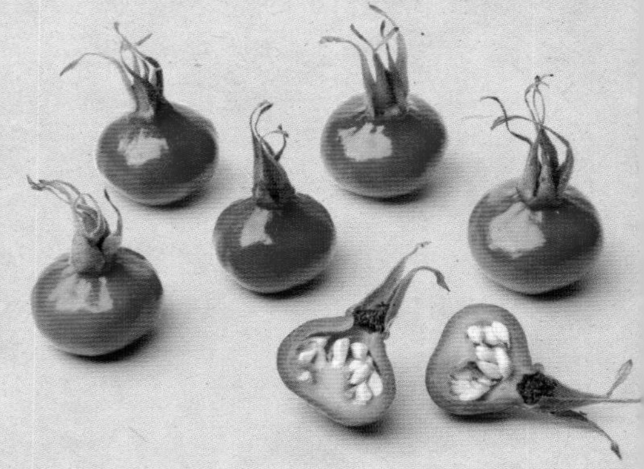

TO BRING LOVE INTO YOUR LIFE

Gather rose petals (dried or fresh, conventionally grown or wild, though wild is always a stronger choice when passion is involved) and hold them in your hands. Picture the kind of love you'd like to invite into your life (not a particular person — we have some control, but not that much) and send that picture into the petals. Place these in a small pouch; keep it close to you during the day, and then sleep with it under your pillow at night.

FOR A NEW RELATIONSHIP

Brew a cup of rose petal tea, lace it with honey, and share the cup with your significant other at the beginning of your evening. This will instill harmony and clear sight — in other words, if you're right for each other, the relationship will progress smoothly and with joy. Conversely, if this isn't the person for you, you'll see it and release the relationship with grace and little or no attachment.

FOR OTHER TYPES OF LOVE

Roses aren't just for bringing romantic love into your life; you can use them to manifest any kind of love. For example, in cases of infertility or estranged relationships, use them as above, bringing a different picture to mind. Ask for help in mending a relationship or in bringing new life into the world (remember, magic works as it works; in regard to infertility, for example, you may find the opportunity to adopt a child instead of conceiving one — we must be open to all possibilities).

TO INSTILL PEACE AND HARMONY

Rosehips, too, have their own special magic. If there has been much disharmony or upheaval in your life, charge a handful of rosehips with peace and harmony, then tuck them around the house, especially in areas where discord has been especially strong (oftentimes, this is the bedroom, which represents relationships). Under the pillows is another good place — here the magic can blend with the subconscious during sleep. Also, try placing them in windows and doorsills to ensure that harmony stays within and discord without.

FOR PROPHETIC DREAMS

Roses have also had a long association with prophesy and foresight. To encourage prophetic dreams, have a cup of rose petal tea before bed and keep your journal nearby (these visions dissipate quickly until you get the hang of holding on to them). You can also try burning rose petals as incense to increase gifts of prophesy and clairvoyance. Light a charcoal disk and sprinkle the dried petals on top. Meditate as you breathe the scented smoke.

FOR BEAUTY

Finally, try rose magic to instill beauty in yourself — inside and out. Roses work their magic by increasing our self-confidence and acceptance of ourselves, not by radically and unrealistically changing our features overnight. Stand before a mirror and really look at yourself. Try to empty your mind of all judgment and simply observe. Add a few drops of rose essential oil or burn some rose incense. Inhale the aroma and imagine any doubts about your appearance dissolving on the exhale. Confirm that you are beautiful (*know* it, even if you don't yet *feel* it). Try this every day for a week and be open to your own beauty. You may quickly find others confirming this newfound knowledge of yourself. Feel free to repeat this spell anytime doubt begins to creep in.

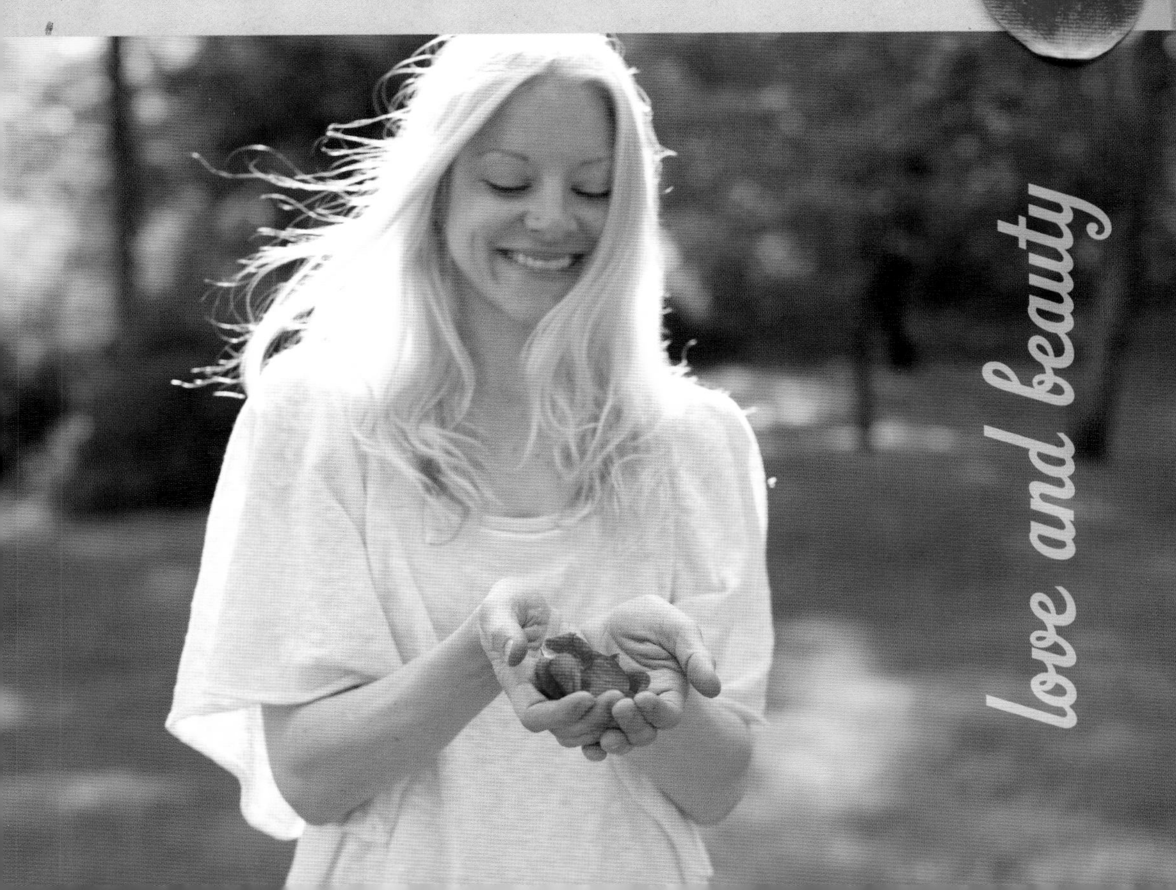

TEAS

Base tea. One batch of rose petal tea can have many uses. For your base infusion, pour 1 cup boiling water over 2 to 4 teaspoons of dried rose petals. Cover and steep for 10 to 15 minutes. Apply that base tea to any of the following:

Cough and cold remedy. Blend the base tea with 1 or 2 teaspoons of honey (a natural sore-throat soother and cough suppressant), plus a dash of lemon and/or brandy to taste. Both the lemon and the brandy are optional, but they do wonders for a stubborn cough, especially one that's kept you up for a few nights.

Digestive tonic. When you're under the weather (you know, below the belt), a strong tea full of tannins is helpful in treating diarrhea and bladder infections. Use a teaspoon more of the dried herb than usual and drink a cup without milk or sweetener. Repeat every 45 minutes to an hour, as needed. If the diarrhea is especially uncomfortable, you may bring on faster relief by adding a dash of black tea to the rose petals.

Rosehip tea. Use 4 teaspoons dried hips or 4 tablespoons fresh per cup of water and simmer on low heat for 5 minutes. This makes a tangy, sour tea loaded with vitamin C. For a little variation, pour this hot infusion over 1 teaspoon spearmint leaves or toss a little ginger in with the hips while simmering. This tea is great chilled or heated, depending on how you feel. But let me tell you, there's nothing like rosehip and ginger tea laced with stevia and a splash of vanilla almond milk in the midst of a snowstorm . . . bliss!

BODY CARE

Dry Skin Soother

Smooth this on your face at night, after exposure to sun or wind, or anytime the skin feels tight and dry. Or, for an easy fix, you can add a few drops of rose essential oil to the moisturizer you already use.

- **1 ounce jojoba oil**
- **8 drops rose essential oil**

Blend the oils and apply!

Makes 1 ounce

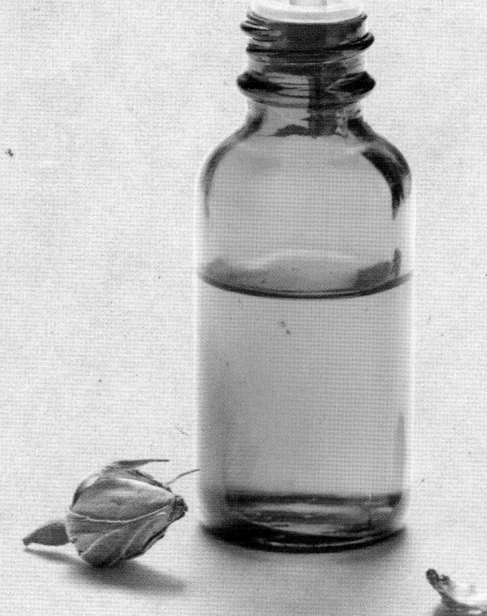

Rose and Coconut Body Scrub

This scrub exfoliates the skin and moisturizes at the same time — perfect for the dryness that's a by-product of climate-controlled environments.

- **½ cup coconut oil**
- **⅓ cup sugar of your choice (brown sugar is always nice and a bit different)**
- **½ cup dried rose petals**
- **1 tablespoon rose-infused oil (optional)**

1. Mix the coconut oil, sugar, and rose petals in a bowl (I like to use my hands to mix — they get moisturized and exfoliated as I work). If the scrub is too oily, add more sugar. You want to be able to scoop this and spread it on your skin, so it's really up to you to decide the consistency. Too grainy? Add some of your rose-infused oil. Mix it up.
2. Scoop your scrub into a half-pint mason jar. Cap your jar, and go on being fabulous.

Makes 8 ounces

ROSE AROMATHERAPY

With diffuser. We've already talked a bit about the nerve-soothing (not to mention warm-fuzzy-inducing) benefits of the rose essential oil. So if you're feeling stressed or anxious, add a few drops of oil to an aromatherapy diffuser (or sprinkle a few drops into hot water), sit back, and relax.

For pulse points. Add a few drops of rose essential oil to a carrier oil (such as almond, apricot, or jojoba) and apply to the pulse points (incidentally, you can try this same oil on skin suffering from eczema).

As steam. Simmer a handful of petals on the stove and let the aromatic steam disperse through the house.

In a bath. Try adding the essential oil to a warm bath, and enjoy the simultaneous relaxation and uplifting action of the scent — not to mention the skin softening and soothing qualities of the rose.

On a charcoal disk. Light a disk, and when it's glowing, sprinkle a few dried rose petals on top.

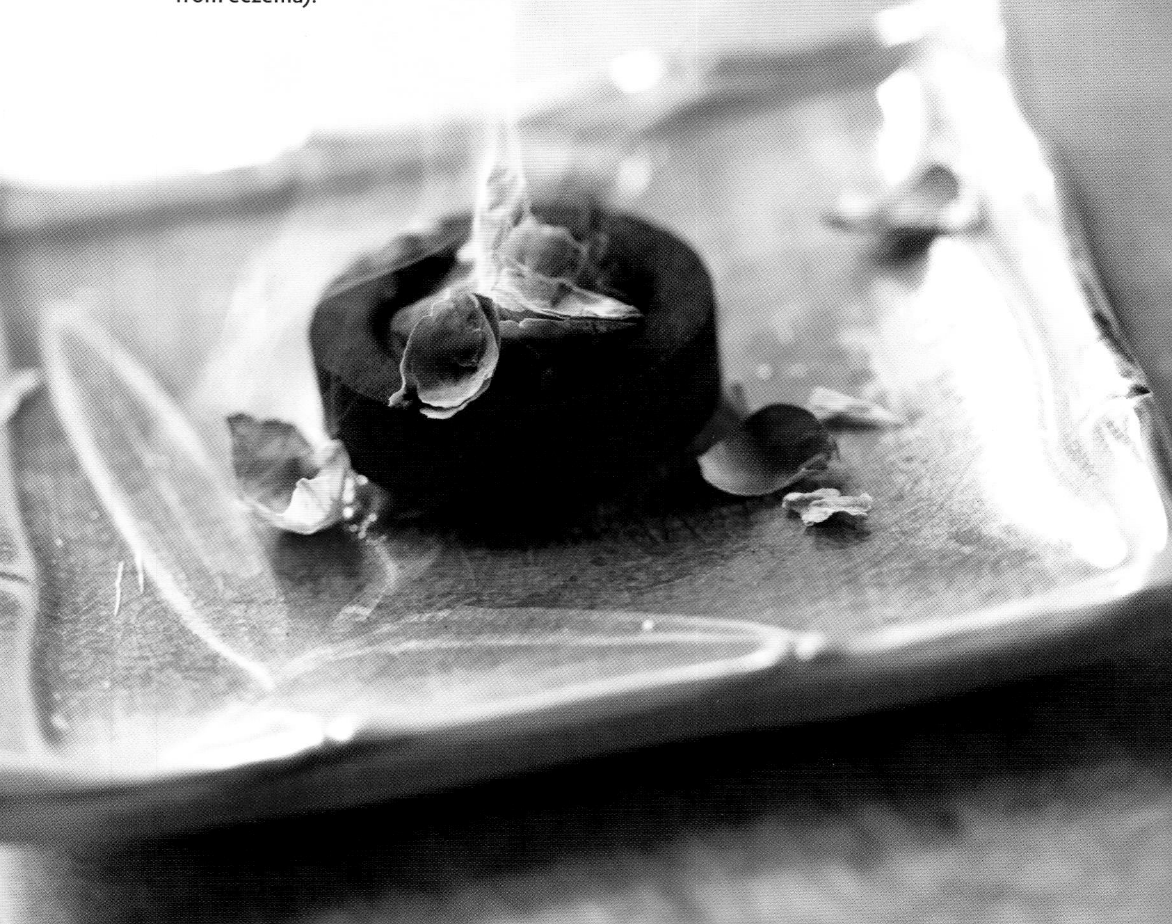

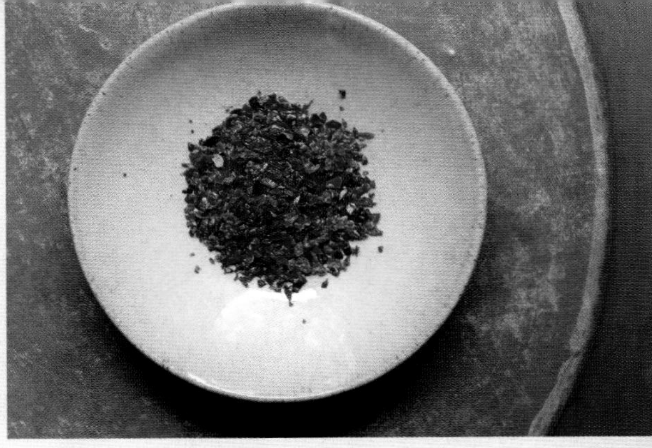

Rose Soap

This is an easy way to make soap (without having to get into all that caustic chemistry). A by-product of vegetable oil, glycerin is a wonderful substance that actually draws moisture to the skin.

- **1 pound glycerin soap or a 1-pound melt-and-pour kit**
- **1 teaspoon powdered soy milk**
- **3 drops vanilla extract**
- **1 tablespoon ground rosehips**
- **4 drops rose essential oil**
- **2 drops essential lavender essential oil**
- **1 tablespoon rosehip-infused almond or coconut oil**
- **7 teaspoons dried rose petals**
- **4 4-ounce soap molds**

1. If using glycerin soap, grate the bar with a cheese grater or food processor (use the grating setting). If using a melt-and-pour package, skip to step 2.
2. Boil water in the bottom of a double boiler, or boil a pot of hot water and place a Pyrex bowl over it to create a double boiler. Put the grated glycerin soap into the top of the double boiler or the Pyrex bowl and allow it to melt completely. Remove the bowl from the heat.
3. Stir the melted glycerin soap, and add the soy milk powder, vanilla extract, and rosehips. Stir until mixed thoroughly (just a note from experience: it's probably a good idea to use potholders here). Add the rose, lavender, and almond oil or coconut oil, as well as 4 teaspoons rose petals. Stir the blend until it is mixed all the way through.
4. For a little added sass, sprinkle a couple of teaspoons of rose petals into your soap molds before carefully pouring in the mixture. Pour in the mixture, filling each mold to the top (if you like, press the remaining rose petals into the top of your soap), and allow the soap to harden. Once completely solid, the soap can be popped out of the molds (press gently on the back of the mold). If the soap sticks, run the mold under hot water for a few moments; alternatively, put the molds in the freezer for a few minutes — no more than 15 — to help magically loosen up those soaps.

Makes 4 bars

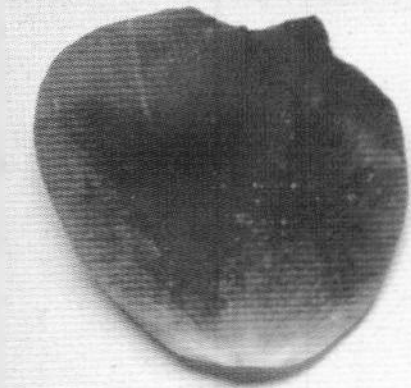

Rose Facial Clay

There's not much that's more healing or detoxifying than a good clay mask. It's super-easy to create your own, and you can use pretty much any flower (including chapter 1's chamomile) if you like. This recipe is definitely not set in stone — you have to experiment and do a little trial and error. But once you have adjusted the recipe to your satisfaction, make sure you write down your ingredients and ratios. Make a huge batch and fill a bunch of jars — this stuff has a really long shelf life. You can give some away as gifts as well! Need to find clay? See the Resources.

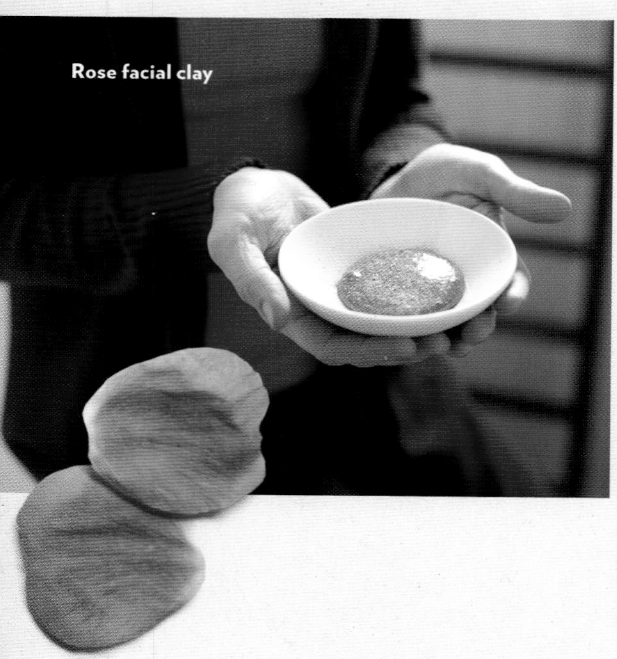
Rose facial clay

2 tablespoons powdered French green clay (for oily/troubled skin), bentonite clay (for serious healing), or white cosmetic clay (for sensitive, dry, or mature skin)

1 teaspoon powdered rose petals (could also include powdered lavender and powdered chamomile)

1 tablespoon glycerin

1 teaspoon raw apple cider vinegar

1 teaspoon jojoba or almond oil (optional, but include for dry skin conditions; use water if you're omitting the oil)

5 drops rose essential oil or 3 drops rose oil, 1 drop lavender oil, and 1 drop chamomile oil

1. Sterilize a 4-ounce jar by boiling it for 10 minutes in a water bath, or run it through your dishwasher.
2. Stir together the clay and the dried herbs. Add the glycerin, vinegar, and jojoba or almond oil (or water if not using oil). Stir to mix well. If it's too soupy, sprinkle in more clay. Not spreadable? Pour in a dash more oil or water.
3. Add the essential oils of your choice and stir. Then apply a thin layer to your face, put your feet up, and relax for 10 to 15 minutes. Rinse with warm water and pat dry. Go out and show off your radiant skin (optional, but highly recommended).

Makes 2 to 3 treatments

FOOD

Rosehip Syrup

Syrups are really wonderful ways to take herbs — especially for children and those who feel unwell. Rose-infused honey or sugar syrup is especially soothing, anti-inflammatory, and antibacterial. This is a variation on a recipe the British Ministry of Food released in 1943 (rosehips have something like 20 times the amount of vitamin C as do the same amount of oranges).

2 pounds fresh rosehips or 1 pound dried

1 cup sugar (I prefer organic brown)

1. Fill a large pot with 6 cups water and bring to a boil.
2. Add the rosehips, reduce the heat to low, and simmer 1 hour or until the rosehips are tender.
3. Filter the mixture through a jelly bag or a colander lined with several layers of cheesecloth. You might want to strain this liquid again, through fresh layers of cheesecloth, in order to remove all those small hairs that cover the seeds. (Let me tell you — it's hard to treat a sore throat when you have a bunch of little hairs irritating it on the way down.) You could even pour this mixture through a coffee filter one last time. Then see the Rosehip Fruit Leather recipe on the next page for a way to use up this puréed goodness!
4. Pour the juice into a saucepan and boil over high heat, adding the sugar. Let this boil for 5 minutes, uncovered. This will reduce the volume slightly and make the liquid more syrupy.
5. Sterilize 6 half-pint mason jars by boiling them for 10 minutes in a water bath (don't boil the lids; just soak them in just-boiled water for 10 minutes) or run them through your dishwasher — lids, jars, and all. Pour the syrup into the jars (heated jars, to avoid breakage) and seal. You can store them in the fridge indefinitely, or, if you'd rather keep them on the shelf for a few months, process the jars in a boiling water bath for 10 minutes. Take a tablespoon every hour for chronic coughs or pour over pancakes to celebrate getting over the flu.

Makes 6 cups syrup

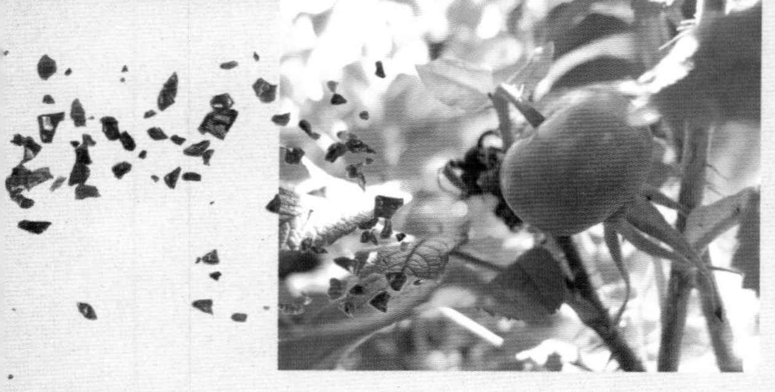

Rosehip Fruit Leather

Remember fruit roll-ups? God, I loved those things — so much sugar! This recipe uses the rosehip purée you ended up with in the rosehip syrup recipe (you know . . . that stuff left over in the jelly bag or cheesecloth) to make your own healthy, fun, and funky fruit rolls.

- **2 cups rosehip purée (see Rosehip Syrup recipe, page 51)**
- **2 tablespoons honey or maple syrup (optional)**

1. Preheat the oven to 200°F/90°C. Line two baking sheets with parchment paper.
2. Add honey or maple syrup, if using, to the purée, and stir to combine. Spread the purée in a thin layer on the lined baking sheets.
3. Slide the baking sheets into the oven. Bake for 3 hours or so, checking on the leather every 45 minutes. The leather is done when it's tacky and pliable.
4. Let cool, then roll it up and cut into strips. Store in an airtight container for a week or two (longer in the fridge).

Makes 24 squares of leather, depending on how large you like them

Rose-Infused Bourbon Balls

My great-aunt Lois had a gift for confections.

- **½ cup bourbon**
- **2 tablespoons dried rose petals**
- **3 cups vanilla wafers (store-bought or homemade), ground**
- **1 cup ground walnuts**
- **1 cup rose-infused sugar (follow the chamomile-infused sugar recipe, page 32, using rose petals)**
- **1½ tablespoons corn syrup**
- **1½ tablespoons cocoa powder**

1. To make rose-infused bourbon, steep the dried rose petals in the bourbon. Store in a cool, dark place for 2 weeks. Shake daily and strain before using.
2. In a large bowl, mix together the rose-infused bourbon, vanilla wafers, walnuts, sugar, corn syrup, and cocoa powder. Shape into balls and roll in rose-infused sugar. Eat, give away, or store in an airtight container (in the fridge, if it's hot in your kitchen).

Makes about 3 dozen

Rose Butter Cookies

Butter cookies are the quintessential cookie, in my opinion. Even when I started substituting vegan butter in these recipes, nothing really changed. Ah, the wonders of the modern age.

- **1 cup butter (vegan or dairy)**
- **1 cup rose-infused sugar (follow the chamomile-infused sugar recipe, page 32, using rose petals)**
- **1 egg or vegan egg substitute**
- **½ teaspoon vanilla**
- **2 cups organic unbleached flour**
- **¼ teaspoon salt**
- **1 teaspoon baking powder (aluminum-free)**
- **Rose-Infused Buttercream Frosting (recipe follows)**

1. In a large bowl, cream together the butter and sugar and beat until light and fluffy. Be patient — this step is important, and I almost always rush it. Beat in the egg and vanilla.
2. In a medium bowl, sift together the flour, salt, and baking powder. Gradually add the dry ingredients to the butter and sugar, stirring to mix. Chill the dough for about 3 hours.
3. Preheat the oven to 400°F/200°C and line a baking sheet with parchment paper.
4. Roll out your dough on a floured cutting board (or roll between two sheets of parchment paper — my preferred method) to ⅛-inch thickness. Use cookie cutters or the rim of a glass — lightly greased — to cut out cookies. Place the cookies on the baking sheet and bake for 6 to 8 minutes.
5. When cool completely, top with Rose-Infused Frosting.

Makes 4 dozen cookies

Rose-Infused Buttercream Frosting

- **½ cup salted butter**
- **1 pound confectioners' sugar (approximately 3–4 cups, to be beaten in gradually)**
- **2–4 tablespoons milk (vegan or dairy)**
- **1 teaspoon rose water**
- **3–4 drops red food coloring or beet juice (optional)**

1. Allow the butter to soften on the counter for 20 to 30 minutes. Cream the room-temperature butter with ½ cup of the confectioners' sugar and just enough milk to make the whole thing start mixing. Beat in the rose water.
2. Keep adding the confectioners' sugar and the milk, beating on high, until you have a good frosting consistency. Add a few drops of the red food coloring or a little bit of beet juice (it won't add a beet flavor) to dye it pink, if you'd like.

Makes about 4 cups

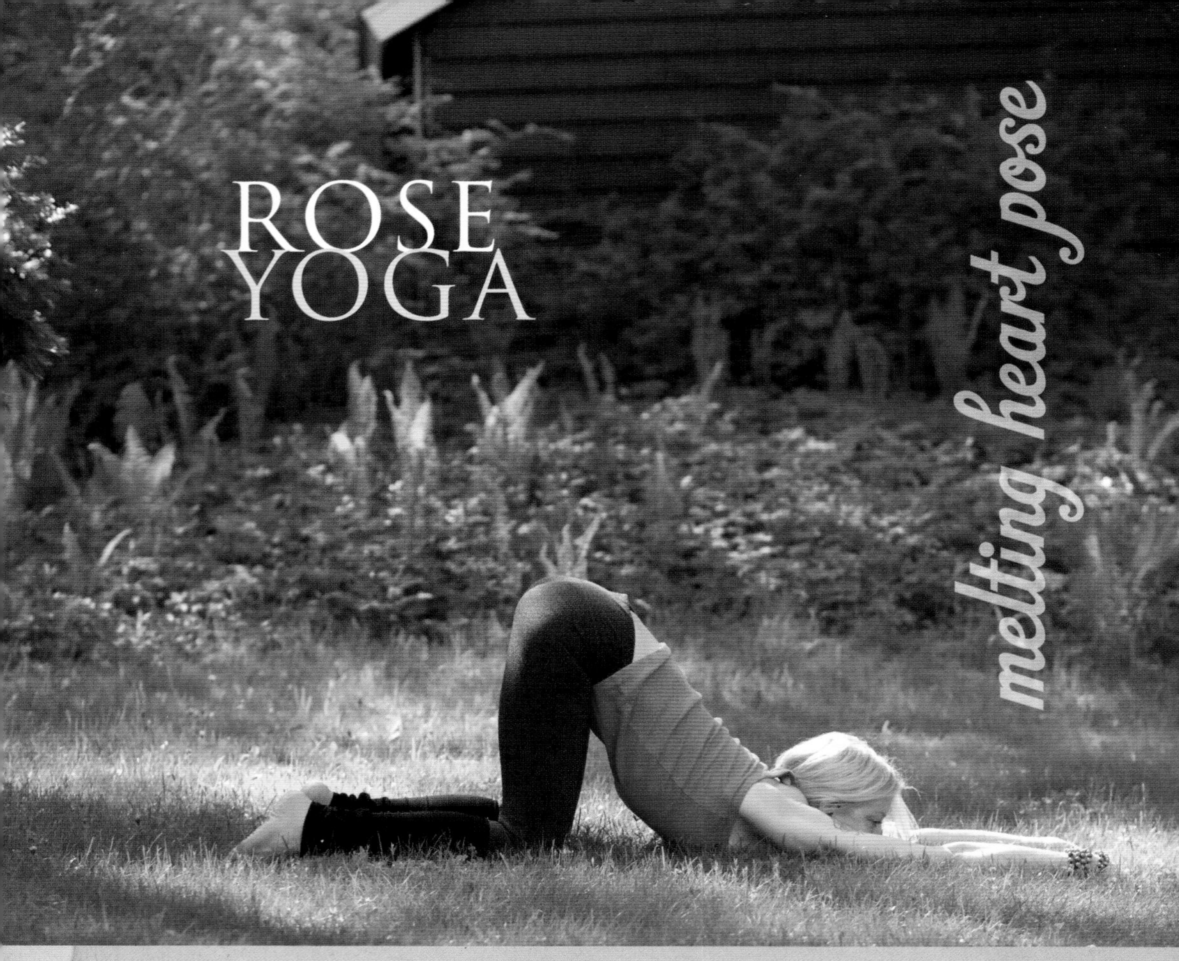

Rose is all about the heart, as we've seen. So, let's get in touch with that heart in one of my favorite poses: Melting Heart Pose (*Anahatasana*).

Starting position. Start on all fours. Make sure that your wrists are beneath your shoulders, knees below your hips. Inhale. As you exhale, leave your hips where they are (you'll really be sticking your bum up in the air; I know . . . graceful) and start to walk your hands toward the front of your yoga mat. Keep going as far as you can.

Moving into Melting Heart. If you have the flexibility, you can come all the way down onto your chest (hips are still straight up over your knees) and rest your chin on the mat. This is Melting Heart Pose. If your heart doesn't quite touch the mat, let it hover and bring your forehead to the mat. If neither of those is an option for you, then don't walk your hands

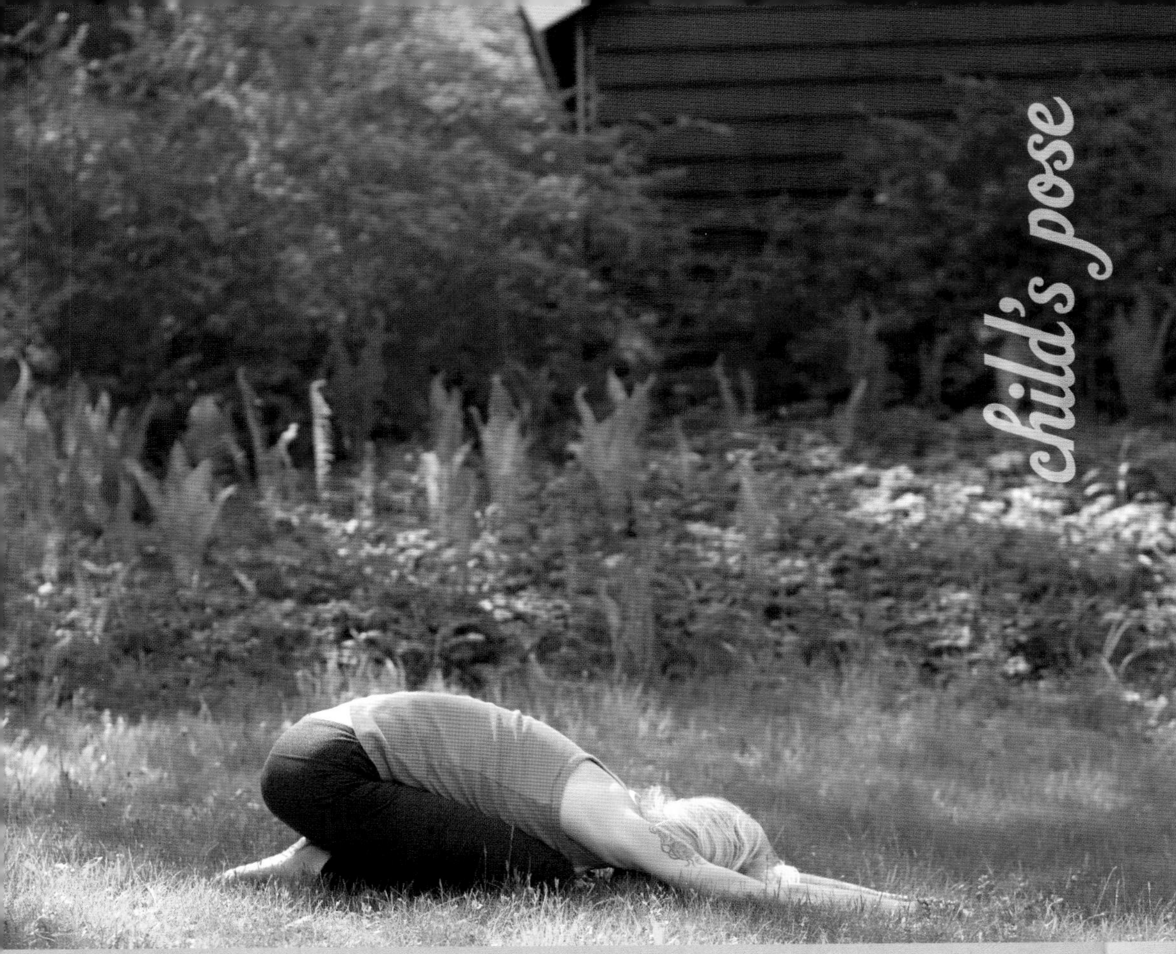

all the way down. Come to your forearms and stop there. Breathe deeply into your heart and back. Stay as long as you wish.

Finishing. Child's Pose (*Balasana*) is my favorite pose for any situation, ever. It is kind of your go-to stress reliever. Inhale. As you exhale, press into your hands and walk yourself back until your hips sit on your heels. Can't sit on your heels? No worries! Just put some blankets or a pillow between your hips and your lower legs and sit on that. Lay your torso along your upper legs. (Not comfortable? Lie on some stacked pillows or blankets.) Your arms can rest alongside your body, fold under your forehead, or stretch out in front of you — whatever is comfortable.

Stay and rest, coming out slowly when you're ready.

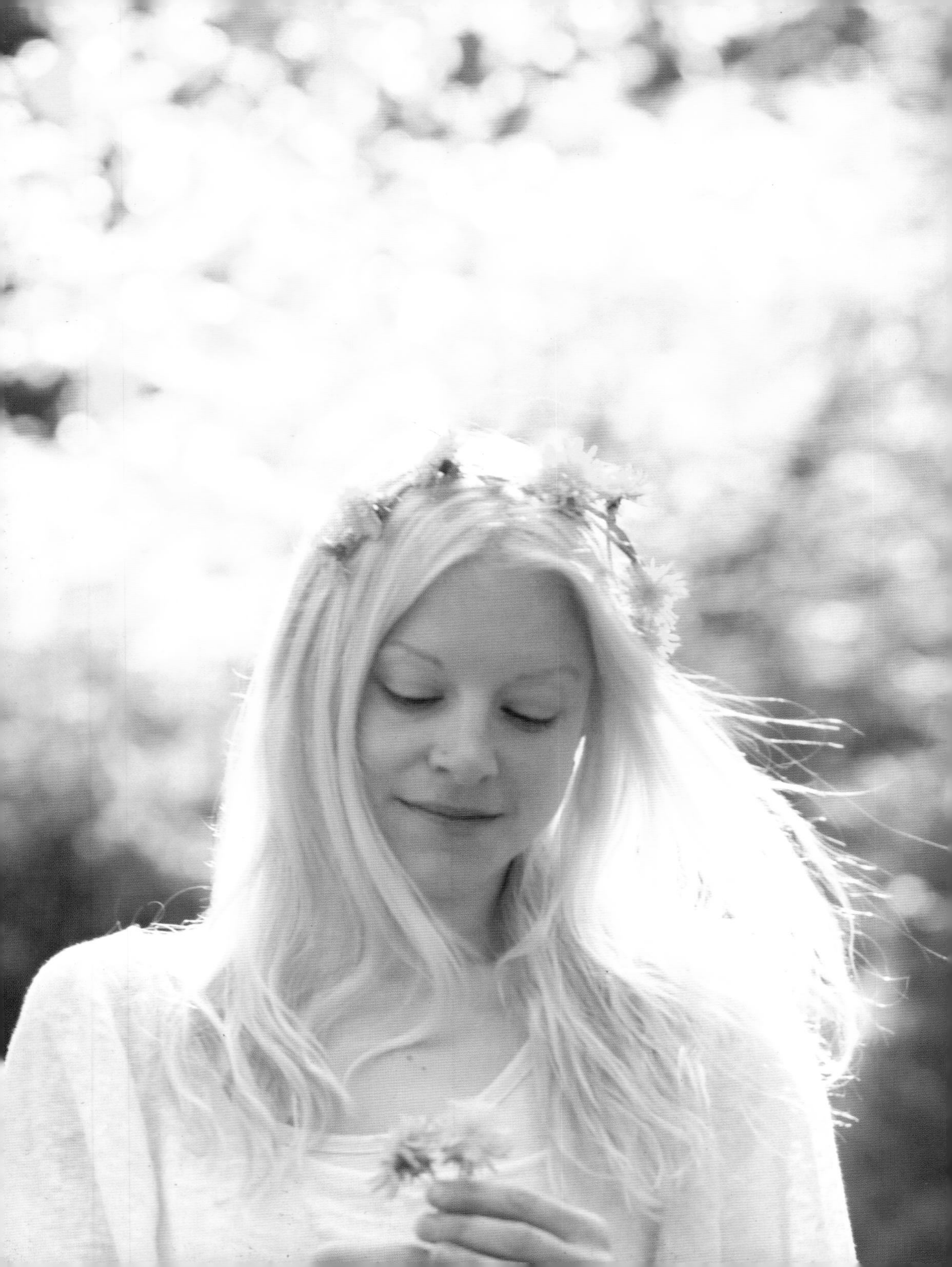

3
Detoxing with DANDELION

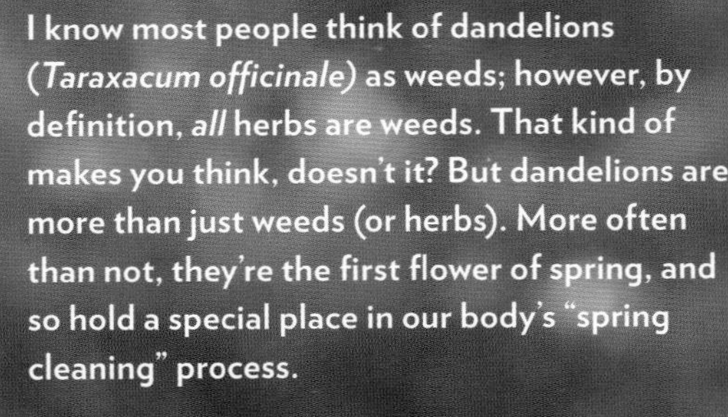

I know most people think of dandelions (*Taraxacum officinale*) as weeds; however, by definition, *all* herbs are weeds. That kind of makes you think, doesn't it? But dandelions are more than just weeds (or herbs). More often than not, they're the first flower of spring, and so hold a special place in our body's "spring cleaning" process.

Just as we sort of neglect giving our homes a good cleaning during the winter, our bodies do the same. During the cold months we conserve energy and naturally slow down; evolutionarily speaking, we just don't get inspired to really move during the winter. (Besides, isn't one of the joys of winter the ability to curl up on the couch with a warm blanket, a book, and hot chocolate? Yes! Heaven!) Our metabolisms slow down to conserve energy, food, and warmth, so the detoxing organs (the liver and kidneys) get a little sluggish, too.

Then spring appears and we get all revved up again. We can't wait to rid our living space of any dust, clutter, and grime. That urge to clean is really a manifestation of what's going on inside our bodies; our winter-logged systems want that same kind of airing out. Dandelion supports the body as it rids itself of stored metabolic wastes, toxins, and excess fat.

Dandelion is practically an herbal apothecary all unto itself: as a powerhouse liver and kidney tonic, it acts as a diuretic, so wastes are removed quickly from the body. As a bitter herb, it stimulates the digestive system, causing you to absorb nutrients from your food more efficiently so that less metabolic waste is generated. This means that the liver can focus on the really important tasks, like helping to rid the body of excess fat stores. And, like all early spring greens, dandelion leaves are loaded with vitamins and trace minerals — something the body has traditionally lacked over the winter.

But you don't have to wait around until March to start "spring cleaning" your body. The lovely things about dandelions are that they bloom multiple times during the growing season, *and* the entire plant — flowers, leaves, roots, and all — dry and keep easily and beautifully for use throughout the colder months. No matter what time of year it happens to be, a little nutritional boost is always a good thing.

If you harvest dandelions, be sure that they are at least 100 yards away from a road and contain no chemical fertilizers or pesticides. Also be sure that you have permission to harvest if you aren't on your own land (a universal truth that I've discovered — no one will begrudge the loss of their dandelions; in fact, people will call and beg you to come to their house and harvest). Gather only young leaves to avoid bitterness. If the flower bud has already formed, cut the plant to the ground and wait for new foliage to appear, then harvest and cut to the ground again. You can do this a few times before the leaves get too bitter. Let some flowers bloom, however; they are good for bees and various syrups and dandelion wines. You can eat the leaves raw or steamed, or dry them for brewing up later as tea.

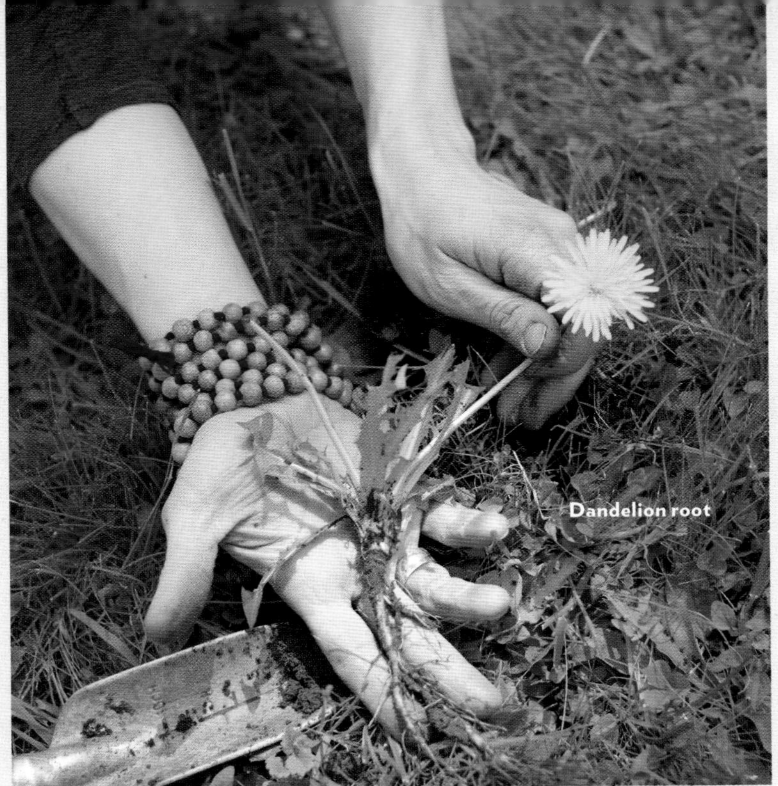

You can gather dandelion anytime during the growing season, but gather roots, which are especially healing for the liver, after the first frost, when the nutrients have collected in the root. The long taproot is easiest to dig when the weather is wet and the soil is soft. See dandelion "coffee" box on page 65 for how to roast and store.

DANDELION

Taraxacum officinale

Parts used: Flower, leaves, roots

How to harvest: Harvest anywhere away from roadsides and potential pesticide/chemical fertilizer use

Effects on body: Detoxifying, nutritive, overall general good health

Effects on mind and spirit: Inspires zest and a love for life and offers relief from being overly committed

Safety first: Use with caution if you suffer from gallstones; also, remove the stem, which is quite unappetizing, before using your herb

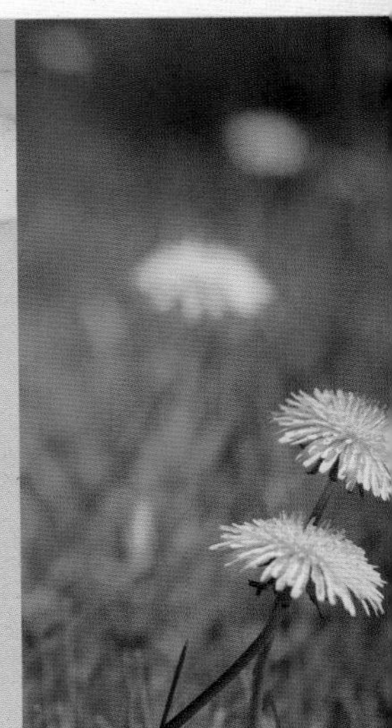

for the Body

As I've already declared from the proverbial rooftops, dandelion is a superhero tonic for the liver, kidneys, gallbladder, pancreas, spleen, stomach, and digestive system. It also helps reduce inflammation related to hepatitis and cirrhosis. Furthermore, dandelion is very high in vitamins A and C, beta-carotene, potassium, iron, and copper. (In other words, dandelion is a major nutritional jump-start for your body after a winter of heavy meals and maybe just a little too much eggnog.) Dandelion serves as a tonic for your whole body, helping correct elimination problems such as constipation, gallstones, indigestion, sluggishness, and fatigue. It also helps fight skin problems and may ease the impact of diabetes by helping to regulate low blood sugar and lowering cholesterol.

Okay, so, where do you start? Well, you can begin by simply adding the young greens to your salads, or lightly steaming or sautéing them. If those options aren't that appealing to you, try a tea. But, a few notes: As a strong diuretic (which means it helps clear waste and excess fluid from your system — great for relieving bloating, by the way), dandelion shouldn't be ingested at the same time as other medicines; otherwise, those drugs will flow right out of your system. Aim for a dandelion-free window of 30 minutes before to 60 minutes after ingesting any drugs or medications. And, as always, talk to your healthcare provider before taking any herbs.

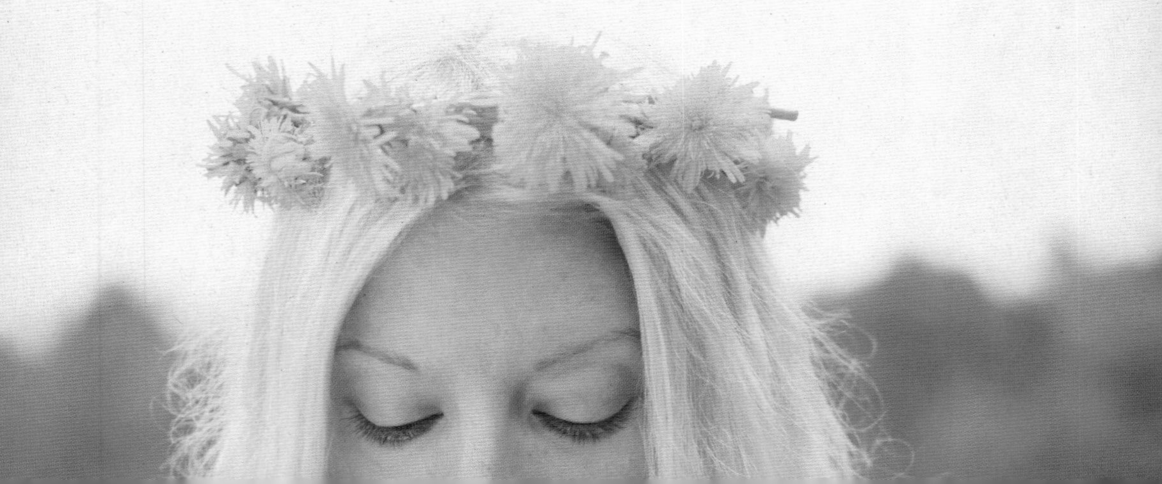

for the Mind

Remember how keenly flower essences work with the mind? (See box on page 22 if you don't.) Since dandelion is so prolific, it's quite easy to harvest enough blossoms to make your own flower essence (see Appendix I). Dandelion essence inspires a natural intensity and love for life — just looking at how prolifically and often the cheerful dandelion blooms is definitely proof enough! However, dandelion will also help you if you tend to find yourself compulsively busy, overly committed, or overly scheduled. This essence is great for anyone — children included — feeling overwhelmed by the amount of activity and responsibility in their lives, especially when that activity level is self-inflicted.

When you become addicted to activity and have a hard time sitting still or being with yourself, your body is sending out the call for dandelion essence. Tension can result when the mind wants to remain busy but the body needs to relax. Dandelion teaches us to listen to our innermost needs — the needs of the heart, not of the head. A few drops under the tongue, and in no time you're lying in your hammock with a book and a cup of tea (or, just maybe, a margarita), wondering why the heck you didn't try this relaxation stuff ages ago.

And if those addictions, anger, and frustrations arise and once again you feel that you're unable to get your life under control or are overwhelmed by what life is throwing at you (or what you have inadvertently invited life to throw at you), pick up your essence bottle. Breathe. Add a few drops to a thermos of water and sip throughout the day.

for the Spirit

The beautiful thing about dandelions is that they can bloom anywhere — city, countryside, between cracks in the sidewalk, on roadsides, and in wastelands. They are a constant reminder of how tenacious, determined, and renewable nature is. When you're feeling lost, alone, or unable to grow or express yourself, go on a dandelion hunt. Sit by the plants and just commune with them for a moment. Ask permission to pick a few blossoms; give thanks, and take them home. Place the blossoms in a bright vase where you can see them on a daily basis. Allow them to remind you of how easily you can persevere as long as you open yourself up to natural forces and let your true self blossom as brightly and relentlessly as the dandelion.

Similarly, use dandelion magic when you're going through a change in life — physically, emotionally, or hormonally (e.g., pregnancy or menopause). Think of how the dandelion goes from simple green leaves to bright yellow flowers to the fluffy seed pod that blows so blissfully in the breeze. Each of the dandelion's stages of development is radically different from the last, yet it moves swiftly and gracefully through each.

As for magical associations, dandelion is linked with the planet Jupiter (the planet which represents hard work), but it is also associated with the sun and the moon (the yellow flower, the sun, and the seed puff, the moon). Its element is air, and it is associated with the feminine.

DANDELION MAGIC

FOR ANXIETY

Feeling anxious? Stressed? Worried? Gather dandelion flowers to cheer you up or spend an afternoon blowing the seed heads, scattering your worries, fears, and inhibitions to the wind.

FOR LONELINESS

When separated from a loved one, gather as many seed heads as you can, and instill each with messages and wishes of love for those absent. Blow on the flower, scattering the intention-laden seeds to the wind and to those far away.

FOR PSYCHIC POWERS

Looking for a magic potion? It is said that drinking dandelion root tea promotes and aids the development of psychic and clairvoyant powers. If this is your bag, try drinking a cup nightly, about an hour before bed to inspire prophetic dreams (and, seriously, be sure it's an hour or more before bed; any closer and that diuretic dandelion power will have you up several times that night . . . trust me). Alternatively, leave a cup of steaming tea by your bedside to invite inspiration, creativity, and problem-solving while you sleep.

FOR TRACKING TIME AND WEATHER

For a truly natural (and magical) clock and weather chart, keep an eye on the dandelions in your yard. They almost always open at 5 A.M. and close at 8 P.M. If dandelion blossoms close during the day, expect rain to fall.

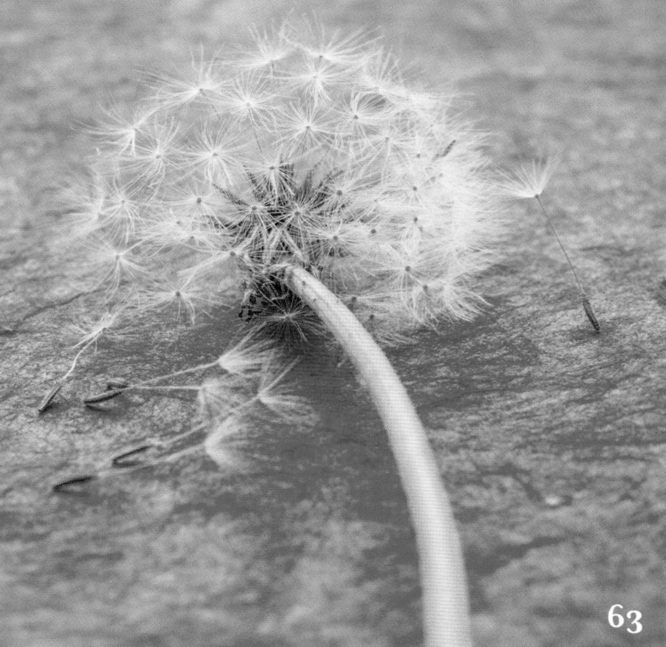

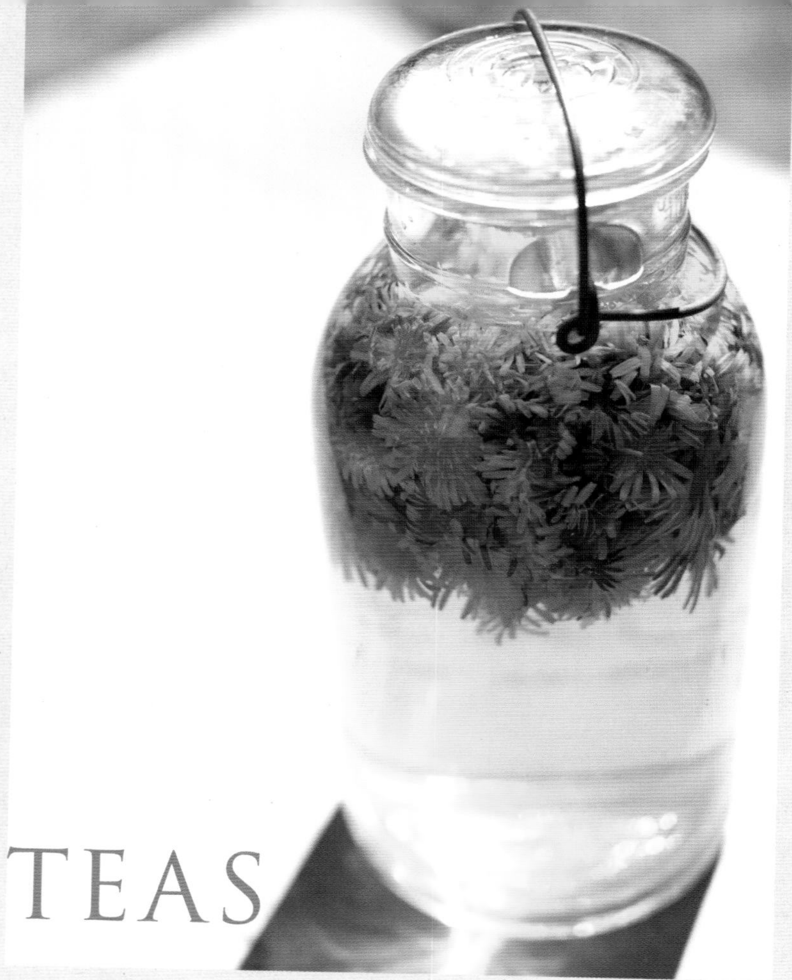

TEAS

Nutrient-dense tea. Rinse one handful of young dandelion leaves under cold water. Chop the leaves roughly and put in a preheated mug. Pour boiling water over the leaves, cover, and steep for 10 minutes. Drink as much of this as you like — it's a wonderful nutritive to restore the body after a long illness or a long winter!

Dandelion sun tea or lemonade. If you have a lot of dandelion blossoms in your (pesticide-free) yard, choose a sunny morning and harvest a quart or two. Place the blossoms in a clear glass quart jar, and fill with tea or lemonade (or juice of choice). Put the jar in a sunny spot for a few hours, then strain and drink.

Digestive tea. You'll need 1 ounce of dandelion root (if you harvest your own, be sure to rinse it under running water and scrub with a sturdy brush in order to remove loose dirt), 1 ounce of dandelion leaves, 1 teaspoon of fennel seeds, and 1 teaspoon of peppermint or spearmint leaves (optional, and exclude if you're making this tea for children).

Simmer the dandelion root and fennel seed in 1½ cups water for 10 minutes. Strain and pour over the dandelion and mint leaves. Let this steep for 10 more minutes, then strain. Drink this tea 20 minutes before or after every meal to stimulate gastric juices and ease digestion.

Detox tea. You can drink this tea to detoxify the body, or use it as a facial wash to help detox and tone the skin. You'll need 1 ounce of each of the following: dandelion root, burdock root, dandelion leaves, red clover blossoms, and nettle leaves.

Simmer the burdock and dandelion roots for 10 minutes in 2 cups water. Strain the tea over the leaves and blossoms and steep for another 10 minutes and strain again. Drink as much of this daily as you like. If using it as a toner, add 2 tablespoons apple cider vinegar — it helps kill bacteria and acts as an astringent — and stick it in the fridge.

DANDELION "COFFEE"

If you've given up (or want to give up) coffee, then you can use roasted roots in place of coffee grounds for an awesome (and medicinal!) herbal "coffee." Carefully wash the roots, chop them, then roast in a 250°F/120°C oven, occasionally turning the pieces until they are dry and aromatic. This can take a few hours; keep checking the roots, taking care not to burn them. You can store these for several months in a clean, airtight container at room temperature. (You can also buy pre-roasted root, if you prefer.)

Take 1 tablespoon of your roasted dandelion root and simmer it in 1 cup water for 10 minutes. Change the amount of root used depending on your personal taste. Doctor it up as you would your favorite coffee. You can also use this to make mochas, lattes, mocha-lattes, and what-have-you.

FRESH ROOT SALVE

If you have some dandelion root on hand, you can put that to use as-is. The fresh root, when cut, will exude a milky, sappy substance that you can apply directly to the skin to relieve and heal burns, stings, acne, calluses, and warts.

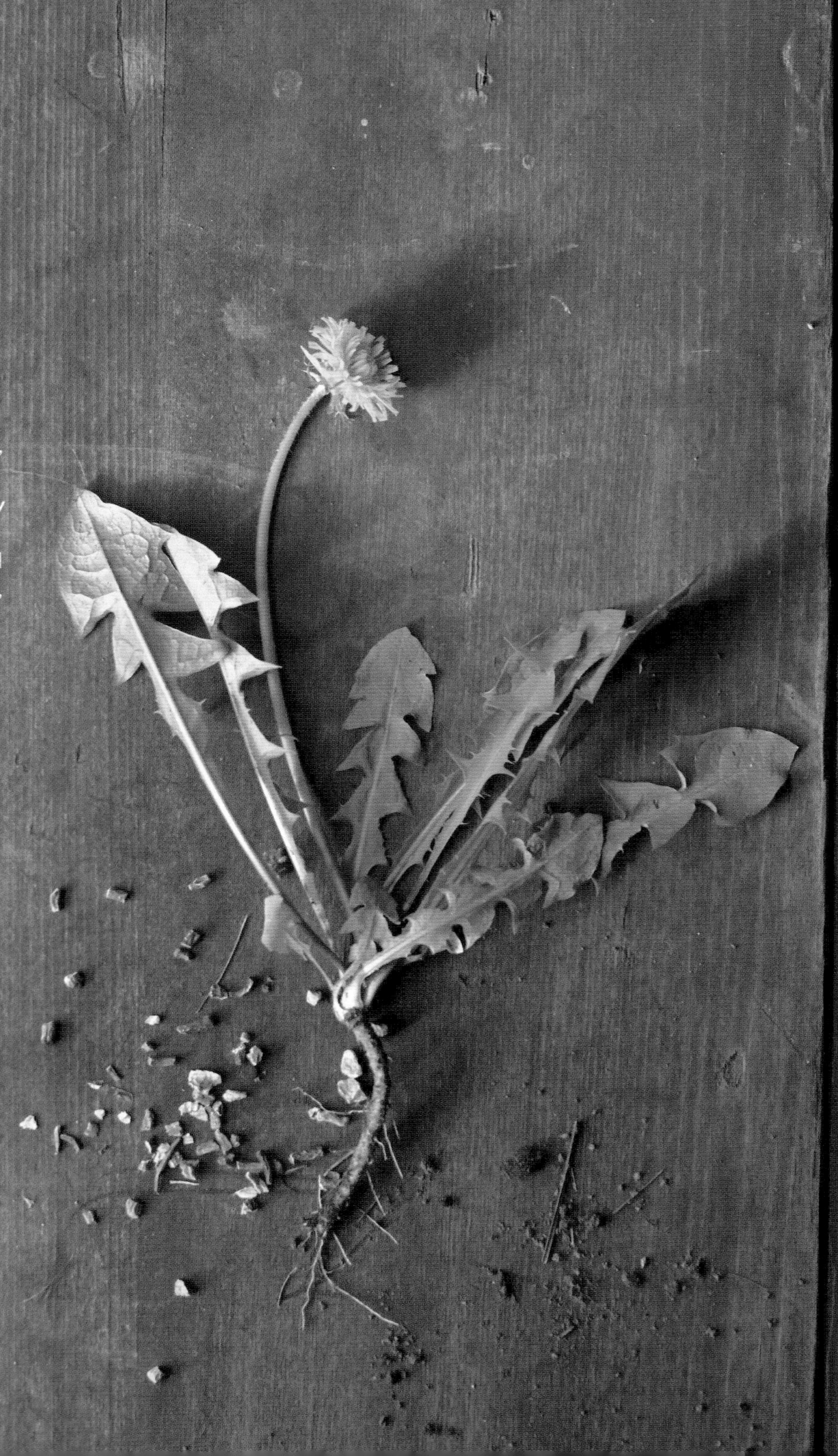

BODY CARE

recipes

Dandelion Toner

Dandelion is a wonderful detoxing agent for the skin. Brew up this toner to cleanse skin, get rid of impurities, and help heal outbreaks. Also try your hand at making dandelion oil to rub on sore muscles, and dandelion salve to use on cracked, dried skin or acne outbreaks (see Appendix II and Appendix III for recipes).

- **½ cup apple cider vinegar**
- **½ cup distilled water**
- **1 handful dandelion greens and flowers, chopped**
- **2 teaspoons loose green tea or 2 bags of green tea**
- **3 drops essential oil (rose, orange, or lavender)**

1. In a small jar, combine the vinegar, distilled water, greens, and flowers. Seal the jar, shake, and store in a dark place for 2 weeks, shaking daily.
2. Strain out the herbs and pour into a sterile bottle.
3. Brew a strong cup of green tea. Steep for 5 minutes, then add to the toner, straining if using loose tea.
4. Add the essential oil and shake. Store in the fridge and use daily, applying with a cotton pad to your face and throat.

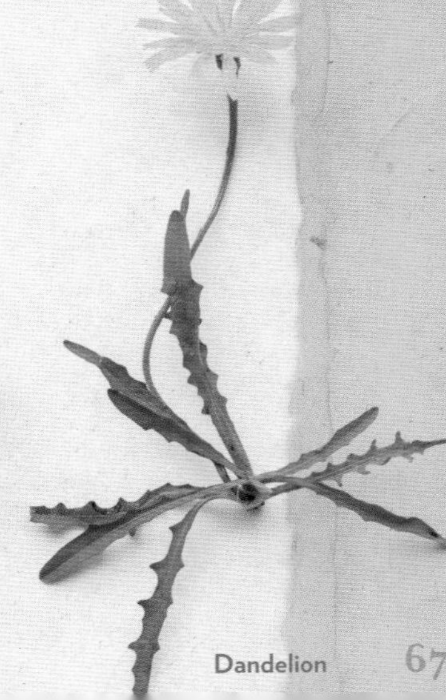

FOOD & DRINK

Dandelion Salad with Cranberries and Warm Balsamic Vinaigrette

Use dandelion flowers fresh in this salad for color and interest. Or, as a great side dish, dip the flowers in a batter of your choice and fry up into dandelion fritters, or steam them and add to vegetable side dishes.

- **3 tablespoons extra-virgin olive oil**
- **3 cloves garlic, minced**
- **¼ teaspoon salt**
- **½ cup nuts, chopped (walnuts or hazelnuts are especially good in this recipe)**
- **1–2 tablespoons balsamic vinegar**
- **2 cups fresh dandelion greens, cleaned, patted dry, and chopped**
- **2 tablespoons dried cranberries**
- **Dandelion blossoms for garnish**

1. In a medium skillet, heat the oil over medium heat. Add the garlic, salt, and nuts, and sauté for a few minutes. Remove from the heat and add the vinegar. Pour the mixture into a bowl and whisk together.
2. Pour the dressing over the clean greens. Sprinkle the dried cranberries on top and add the fresh blossoms.

Heirloom Carrot and Dandelion Green Casserole

This recipe comes from my Great-Aunt Lois. It's the ultimate comfort food, but I like to gourmet-it-up with some colorful, heirloom carrots, dandelion greens, and a really good, deep cheese like a Spanish manchego.

- **4 cups chopped carrots**
- **4 tablespoon butter or vegan butter**
- **½ cup chopped onion**
- **½ cup chopped red, yellow, or orange peppers**
- **½ cup milk, nut milk, or cream**
- **1 cup dandelion leaves**
- **½ cup chopped olives (your choice)**
- **Salt and pepper to taste**
- **⅓ cup grated cheese (I like Spanish manchego; if you want a vegan option, choose a vegan cream cheese rather than a block cheese — those don't melt well, in my experience)**

Recipe continues on page 70

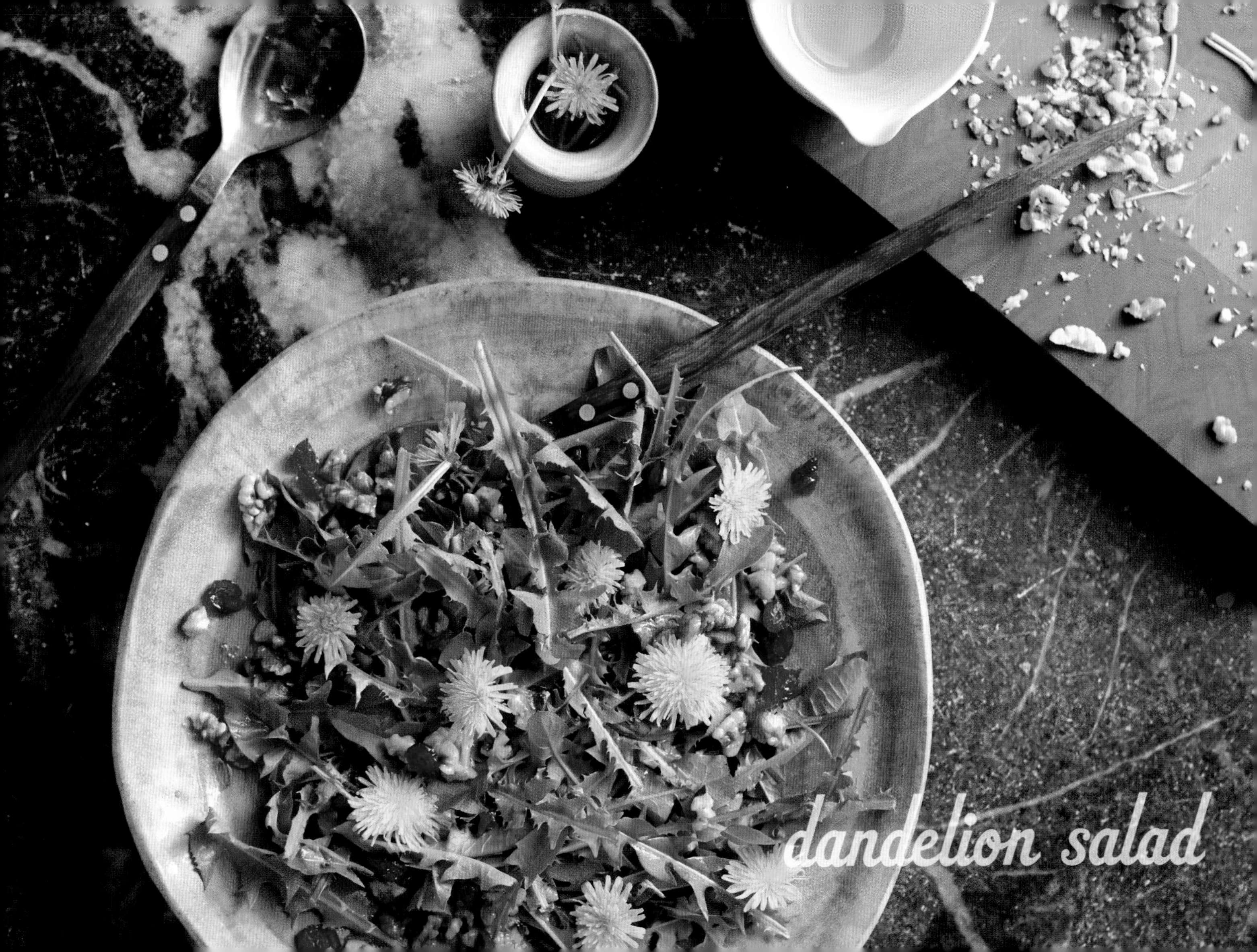
dandelion salad

1. Preheat the oven to 400°F/200°C. Lightly steam the carrots (just this side of done, so maybe 7 minutes in the steamer).

2. Meanwhile, in a medium skillet, melt the butter over medium heat. Add the onions and peppers and sauté for 5 minutes. Add the milk, steamed carrots, dandelion leaves, olives, and salt and pepper to taste, and sauté for 5 more minutes. Stir and pour into a shallow 2-quart baking dish.

3. Sprinkle the cheese (or cube and drop the cream cheese) on top and bake for 15 minutes. Serve hot over rice, burgers, or baked tofu, or just on its own.

Serves 4

Dandelion Syrup

Dandelion flower syrup is a great way to get the benefits of this early spring tonic into the little ones of your household. Use to sweeten hot drinks, on its own, or as a syrup for French toast or pancakes. Using honey instead of sugar makes this a marvelous cough and cold remedy.

- **1 cup dandelion flowers**
- **2 cups sugar (preferably dehydrated cane juice or Sucanat) or honey**
- **1 slice citrus fruit (any kind), cut with rind on (for flavor) or ½ cup berries of choice**

1. Steep the dandelion flowers in 3 cups hot water overnight.

2. Strain the dandelion water into a saucepan and add another cup of water. Add the sugar (or honey) and the fruit. Bring to a boil over medium heat and simmer 15 to 30 minutes or until the liquid thickens. Strain and store in the fridge.

Makes approximately 2 cups syrup

Dandelion Wine

Can you think of a better way to get your herbs than in wine? I think not. The best part? Opening a bottle and enjoying a glass of dandelion wine on a cold winter's night, remembering the bright yellow bounty of your first spring harvest.

- **2½ quarts tightly packed dandelion blossoms, picked in full bloom**
- **3 quarts sugar**
- **1 pound seedless raisins**
- **1 orange**
- **1 lemon**
- **½ teaspoon cake yeast**

1. Wash the blossoms well and drain. In a large pot bring 4 quarts water to a boil. Add the blossoms to a 1-gallon glass or ceramic container with cover and pour the boiling water over them. Let stand overnight.

2. Strain out the blossoms and discard them. Return the liquid to the container and add the sugar. Stir well.

3. Chop the raisins, orange, and lemon and add them to the liquid. Add the yeast to the mixture. Cover and let stand at room temperature until

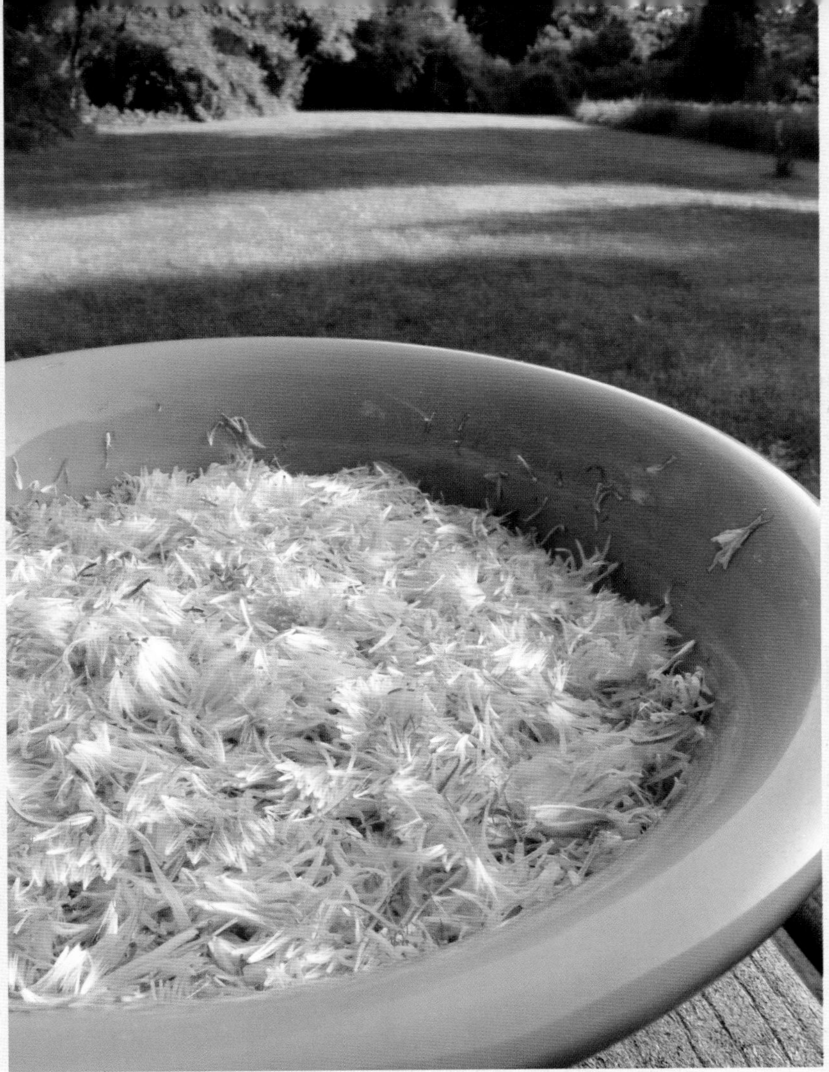

thoroughly fermented (you'll notice that the liquid will start to bubble and foam — this is a good sign; when it stops bubbling, you'll know fermentation is complete). Check on and stir your mixture daily. Store the covered container at room temperature in an out-of-the-way place.

4. Strain the fermented wine and bottle it, corking loosely. After 3 days, push the corks in tightly. Let the wine age in the bottles for at least 6 months before drinking.

Makes 16 cups

Stuffed Mushrooms with Dandelion Greens

My dad used to make these stuffed mushrooms and they are a-m-a-z-i-n-g. The addition of some healthy, slightly bitter dandelion greens is the perfect foil for the rich cheesy buttery-ness of these guys.

- **⅔ cup olive oil**
- **2 cups fresh dandelion greens, washed and patted dry**
- **¼ cup grated onions**
- **⅓ cup grated (fresh!) Parmesan cheese (skip if making vegan 'shrooms)**
- **½ cup crushed breadcrumbs (for extra pizazz you can toast some bread slices brushed with olive oil and garlic and then pulse them in a food processor or blender)**
- **1 teaspoon chopped, fresh parsley**
- **¼ teaspoon dried oregano**
- **¼ teaspoon black pepper**
- **1½ pounds baby portabellas, cleaned (retain stems if you like — just chop them up and mix them in with the stuffing)**
- **Lemon juice**

1. Preheat oven to 350°F/180°C. Line the bottom of a covered 2-quart baking dish with parchment paper.
2. In a medium skillet, add 1 tablespoon of the olive oil and lightly sauté the greens over medium heat for about 5 minutes.
3. In a large bowl, combine the sautéed greens, onions, Parmesan (if using), breadcrumbs, parsley, oregano, pepper, and the remaining olive oil. Mix well.
4. Brush the mushroom caps with lemon juice. Using your clean hands, stuff the caps with the mixture. Place the stuffed caps on the lined baking dish and bake, covered, for 25 minutes.

Serves 4

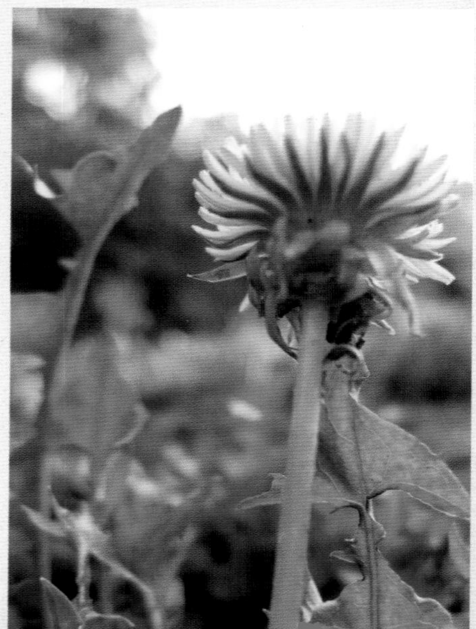

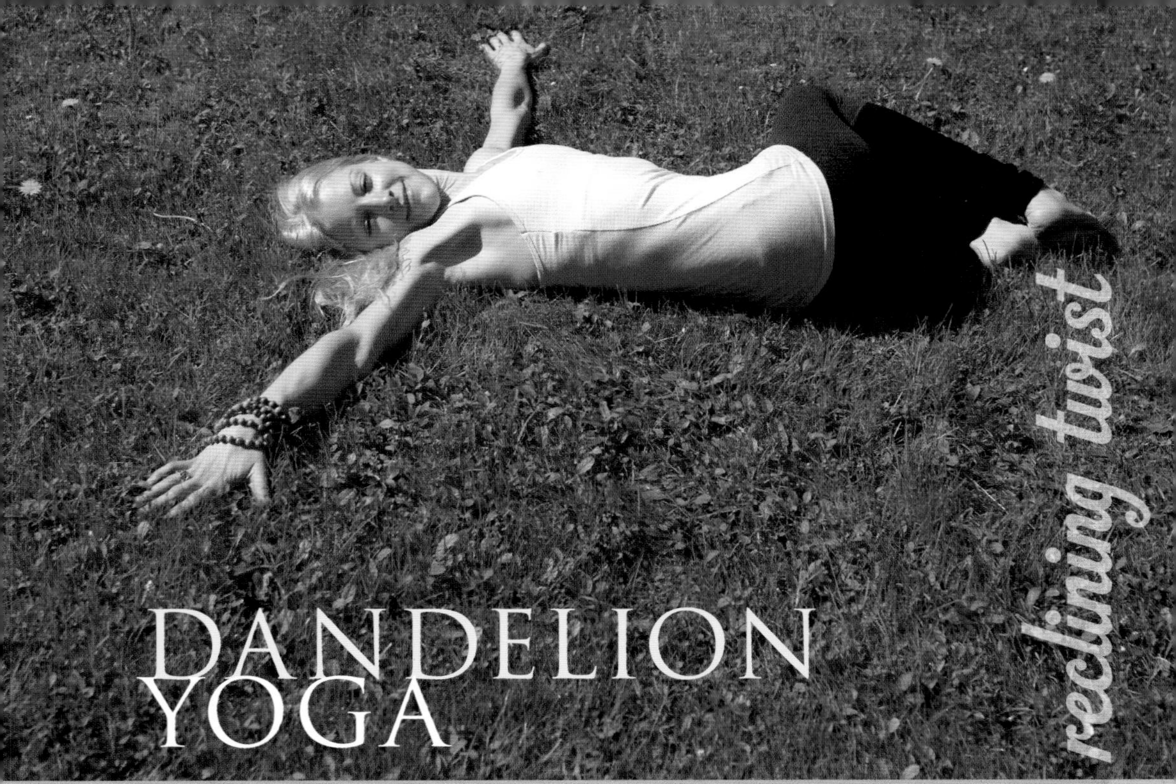

DANDELION YOGA

Since dandelions are all about detoxification, we'll work with a twist known as Reclining Twist or Twisted Roots. This pose works well to detoxify the internal organs and is wonderful for digestion and for spinal health. The twist, plus the pressure of breathing deeply into the belly, helps to squeeze out all of the old blood and toxins. And when you untwist, all the fresh blood and oxygen are allowed to rush back in.

Starting position. Lie on your back with your knees bent, feet planted on the floor. Stretch your arms out to your sides in the shape of a T.

Twisting. Inhale. As you exhale, let your knees drop to the left and turn your head to the right. Try to get that right shoulder as close to the mat as possible. This is Reclining Twist. If this is pretty easy for you, bring your knees back to center and cross your right leg over the left, then drop them again to the left. Stay as long as you like. When you're ready, bring your knees to center on an inhale, switch the crossed leg, exhale, and drop them to the other side.

Finishing. Hug your knees into your chest and rock gently if it feels good. Breathe and stay here as long as you like.

4

Adapting with HOLY BASIL

Sometimes life is just, well, too lifelike. You know what I mean? You *want* (no, you *need*) to sit down on the couch, porch swing, beanbag, cushion, or hammock, and just relax. You want a good book, film, magazine, or moment of silence just to *be yourself*, to be *by* yourself. Am I right? I know you know the feeling; I can't be alone on this one.

But how often do we allow ourselves just to *do nothing*? I'm not talking the kind of nothing where you're planning your grocery list or taking 10 breaths before coming out from hiding in the bathroom, sidling back to your desk before anyone starts looking for you. I'm talking blissful, rejuvenating, and restorative *nothing*. How often?

I'm going to guess not very.

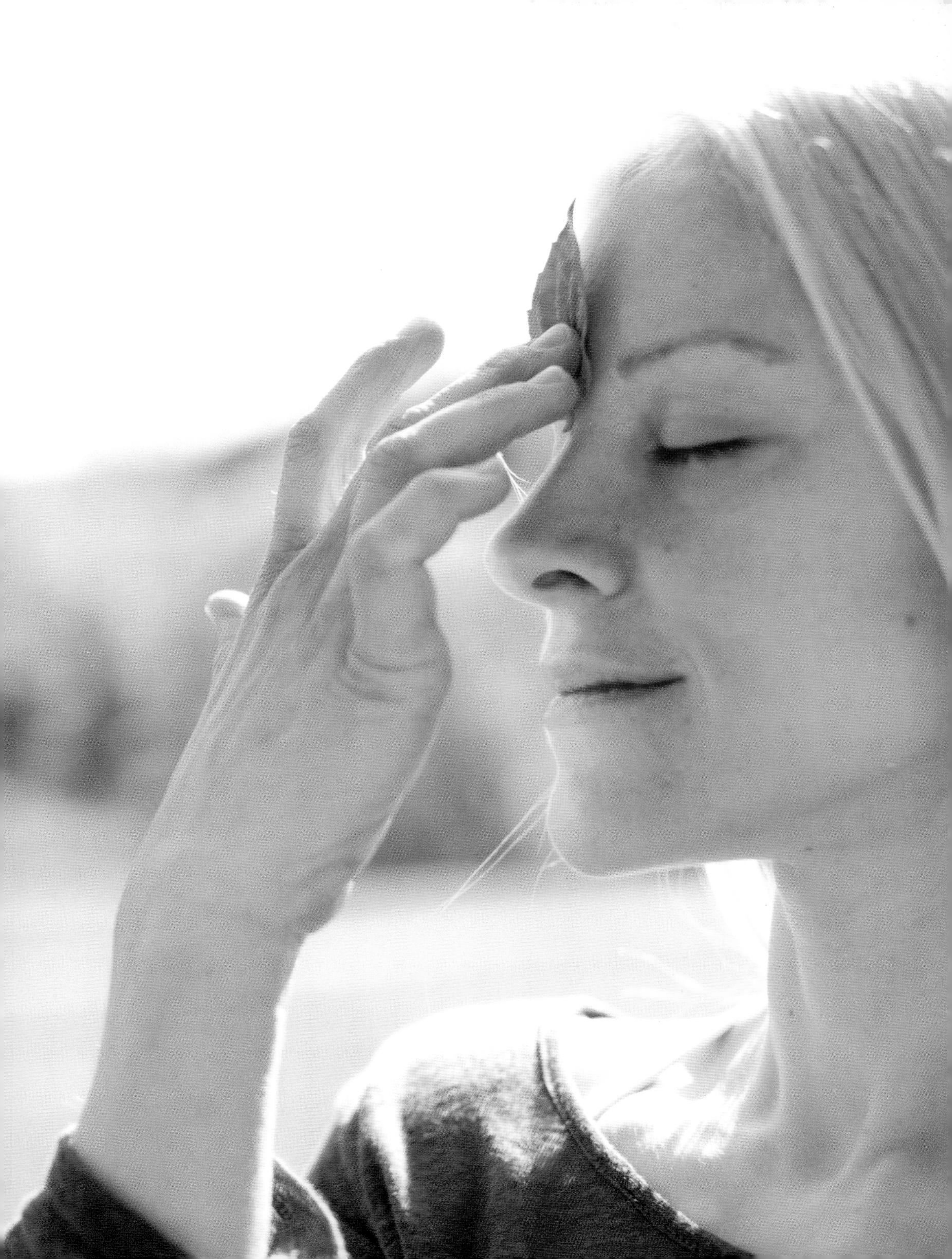

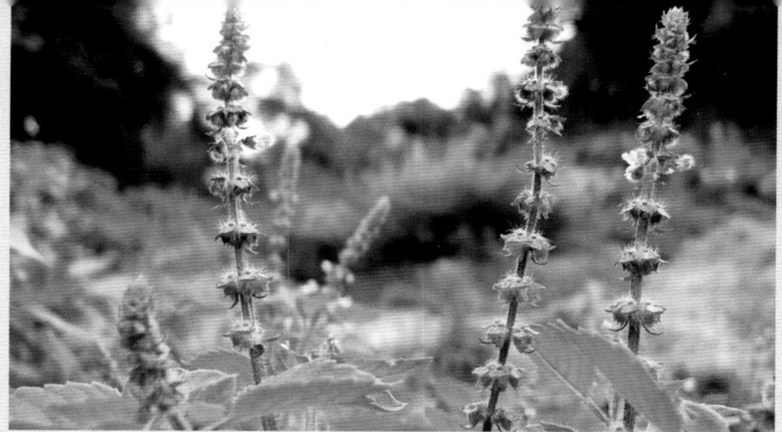

Want a solution? Try holy basil (*Ocimum sanctum*). Also called tulsi or *tulasi*, holy basil is one crazy-awesome healing herb. Considered sacred by practitioners of Hinduism (hence "holy" basil), it has been used in Ayurvedic medicine (the 5,000-year-old medical system in India) as a *rasayana*, or a promoter and protector of long life.

So what's the difference between holy basil and culinary basil (*Ocimum basilicum*)? Though there are more than 40 varieties of culinary basil (including cinnamon basil, lemon basil, Thai basil, purple basil, and licorice basil, to name a few), all of the culinary varieties are used mostly for their savory characteristics. Although their medicinal qualities aren't quite as developed as holy basil, culinary varieties can be used to treat inflammation and headaches.

There are also cosmetic differences between the two herbs. Holy basil's leaves are rather coarse and sport a grayish-green color with ridged edges while culinary basil's leaves are shiny, green, and smoothly rounded. Culinary basil's flowers are white while holy basil's are a lovely lavender. What about the scent? Think of holy basil as the sweet one and culinary basil as slightly spicier. It's due to these subtle differences in chemical make-up and the way these constituents work in the body that holy basil has been vaulted into the medicinal realm.

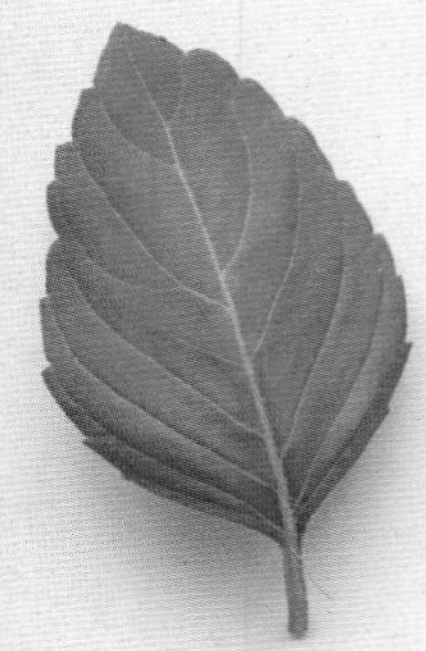

Holy basil, just like her sister basils, is an annual that will grow well only in warm (think Mediterranean) environments. While it might grow wild in places like India, most of us have to cultivate this herb indoors or in our gardens. It can become invasive, so if you are planting it in the garden, keep it in containers if you don't want to risk a takeover. If you can let some of it go to flower, though, bees and butterflies will love you forever.

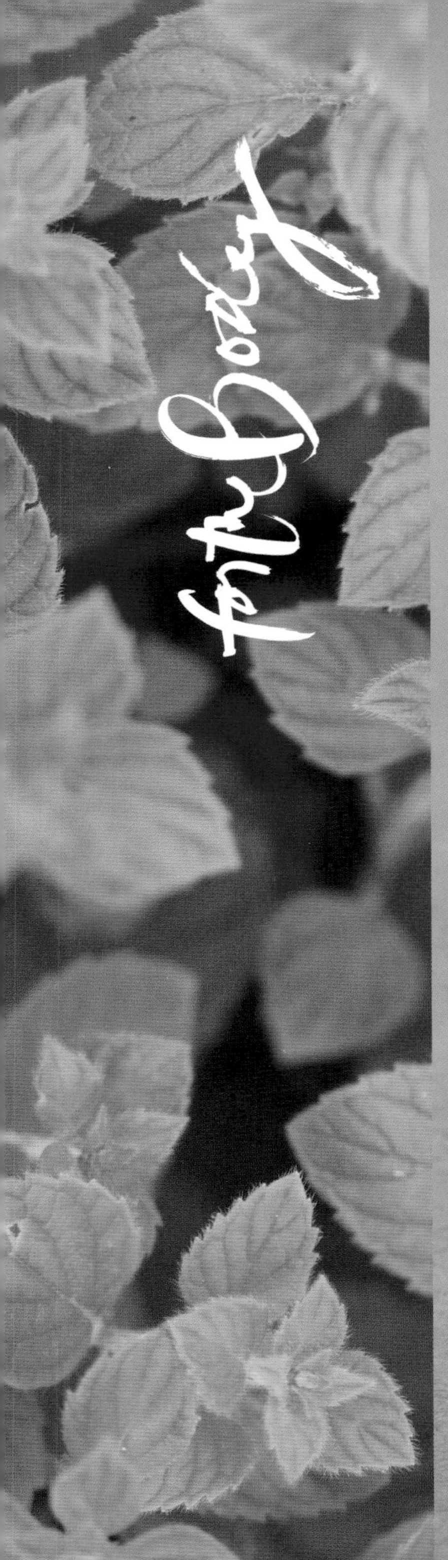

Holy basil, like many herbs, is an adaptogen. Basically, an adaptogen is any herb that protects the body against stress — physical, mental, or emotional; adaptogens beat stress by helping to shield and protect the nerves.

You know that expression, "My nerves are shot"? We say that because that's how it is: when we're stressed or tense for long periods of our lives, our nerves become sensitive, careworn, and sparky. In other words, it doesn't take much to frazzle us. But if you take holy basil, it's as if your nerves are coated in a warm, mossy, über-protective coating that shields them from stress. The beauty of this particular herb is that it can soothe anxiety and the stress response without making you drowsy during the day, but it will leave you calm enough to sleep deeply at night.

Just because it's called "holy" doesn't mean that it is completely dissimilar from its fellow basils. All herbs in the basil family are wonderful for treating skin issues. Simply macerate (chew or use a mortar and pestle) the leaves, and apply as a poultice to burns, bites, and stings. The leaves will draw pain and itching away from the affected area.

When taken as a tea, holy basil can also help calm coughs, reduce fever, and soothe sore throats. It can strengthen the kidneys and, if kidney stones are present, will help to expel them if you drink the juice or tea regularly for six months. It will also strengthen the liver, aid digestion, relieve cramps, and regulate hormones. And, like all basils, the tea makes a wonderful eye bath (cool it first, obviously!) to treat night blindness, exhaustion, and allergy eyes.

Note: All varieties of basil, including holy basil, are considered safe. However, holy basil hasn't been tested for its effects on embryos, so it's best to avoid it while pregnant. Also, it's thought to reduce fertility in women (only while you take it — not permanently), so if you're trying for a wee one, best to skip the holy basil.

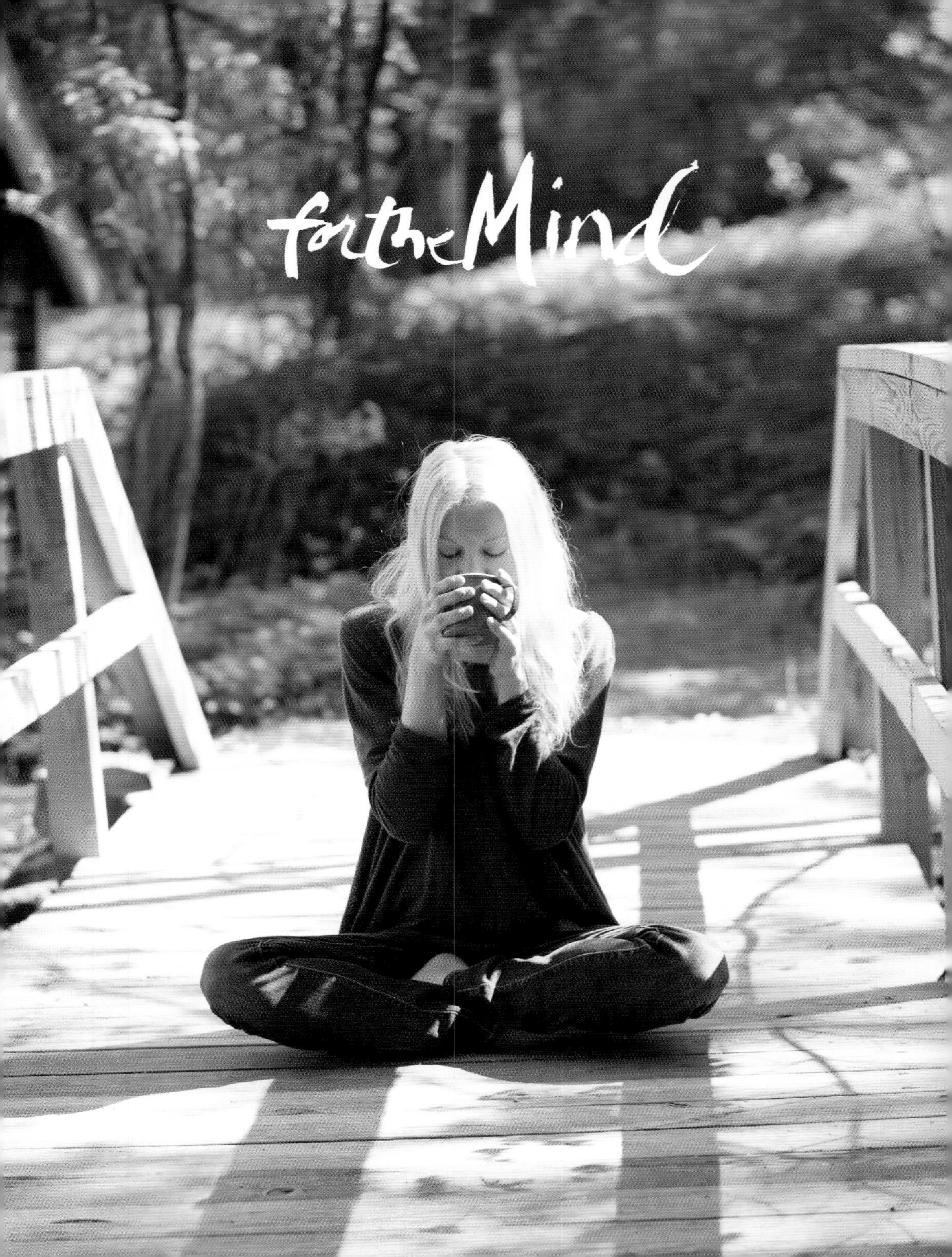
for the Mind

Holy basil has wonderful benefits for the mind. It boosts blood circulation to the brain, promoting memory, aiding retention, and enhancing mental longevity. Try sipping some tea while studying or before a big test or presentation. Inhale the steam of the tea as you prep and let the mind soak it in, just like it's soaking in all that new information you're trying to cram in there.

It's also a gentle antidepressant, and it regulates hormones and eases panic attacks. Even if you don't suffer from chronic depression, turn to holy basil in times of stress, loss, change, or anxiety. Holy basil lowers cortisol levels (that stress hormone you feel as anxiety in the belly and that seems to find us and hound us once the sun sets), helping you sleep when stress is driving you right out of your mind. It lifts the spirit and promotes a brighter outlook.

I carry around a little vial of holy basil essential oil if I think I'm going to be in a situation that will seriously stress me out (parties where I don't know anyone, a new yoga class I'm teaching, first day on a job, meeting new people . . . you get the idea). I'll take a sniff of the essential oil, and things will just sort of magically balance. Alternatively, you can mix a few drops of essential oil with a carrier oil (like almond) and rub them on your pulse points.

Try taking the holy basil flower essence when you're seeking spiritual renewal, you need help quieting the mind (in meditation, for instance), or you just can't seem to lift yourself out of the procrastination habit; this herb is all about new beginnings and brighter outlooks. And, speaking of new beginnings, it's hard to have one if you're still stuck in the past. So, take this flower essence if there's something you want (or need) to release and move past. Holy basil moves your awareness from your head (where anxiety lives) to your heart (the home of comfort, love, and security). Sound a bit out there? See for yourself. Take this essence for a couple of weeks and find out if it changes your outlook.

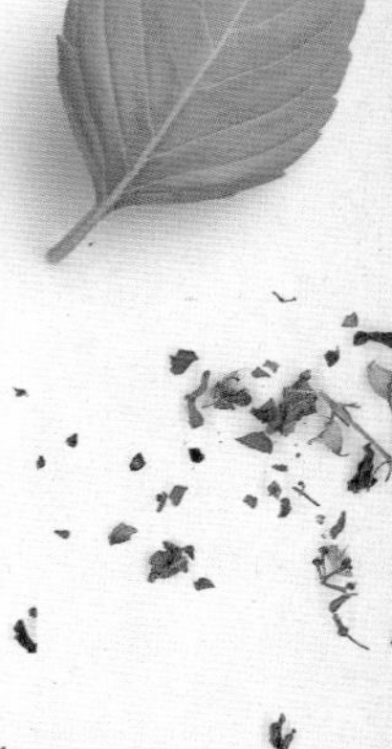

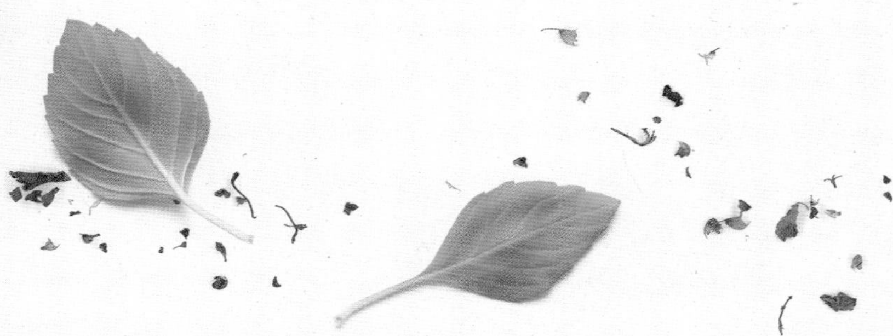

for the Spirit

Traditional Western magic focuses on basil, but holy basil has its own kind of divinity, at least in Eastern spirituality. Holy basil is considered sacred to the Hindu god Vishnu, who is, basically, the protector of creation, love, and mercy, and, really, just keeps everything moving smoothly. According to myth, he also incarnates as a human from time to time, when the scales are tipped more toward the evil side of things. Talk about a stressful job, right? No wonder the poor soul found the need to create holy basil and hold it sacred. Practicing Hindus use holy basil in meditation rituals and prayer, and ingest the herb to bring energy and purity into the body and mind.

Basil itself has a masculine attribution (fits nicely with the holy basil/Vishnu connection), and its element is fire. It's good to invoke the soothing scent of basil when there has been disharmony between people. Looking for love? Add basil to incense in order to scent your home and clothing.

I've focused on holy basil in this chapter because it's been such an influential herb for me — healing, inspiring, and fun to work with. However, if you can't get your hands on holy basil, you can substitute one of the many varieties of culinary basil for any of the recipes that follow. Just note that the stress-relieving effects won't be quite as strong, and the flavors and scents will vary.

HOLY BASIL

Ocimum sanctum

Parts used: Leaves
How to harvest: Snip top leaves consistently in order to encourage bushy growth; pinch off flower stalks to inhibit bolting
Effects on body: Antioxidant, calms coughs, eases the pain of bites and stings
Effects on mind and spirit: Soothing, calming, anti-stress, antidepressant, courage-inducing
Safety first: Avoid while pregnant or while trying to conceive

aromatherapy

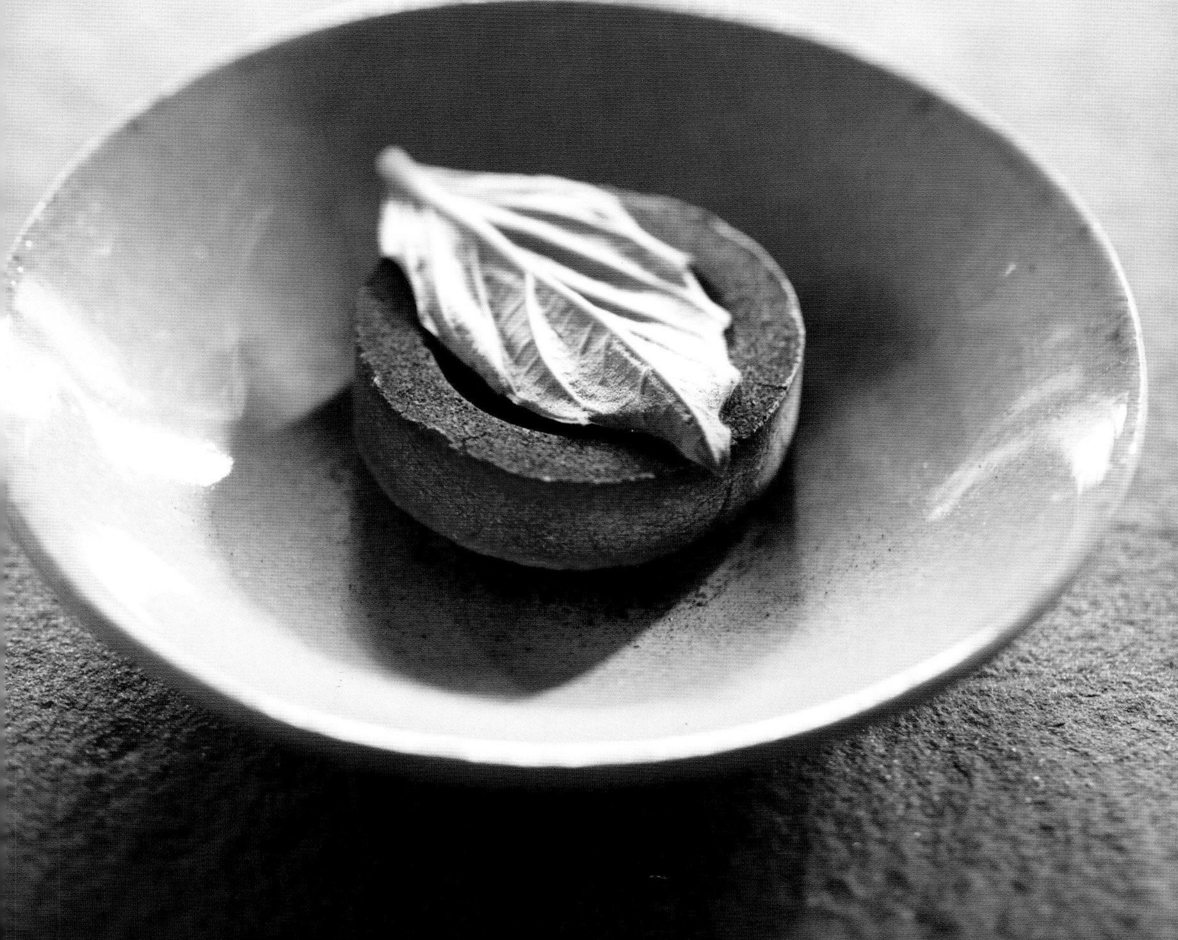

HOLY BASIL AROMATHERAPY

Stress relief. What we're ingesting from this tea is important, but its aromatherapy quotient is almost as important. Before drinking your holy basil tea, find a quiet place to sit. Inhale your brew deeply. Close your eyes. Go wherever the mind takes you (as long as it's peaceful; if not, keep inhaling the steam). Open your eyes. Sip your tea mindfully, savoring your drink and the moment. This peace exists within you all the time. Sometimes you just need a little help reacquainting yourself with it.

Insomnia relief. If you tend to wake up in the night in an anxiety-ridden panic (I may have experienced this once or twice . . .), keep a little aromatherapy blend by your bedside. Fill a small jar, such as a lip-balm tin, with 1 or 2 tablespoons of carrier oil, such as almond oil. Add enough drops of holy basil so that you can smell it easily. Stop there, or add lavender, chamomile, and/or rose. Take a whiff or rub a bit on your temples for a soothing middle-of-the-night acupressure massage.

Cough and cold blend. A mixture of holy basil and eucalyptus is a wonderful aromatherapy blend for the dratted cold season. Pour 1 or 2 tablespoons of carrier oil (such as almond oil) into a shallow dish. Add 5 drops holy basil essential oil (or more; just make sure you can smell it) and 2 drops of eucalyptus. Go easy with eucalyptus — she can steal the show with just an extra drop or two.

Now, go ahead and inhale the scent of this blend. Nose stuffed up? No worries. Rub the oil on your chest, or dab a bit under your nose (carefully; if your nose is raw, you might want to skip this part). Alternatively, rub the blend on your wrists and temples, keeping away from the eyes.

Cold and flu steam. Heat 2 cups of water on the stove until just boiling. Turn off the heat and pour the water into a heatproof ceramic bowl. Add a few drops each of holy basil, mint, and eucalyptus essential oils. Being careful not to burn yourself, drape your head with a towel and place your face over the steam (if it burns, wait a few moments for the water to cool). Inhale the steam for 10 minutes, then take a break. If the skin around your nose is raw, put a little moisturizer on it.

If you don't have the essential oils, you can just cook up a big batch of holy-basil-and-peppermint tea (try 1 tablespoon total of herb per cup), drape your head with a towel, and soak in the steam. You'll have the bonus of being able to drink the tea later. (Don't take eucalyptus internally, though.)

TEAS

Base tea for stress relief. Steep 2 teaspoons dried holy basil leaves (or 4 teaspoons fresh) in 1 cup boiling water in a preheated mug for 10 minutes. This alone should do a great deal for your stress level, especially if you're sipping in a quiet, contemplative state that allows you room to breathe. Sweetness helps, too.

Tea to support your stamina. To your base tea (above), add a little energy: 1 teaspoon dried peppermint leaves or a few cinnamon chips or a cinnamon stick, and 1 teaspoon good-quality green tea. Now you have a spicy, flavorful, energy-filled tonic that will see you through the rest of your day. (This is perfect, by the way, for that inevitable midafternoon slump, otherwise known as the "give me a cookie before I start taking filing cabinets hostage" hour.)

Tea for insomnia. Holy basil is a wonderful pre-bedtime ritual, especially if your insomnia is anchored in anxiety (and that whirling mind thing so many of us experience at night). Straight holy basil tea will be just fine, but skip the sweetener (unless you use stevia) or you'll jack up your blood sugar too much. But better yet, brew your tea in hot milk (for the tryptophan effect), and if you're feeling a bit adventurous, add a dash of chamomile.

Tea for coughs and colds. To your holy basil base tea, add 1 part mint, ¼ part ginger, ⅛ part cinnamon, and/or ⅛ part cloves. Add a dash of lemon juice and honey, and you have a fantastic chest-clearing cough and cold remedy. Add a dash of brandy, if that suits you, to help sleep come and soothe the frazzled nerves illness can bring.

Holy basil hot cocoa. To make a wonderful holy basil hot chocolate, heat 1 cup milk (dairy or non), turn off the heat, and steep 2 teaspoons holy basil for 5 minutes. Strain the milk and put it back into the pan. Add 1 tablespoon good-quality cocoa, a little vanilla extract, and sweetener of choice. Blend and heat.

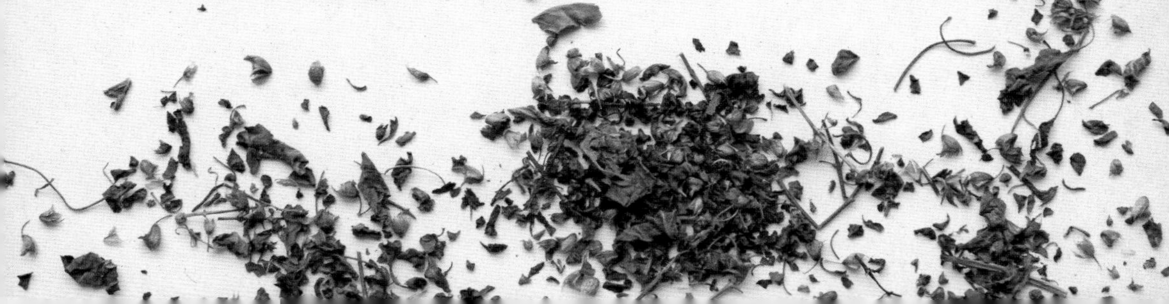

HOLY BASIL MAGIC

FOR SAFE TRAVELS

One of the easiest, and oldest, methods of borrowing a bit of magic from an herb is to simply carry it with you. I like to put a variety of herbs and stones or crystals in a little pouch and tuck it into my pocket. A pinch of holy basil (or even a tea bag!) in your pocket will help protect you during your travels.

In the Hindu tradition, you don't even need to carry the basil with you (which would possibly save you from some grief in airport security); you can simply rub a fresh basil leaf on your forehead, at the point of your third eye (see chapter opener photo). I like to close my eyes and visualize myself arriving safely at my destination, filled with energy and enthusiasm after a long journey.

TO ATTRACT LOVE AND LUCK

There are a few good basil traditions for attracting love and luck. One of my favorites is to rub powdered basil over your and your partner's hearts to keep your eyes only on each other (although, if your partner proves to be a serial wanderer, I'm not sure you want the help of basil to keep him or her around; best to carry a leaf in your pocket to attract new love and luck).

If you've had a disagreement with your partner, or the two of you seem to butt heads, dab a little basil essential oil on the pulse points; the scent is a love perfume and it helps facilitate understanding between two people.

TO DETERMINE THE LONGEVITY OF A RELATIONSHIP

Not sure if you're meant to make it with your partner? Light a charcoal disk (the kind used for incense) and place two fresh basil leaves on it. If they burn to ash quickly, then the relationship you're in (or starting, or hoping for) will be successful. If the basil leaves crackle and jump, you'll have lots of . . . energy . . . in the relationship (whether this is harmonious or disharmonious energy remains to be seen). If the leaves fly apart from each other, well, you probably just don't want to go there.

Another fun tradition I came across helps divine whether or not your partner is faithful (although, good luck trying to do this with any subtlety). Place fresh basil on his or her hand; if it withers, well, you have your answer.

TO ATTRACT WEALTH

A pot of basil in your house, or a plot in your garden, attracts wealth of all kinds. If you own a business, you can slip a basil leaf into the cash register, helping your space attract even more revenue. A Haitian tradition is to create an infusion of basil in water for three days (think sun tea) and then sprinkle the water over your doorstep. This will keep money in and thieves out.

The ultimate house-warming gift? A potted basil plant, for luck.

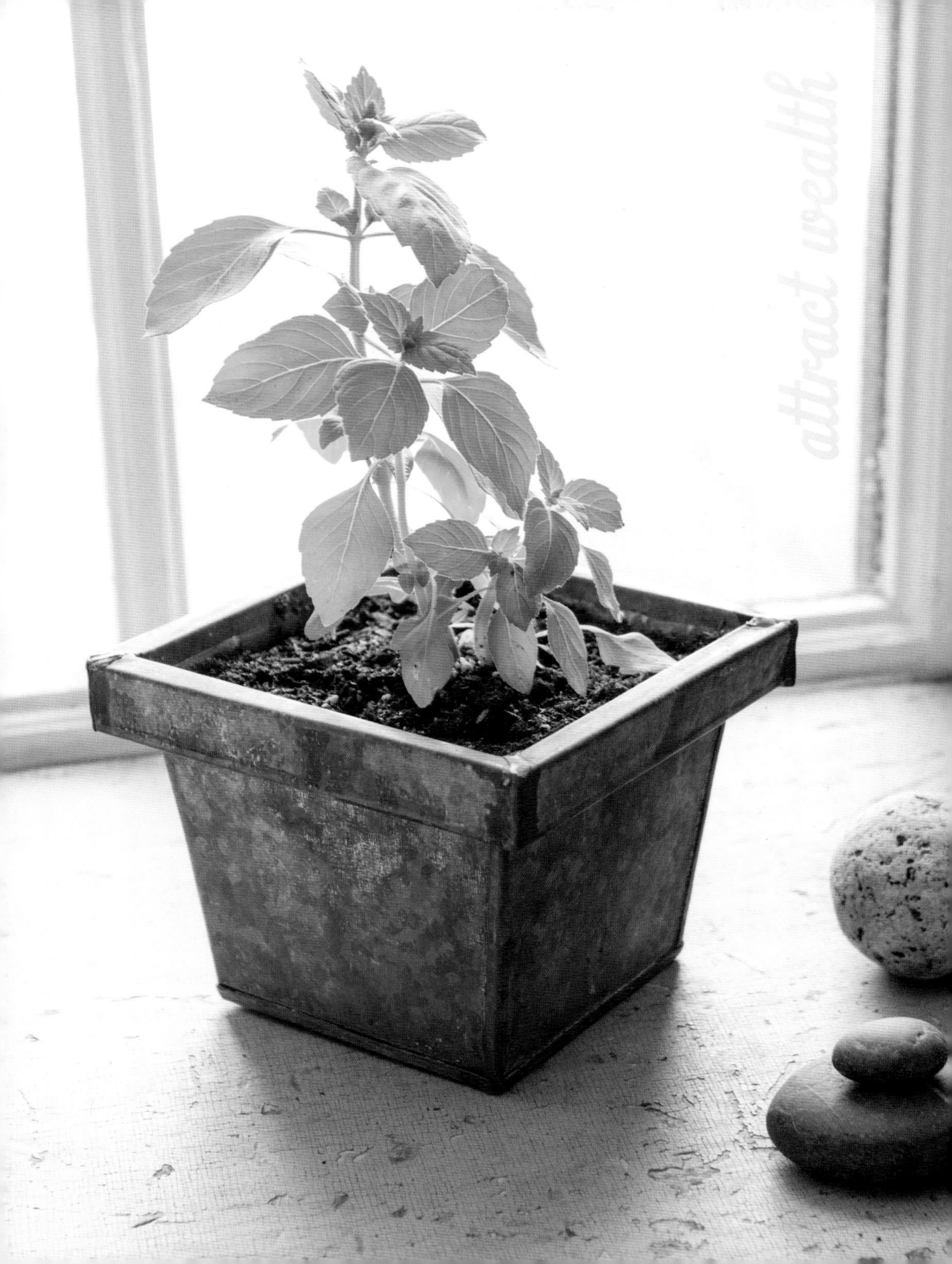
attract wealth

recipes

BODY CARE

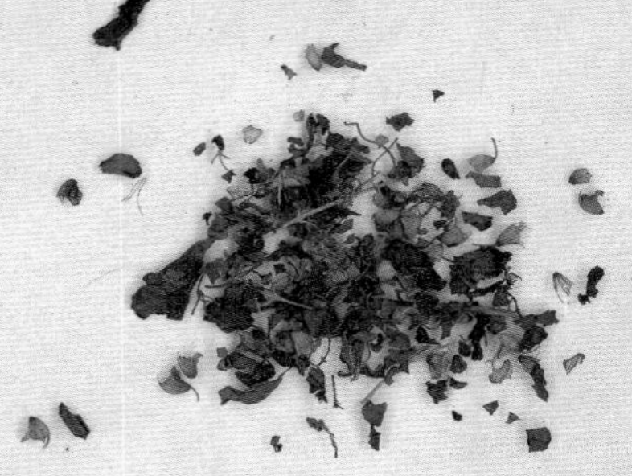

Cough and Cold Chest Rub

Chest rubs work best when they're a tad warm, so feel free to use this as you make it. You can also gently heat the rub by pouring a portion into a glass and then setting the glass over or into a mug of recently boiled water.

- **½ cup good-quality oil (I like almond oil)**
- **3 drops holy basil essential oil**
- **3–5 drops eucalyptus essential oil**
- **1 teaspoon ground ginger**
- **¼ teaspoon ground cayenne (optional; skip if you have sensitive skin)**
- **1–2 teaspoons powdered mustard (optional; it's fantastic for clearing chest congestion)**

1. In a small saucepan, gently heat the oil until warm (not simmering) over low heat. Turn off the heat, and add the essential oils and ginger, and cayenne and mustard, if using.
2. Let steep for 20 to 30 minutes, then reheat over low heat. If you like, strain the heated oil through a sieve to remove all those powdered particulates (optional).
3. Rub the warm oil on your chest. If you wear contacts, wear gloves or take out your contacts with clean hands prior to applying the rub (trust me on this one). Cover the area with an old, soft piece of cotton to keep the chest warm and to protect your clothing. Once the oil cools, feel free to reapply as needed.

Makes 2–4 applications

Holy Basil Mouthwash

The easiest method is to make a strong holy basil tea and keep it in the fridge for use morning and night, but you'll have to discard it after a few days. For a mouthwash with a better shelf life and a stronger cleaning/freshening aspect, try this. You'll still have to store it in the fridge, but it should be good for about a week. Gargle with this, too, for sore throat flare-ups.

- **3 tablespoons dried holy basil**
- **2 tablespoons witch hazel or apple cider vinegar**
- **Peppermint, cinnamon, or clove essential oil to taste**
- **Dash of lemon juice (for whitening)**

1. Bring 2 cups water to a boil. Place the holy basil in a jar and pour the boiling water on top. Let it steep for 15 minutes, then strain. Let cool.
2. Add the witch hazel or apple cider vinegar, essential oil, and lemon juice to the tea, cover, and shake.
3. To use, rinse with the mouthwash and then spit out.

Makes 16 ounces

Kidney Healing Compress

If you suffer from chronic fatigue or mid-low back pain or kidney stones, or you've had a long day (or week, month, or year), are emerging from a long illness, or just feel sort of tired and sluggish in general, this might be a good project for you.

A side note: Keep your compress towels separate from the rest of your towels when doing laundry. The ginger can be potent and could affect the rest of your linens.

3 tablespoons dried ginger or 2 tablespoons fresh ginger

1 tablespoon dried holy basil

2 tablespoons dried dandelion leaves

1. In a medium saucepan, heat about a quart of water over medium heat. Add the ginger, holy basil, and dandelion leaves. Bring to a simmer, then turn off the heat and cover. Steep for 10 to 20 minutes.
2. Strain the water to remove the herbs, and put the liquid back in the pot on the stove. Test the temperature. It should be really warm, but not scalding. Dip a piece of wool or flannel (or a washcloth, whatever) into the liquid and hold it to your face. If you can handle the temperature, then it's ready.
3. Using tongs, dip a kitchen-towel–sized piece of fabric into the water. Using gloves, wring it out. Lie down on your stomach, and have a friend drape the cloth on the bare skin of your mid- to lower back, between where the ribs end and where the top of a pop-star's pants would land.
4. Cover the cloth with a big fluffy towel and/or blanket to keep the compress warm. Now relax until it cools. Reapply as often as necessary or desired. If you have leftover compress water, dump it out. It loses its zing after 24 hours. You can rub a little castor oil (great for toning the organs) into the kidney area after you've ended your treatment.

Makes 1 compress

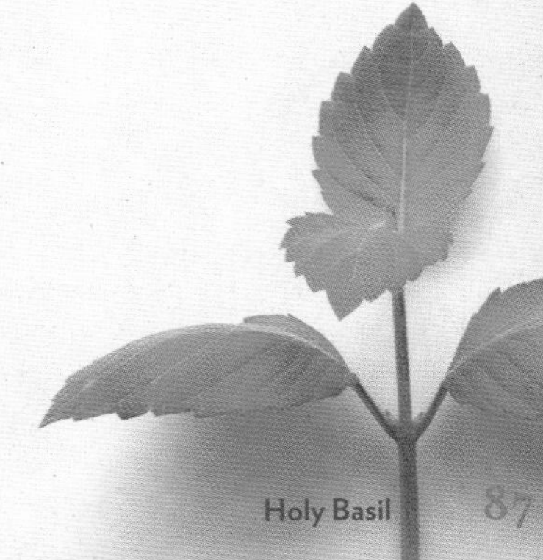

Lemon and Holy Basil Lotion

Blend up this super-easy formula for a lotion that not only soothes sore, tired, and irritated skin, but also lifts and lightens the spirits (and, incidentally, any discoloration in the skin as well). Use this on your lips, face, hands, feet, or wherever.

- **½ cup almond (or similar) oil**
- **1 tablespoon dried basil (holy, ideally, but any will work)**
- **3 tablespoons grated beeswax**
- **3 drops basil essential oil**
- **5 drops lemon essential oils**
- **1 tablespoon honey**
- **⅛ teaspoon baking soda**

1. In a small saucepan, heat the oil just until it's warm (don't boil it), and steep the herb for 10 minutes. Alternatively, just leave the herb in the oil and steep overnight at room temperature. Strain the oil into a small bowl. You should still have ½ cup oil; if not, add a little oil.
2. Return the strained oil to the pan and heat gently. Add the wax and heat until melted. Turn off the heat and let it cool for a few minutes.
3. Add the essential oils, honey, and baking soda, and blend. I like to use an eggbeater, but that's up to you (just don't let anyone lick the beaters). Check the scent and add more essential oils to suit your own taste (so to speak).
4. Pour the lotion into a clean 4-ounce glass or sturdy plastic container (run it through the dishwasher or just wash in hot, soapy water), and let it sit until completely cooled. Once cooled, you can cap it, label it, and store it. If you cap it too soon, condensation might collect, and the last thing you want in a lotion like this is some rogue water!

Makes 4 ounces

Holy Basil and Spearmint Toothpaste

Homemade toothpaste! I love this stuff. I like to use a wide-mouth jar and just dip my toothbrush into it. If you have multiple family members using this paste, get a jar for each of them.

- **⅔ cup baking soda**
- **10 drops holy basil essential oil**
- **Powdered stevia to taste (optional)**
- **5 drops clove, cinnamon, or peppermint essential oil (optional; for taste)**

In a small jar, combine the baking soda, essential oil, and stevia, if using. Mix it up. Add water a bit at a time, stirring, until you have a paste-like consistency. Despite the presence of baking soda (which is a cleanser, whitener, antibacterial, and odor fighter), this is not abrasive to the teeth. It's perfectly safe for veneers, dentures, and sensitive teeth.

Makes around 5 ounces of toothpaste (that's 200+ brushings!)

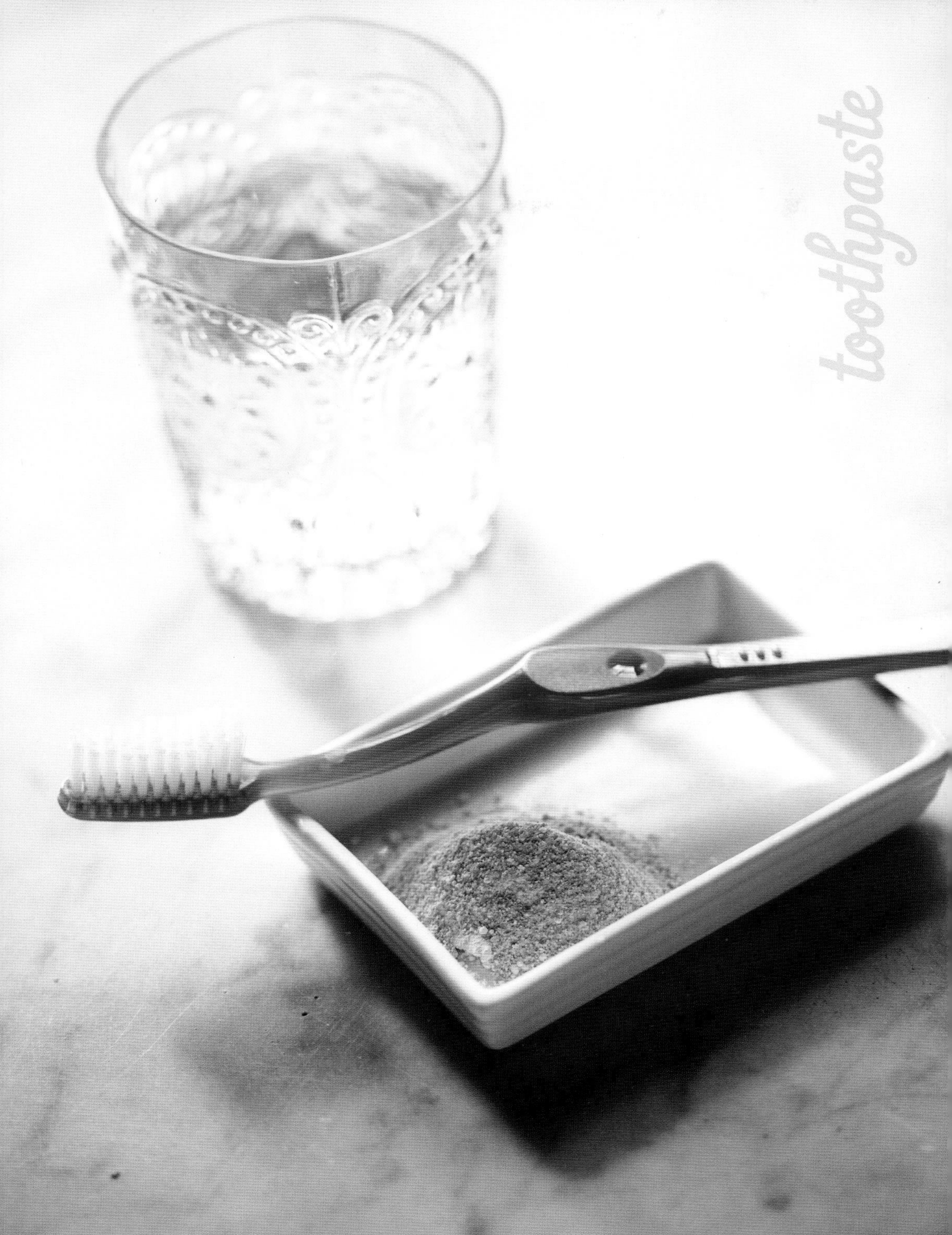
toothpaste

recipes

FOOD & DRINK

Holy Basil Spice Butter Cookies

These cookies come from my grandmother's recipe and are made for accompanying a warm cup of tea. Think a hardy black tea such as Irish Breakfast or even a smoky one like Lapsang Souchong.

- 2 cups organic, all-purpose flour (you may need a bit more if you're using maple syrup)
- ½ teaspoon aluminum-free baking powder
- Pinch of salt
- ½ teaspoon ground holy basil
- 1 teaspoon cinnamon, ginger, cardamom, or pumpkin pie spice
- ½ cup (1 stick) butter or vegan substitute, room temperature
- ¾ cup evaporated cane juice, honey, or maple syrup
- 1 teaspoon vanilla extract
- 1 egg or vegan substitute
- ¼ cup milk (dairy or non-dairy, unsweetened)
- 1 tablespoon chopped candied ginger (optional)

1. Preheat the oven to 375°F/190°C. Grease two cookie sheets or line them with parchment paper.
2. In a medium bowl, combine the flour, baking powder, salt, basil, and spice, and mix well.
3. In a large bowl, cream the butter and sweetener. Add the vanilla and egg, and mix until combined.
4. Add half the dry mixture to the large bowl. The first rule I learned about butter cookies is not to overmix the batter (same thing with muffins, if you're familiar with baking those), so stir gently. Add the milk, then add the candied ginger, if using. Mix just until combined and add more milk if needed. You want to be able to drop this batter from a spoon and have it hold together, not puddle or crumble all over your baking sheet.
5. Drop rounded spoonfuls of batter onto baking sheets and bake for 10 minutes, or until the edges start to brown.
6. Remove from the oven and let cool on baking sheets for a few minutes, then place cookies directly on the rack. Trust me — rushing this process leads to tasty, but crumbling cookies. These will keep for a couple of days at room temperature (though if my own experience is at all common, I doubt they'll last that long).

Makes 3–4 dozen cookies

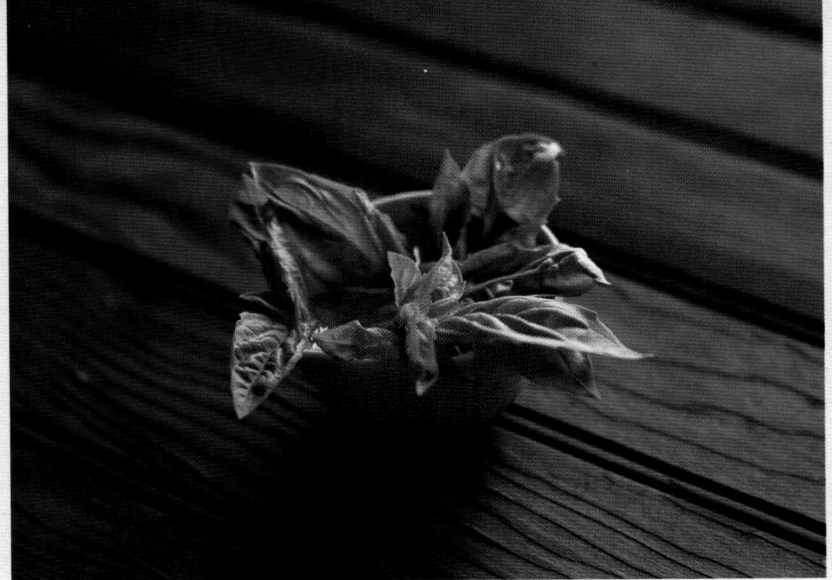

Thai-Inspired Holy Basil Tofu

Basil is a common ingredient in green curries (my favorite curry, personally). Why not replace Thai basil with a dash of holy basil? Serve it over rice, potatoes, quinoa, or whatever grain or starch suits your fancy. Me? I just pour it in a ridiculously huge bowl and eat it that way.

For the paste:

- 1 cup fresh basil leaves or ½ cup dried (use holy basil if you can find it, otherwise Thai basil)
- 2 shallots, chopped
- ¼ cup cilantro (half of that if dried)
- 1–2 tablespoons mint (optional)
- 1–3 Thai green chiles or jalapeños
- ½ teaspoon cumin
- ½ teaspoon white pepper
- ½ teaspoon coriander
- 1 tablespoon soy sauce or shoyu
- 2 tablespoons lime juice
- 1 stalk lemongrass (if you can find it)
- 1 tablespoon fresh ginger, minced (or to taste)
- 3–4 cloves garlic, minced (or to taste)

For the tofu mixture:

- 4 tablespoons good vegetable oil (I use coconut)
- 1 14-ounce package firm tofu (organic, if possible)
- 6 cups cubed vegetables of choice (zucchini, eggplant, bell peppers, kale, broccoli, green beans, onion; perhaps also some green apple, raisins, or nuts)
- ¾ cups coconut milk (light or regular)
- ¾ cups water or veggie broth

Recipe continues on next page

1. To make the paste, combine the basil, shallots, cilantro, mint (if using), chiles, cumin, pepper, coriander, soy sauce, lemon juice, lemongrass (if using), ginger, and garlic in a food processor and blend until you have a paste consistency. You can add a couple of teaspoons of water at a time if you need to.
2. Heat 2 tablespoons oil in a skillet over medium heat. Cube the tofu and add it to the skillet. Sauté the tofu until brown on all sides (alternatively, you can toss the cubed tofu in some oil and bake it at 375°F/190°C for 35 minutes).
3. Heat the remaining oil in a large pot over medium-low heat. Add the vegetables, and sauté 7 minutes or until soft and fragrant. Alternatively — and I do this in the summer, especially — sauté the onion and steam the rest of the vegetables. Sometimes it's nice not to have the heaviness of the oil.
4. Add the tofu and paste to the pot. Stir, stir, stir, for about 5 minutes. Add the coconut milk and water or broth. Cover that bad boy and simmer for about 15 minutes or until the vegetables are done to your liking. Since I like crisp vegetables, I tend to undercook them in step 3 and then cook the full amount of time here, so that all those lovely spices mingle.

Serves 6

Holy Basil and Honey Spritzer

This is a fantastic libation for warm summer days or even celebrations, such as the high fall and winter holidays. You can make this with wine or water, depending on your preference.

- **½ cup fresh holy or cinnamon basil or ¼ cup dried**
- **¾ cup honey or maple syrup**
- **2 cups wine or sparkling water**
- **1 ounce honey liqueur (optional; skip if you're using wine)**

1. Bring 2 cups water to a simmer. Turn off the heat and add the basil. Cover and steep for 10 minutes.
2. Strain the liquid (add more hot water if you need to so that you still have 2 cups), and add the honey or maple syrup. Refrigerate until chilled.
3. Add the wine or sparkling water, stir, and serve. If you're using honey liqueur, pour a little liqueur in each glass, then top with the fizzy sparkling water spritzer.

Serves 4

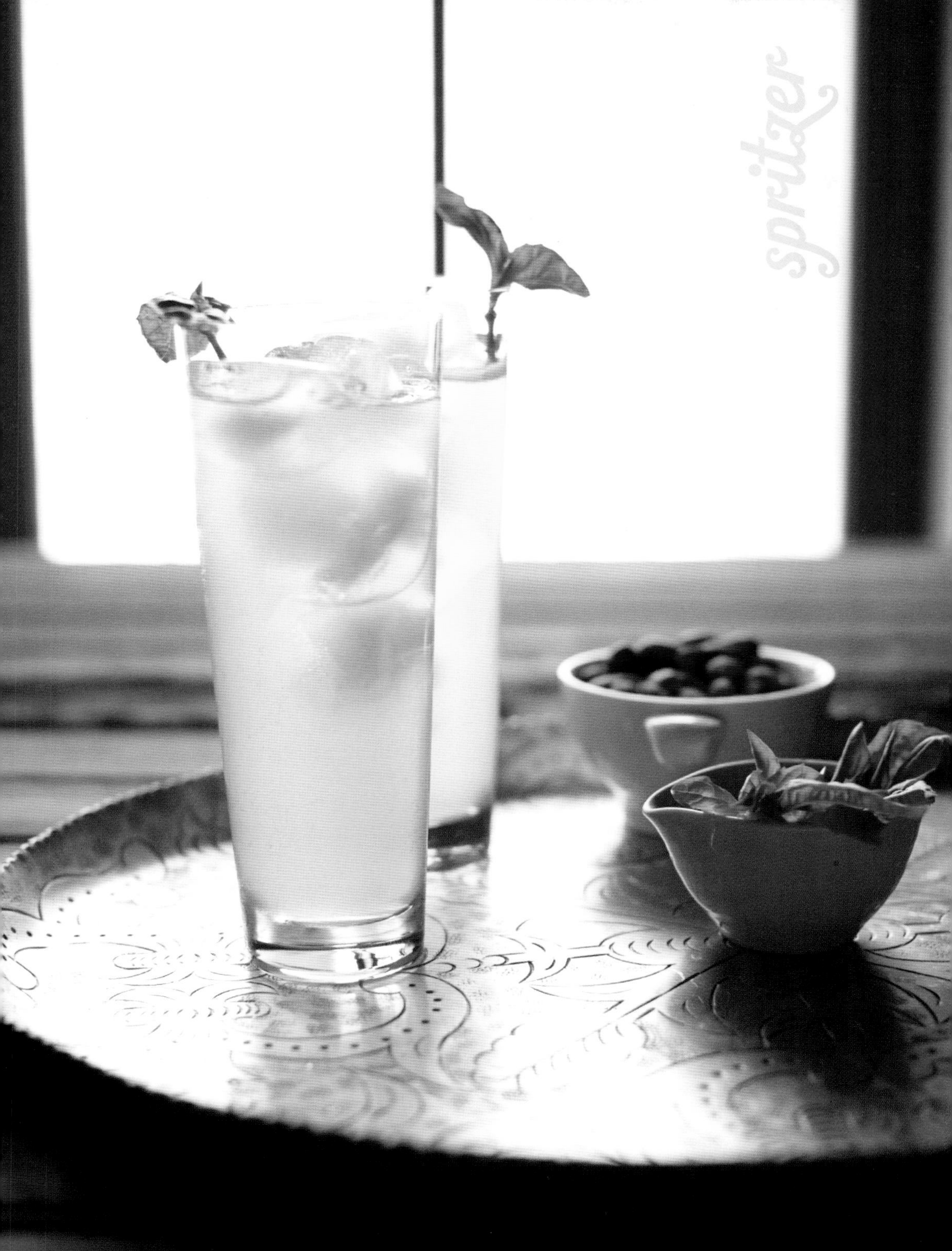
spritzer

HOLY BASIL YOGA

Since the practice of using holy basil is about adapting and finding a way to bring more peace into our lives, our yoga pose is going to aim to do this. When you think about where stress affects your body, you probably think of hunched shoulders, aching stomachs, and bent posture — as if you're trying to disappear into yourself. When I see this in my yoga students, the first thing I want to do is open the heart, the shoulders, and the abdomen. Cobra Pose (*Bhujangasana*) is a great way to do this. The other thing I want to do is place the head lower than the heart with a simple forward bend. Anxiety lives in the head; it's a manifestation of the mind. Grace, peace, and stillness lie in the heart.

Warming up with standing forward bend. So, let's start with a gentle spine warm-up. We're going to begin with the Standing Forward Bend, or *Uttanasana*, as it's known in Sanskrit.

Stand evenly with your feet hip-distance apart and take a few nice deep breaths. First pull the inhale into your chest and heart area. Fill up your lungs and hold your breath (without tension); then let it go and feel your shoulder blades (scapulae) drop down your back. Now take another deep breath and pull it into your belly as well as your heart. Fill up the whole front of your body. Release, and let all that tension and stress release with your breath. If this is all that you have time to do on a given day, then just do this. Standing and breathing a few times will do wonders.

Take one more deep breath and as you exhale, bend your knees slightly and roll your spine down. It doesn't matter how far you go or whether or not you can touch the floor. Just dangle here. Let your head go. Decompress your spine. If you're pretty flexible, try straightening your legs a bit, but don't lock your knees and don't stress your hamstrings. Be gentle. You can also fit your fists inside the crooks of your elbows, folding your arms in a kind of hammock. This adds a bit of weight to the spinal decompression.

All done? Inhale and let your body relax. Exhale, bend your knees, and roll up, so very slowly.

Moving into Cobra. While standing on a mat or carpet, roll back down, bending your knees until you can comfortably drop to your hands and knees. If you have back, neck, or shoulder issues, stay on all fours.

If you're okay to continue, lie on your belly. Align yourself by placing the tops of your feet flat on the floor, forehead on the floor (or on a rolled-up blanket or towel if that's uncomfortable for your neck; your neck should be straight and not at all pained), and hands right under your shoulders. Take a couple of deep breaths.

On your next inhale, pull your belly button in toward your spine to activate your belly muscles, draw your shoulder blades down your back, and press into the floor with your hands. While pressing your hips into the floor, lift your chest as much as you can (but not so much that your hips lift from the floor). Keep that belly drawn in, shoulders down, and neck straight (don't look up, in other words). Take a deep breath to stretch the front of your body. This is Cobra Pose. On an exhale, come back down. Try this three times, if you like; then lie down, turn your head to one side, and relax. Breathe. Turn your head to the other side.

Finishing. Move into Child's Pose (see page 55), and stay there and breathe as long as you wish. When you're ready to come back up, move your hands beneath your shoulders, take a deep breath, and press yourself up through your hands. Sit for a moment if you need to, and then go about your day.

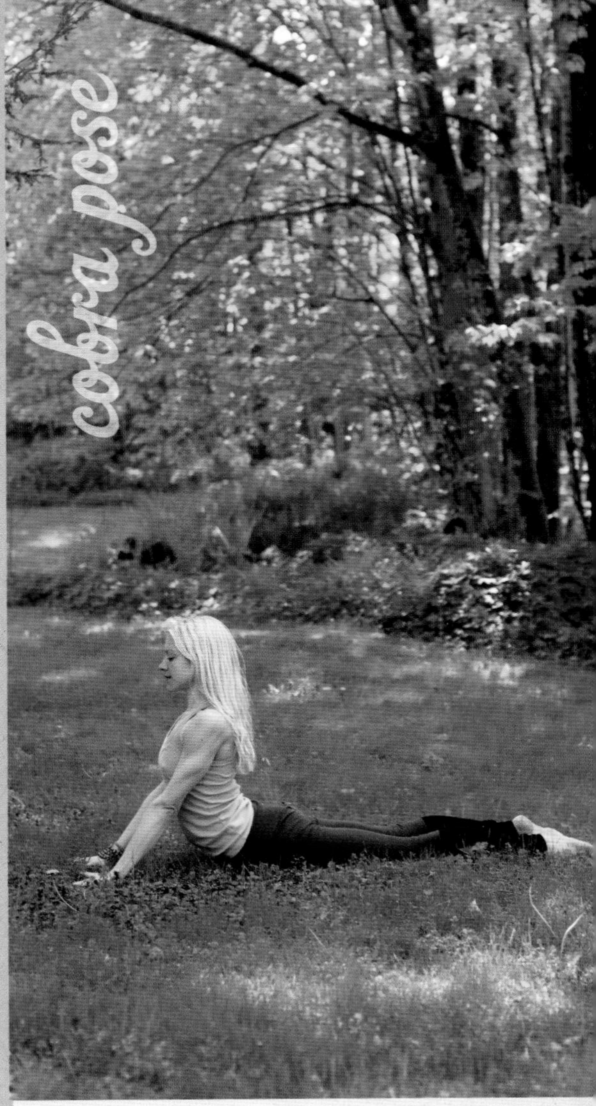

A NOTE ON BREATHING

Many times you'll see the roll-up associated with an inhale. This is fine, but I prefer an exhale because there's less chance of getting dizzy and falling over. It also gives your body time to regulate your blood pressure. If you do get light-headed, however, just roll back down a bit and come up more slowly. Your head always comes up last.

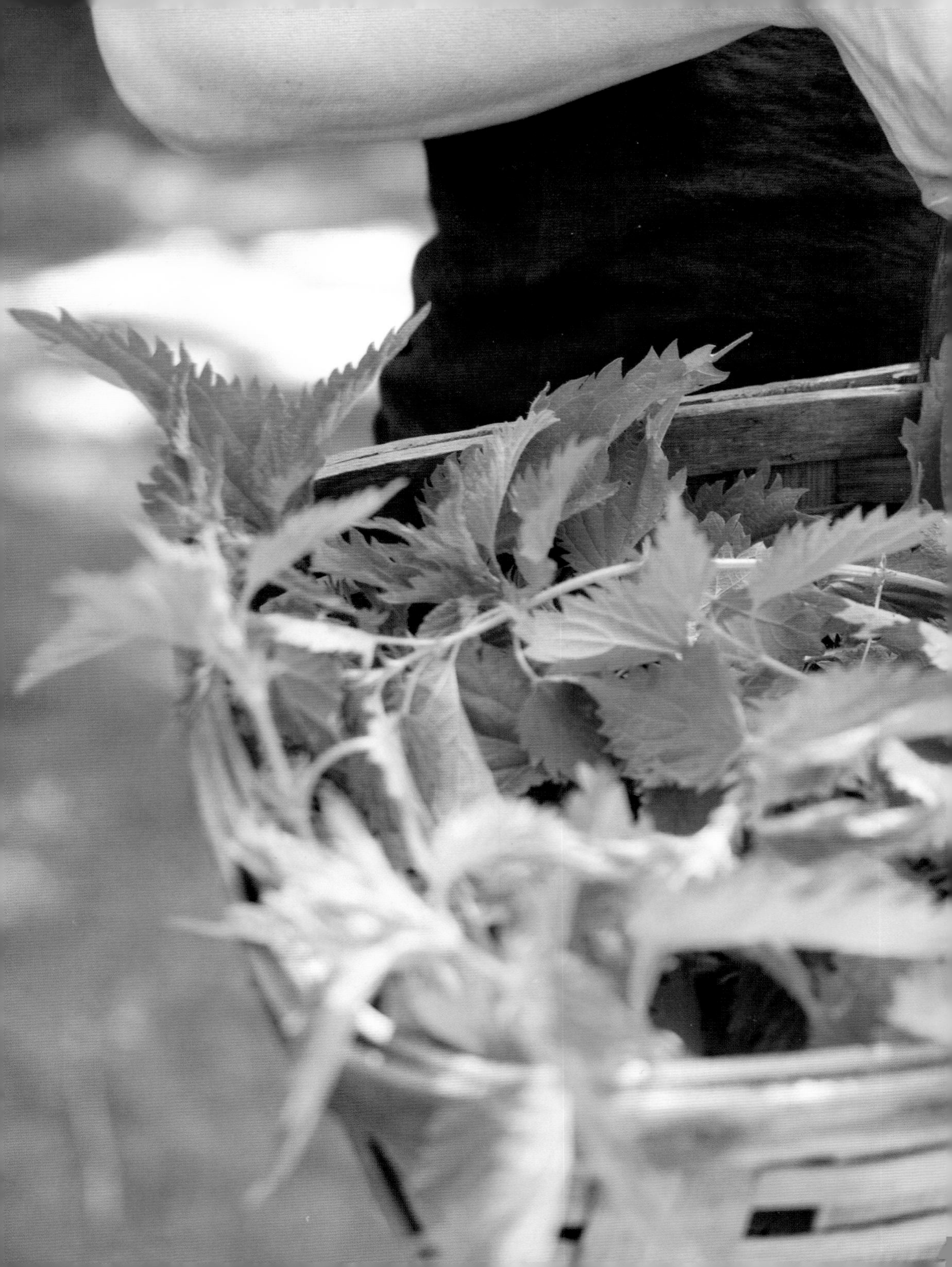

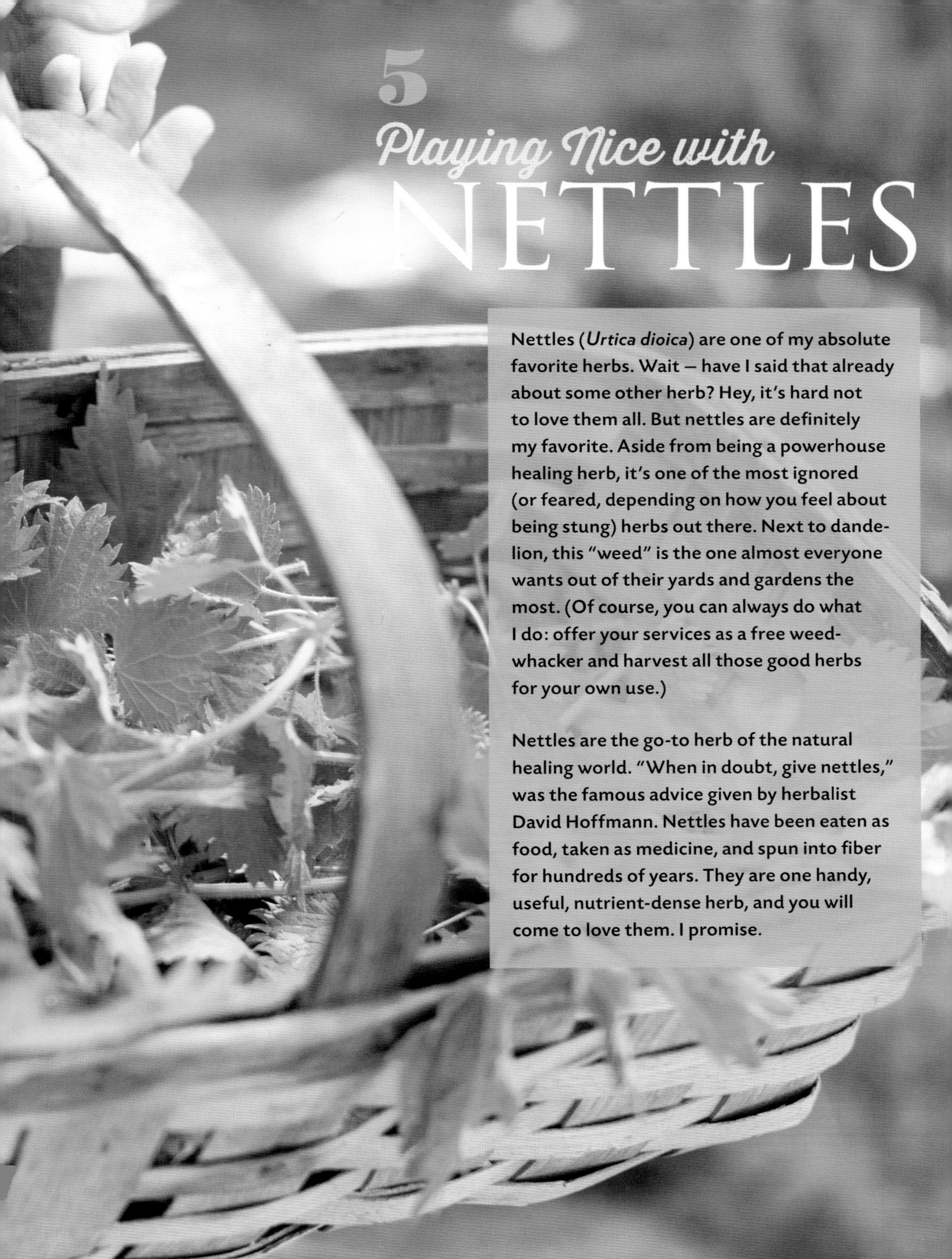

5

Playing Nice with NETTLES

Nettles (*Urtica dioica*) are one of my absolute favorite herbs. Wait — have I said that already about some other herb? Hey, it's hard not to love them all. But nettles are definitely my favorite. Aside from being a powerhouse healing herb, it's one of the most ignored (or feared, depending on how you feel about being stung) herbs out there. Next to dandelion, this "weed" is the one almost everyone wants out of their yards and gardens the most. (Of course, you can always do what I do: offer your services as a free weed-whacker and harvest all those good herbs for your own use.)

Nettles are the go-to herb of the natural healing world. "When in doubt, give nettles," was the famous advice given by herbalist David Hoffmann. Nettles have been eaten as food, taken as medicine, and spun into fiber for hundreds of years. They are one handy, useful, nutrient-dense herb, and you will come to love them. I promise.

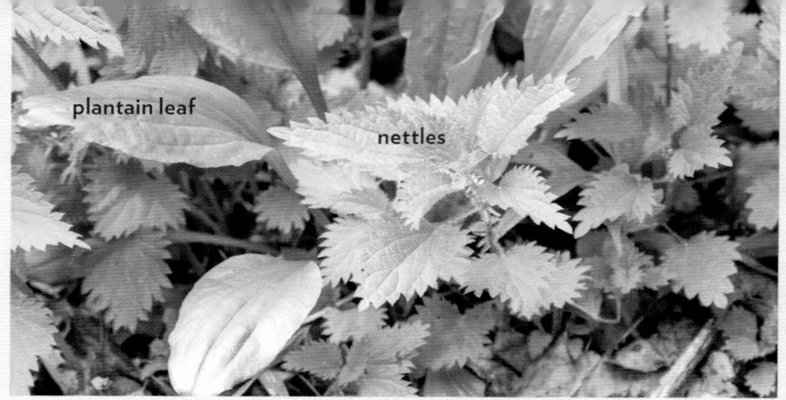

Nettles will grow in the wild pretty much anywhere there's lots of moisture — in river and lake beds, septic systems, swampy areas, manure piles, and compost heaps. Find a patch and harvest in the early spring, before the nettles grow to full size and definitely before they flower. If you cut the plants back after flowering, you can usually coax a second crop later in the summer.

Note: Take a look at the plantain leaf in the photograph above. You'll recognize it; you've probably been stepping on it for most of your life. Plantain is amazing for taking the sting out of nettles (and it just so happens that it often grows near the plant), as well as bites, cuts, and scrapes. Before you harvest nettles, have some plantain nearby. If the stinging is too much, chew up a plantain leaf (yup — chew it) to make a poultice and apply this to the sting. It will provide immediate relief.

NETTLES

Urtica dioica

Parts used: Leaves
How to harvest: Gather in wetlands and wastelands before flowers bloom
Effects on body: Detoxifying, cleansing, and nutrient-dense
Effects on mind and spirit: Eases exhaustion, frustration, and sensitivity
Safety first: Beware the sting — always wear protective gear when harvesting nettles and consume only leaves that have been dried, brewed, or cooked

for the Body

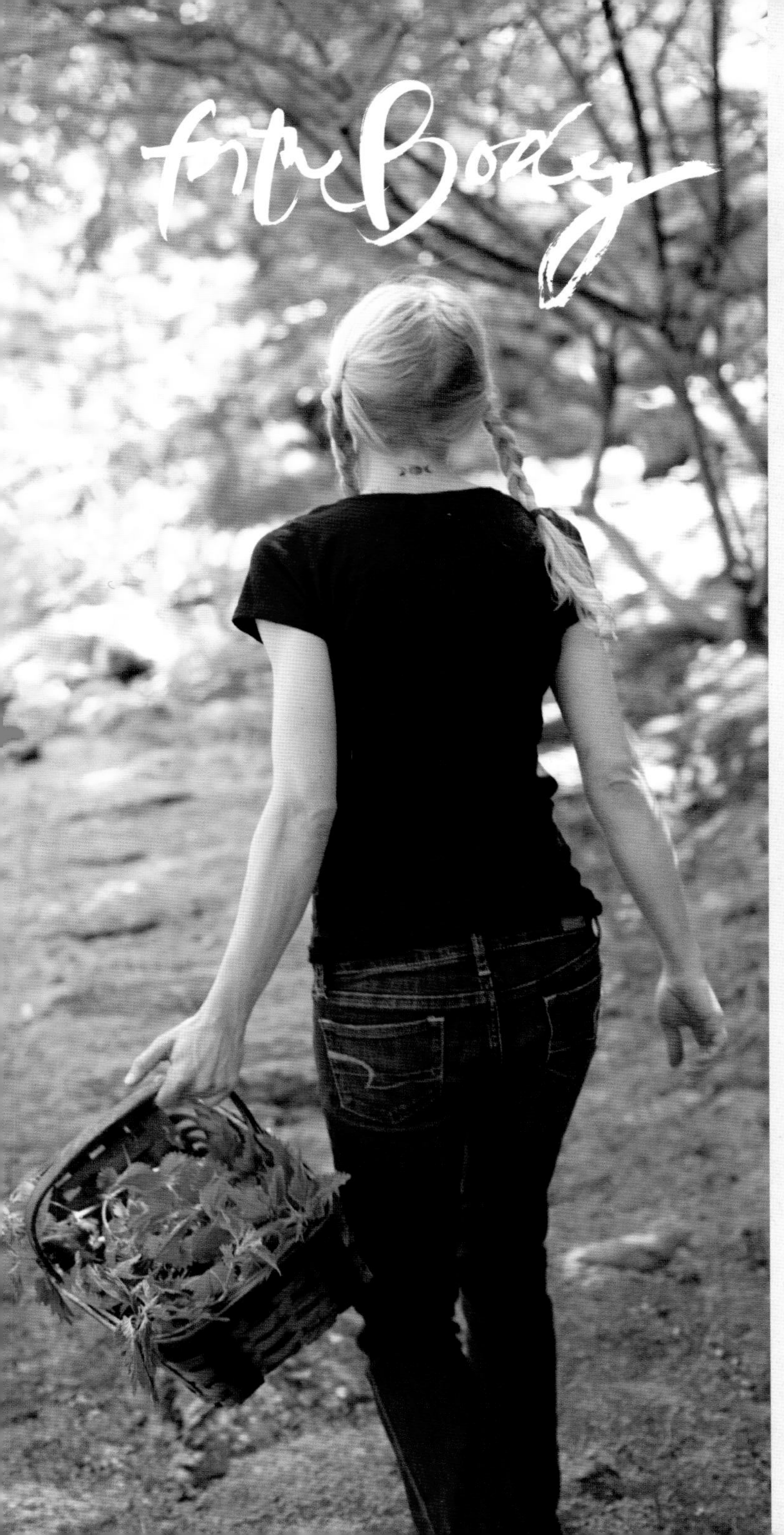

Let's begin with the basics: nutrition. Out of all the herbs we talk about in this book, or, heck, even could talk about (and that's *a lot*), nettles are among the highest in protein. But wait! There's more! Not only that, but nettles even aid in the digestion of proteins (as well as carbohydrates and fats) by building and cleaning the blood, toning and detoxifying the liver, and helping the kidneys become much more efficient.

But it's not just protein we're talking about here, although that's important; nettles are also a really powerful source of iron (pregnant goddesses, listen up), vitamins, minerals, chlorophyll, and fiber. Don't fall out of your seat yet, but nettles also contain an antihistamine that can nip those nasty allergies in the bud (especially the awful itchiness that arises in the eyes, nose, and soft palate).

So how does this bad-boy herb accomplish so much? Well, like all stories worth telling, it's complicated. Let's just say that nettles are closely linked to protein absorption in the body. Nettles facilitate the breakdown of protein into energy and nutrients. When your digestion and assimilation are improved, your energy level, allergic reactions, illness, and stress all get better.

Not only do nettles help digest protein, but they also help rid the body of excess protein. So, if you suffer from gout, arthritis, or overacidity (all those protein-related complications), nettles will help escort those troublesome proteins right on out of the body, bringing relief to acidic conditions. Overeating protein can also cause swelling in the lower extremities, pain in the kidneys, and pale or foul-smelling urine (anyone who has tried a high protein/ low carb diet knows what I'm saying). Nettles will help the kidneys get back on track, removing the excess fluid from the body.

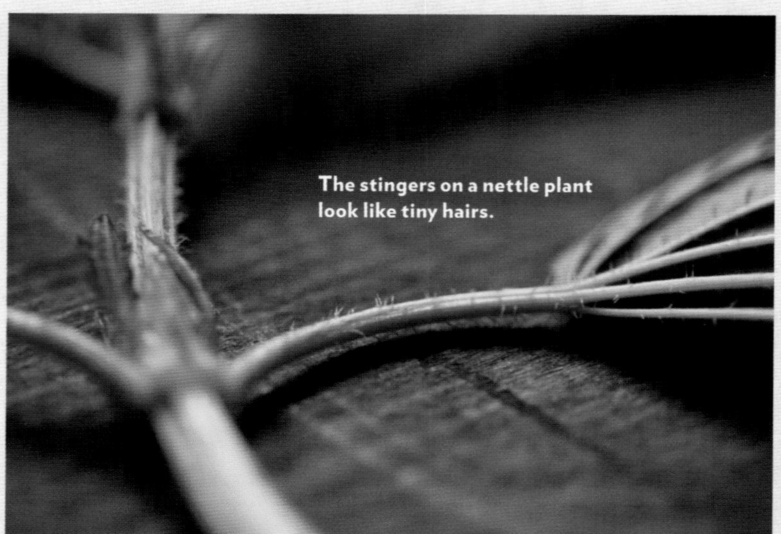

The stingers on a nettle plant look like tiny hairs.

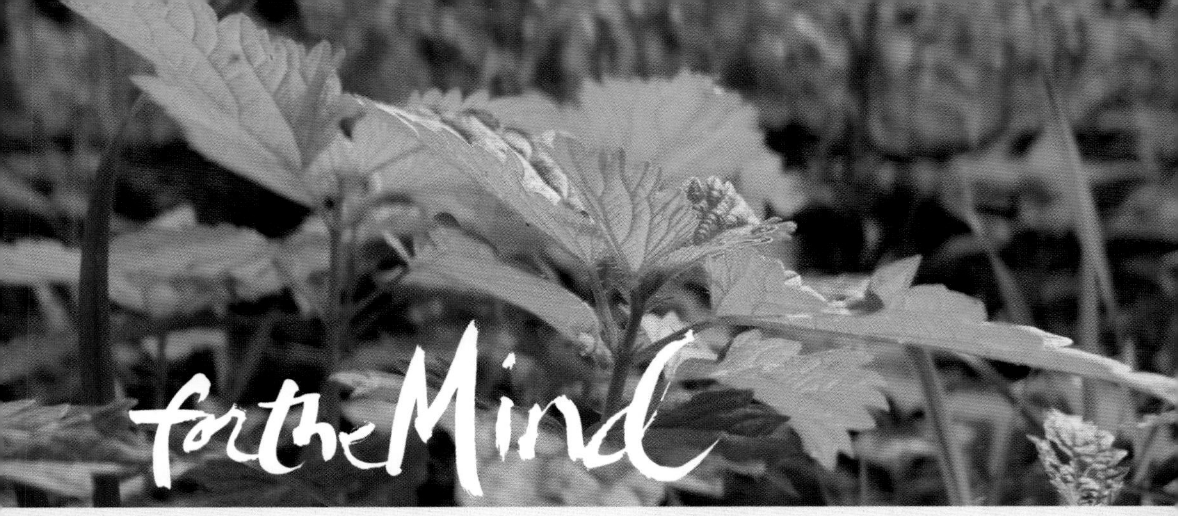

for the Mind

Often, we can intuit a flower's particular essence qualities just by examining the plant itself. Let's begin with the sting. The sting of nettles is sharp and annoyingly difficult to remove (unless you have some nice, chewed-up plantain nearby, of course), but not long-lasting. Therefore, it stands to reason that if you've been "stung" in the past but are still holding onto that grudge, creating a soothing blanket of pity or stubborn chip-bearing, then nettles are probably the remedy for you. Alternatively, if you're easily offended (or feel stung, so to speak) by criticism, others' opinions, or harsh words, then nettles can protect you there, too.

If you've ever seen a field of wild nettles, you were probably impressed by this plant's vast numbers and seemingly inexhaustible ability to reproduce, no matter what the caretaker, gardener, or landscaper tried. Nettles don't care what you want or what you think of them. If conditions are right, they're going to root in and take hold, and there is little you can do about it besides respect their ability to be completely and unfazedly themselves. So, if you're a person easily pushed around, flowing in and out of trends, and susceptible to peer pressure, nettles can help you take root and develop a good defense (maybe not stinging, though; that's a little harsh) to shield you from those outside forces.

Often, too, a plant's flower essence will assist in healing the same physical ailments the plant itself heals. Insomnia, joint pain, frustration (the kind that follows any kind of chronic pain), and exhaustion are all helped by nettles' essence.

for the Spirit

Nettles are what we herbalists like to call an "Old World" plant, meaning it's been around since long before written records were kept, when herbal lore was solely an oral tradition. Nettles, which grow abundantly in Europe as well as North America, were enormously popular medicinally, spiritually, and magically.

Almost across the board, nettles were used for protection against anything — illness; enemies; slander; unwanted spirits, energy, and curses. There's a pretty powerful stinger on that plant, after all. Nettles protect with their sting — a sharp but temporary warning to keep away. Thus, nettles are often used by mothers to protect their (born or unborn) children.

Nettles love soggy, wet ground and make seemingly infertile land, well, fertile. Use nettle magic when you're trying to conceive and to inspire fertility. And, even though nettle is a fertility-inducing herb, it's associated with masculine energy (men, after all, are involved in this fertility business, too). Its planet is Mars and its element is fire.

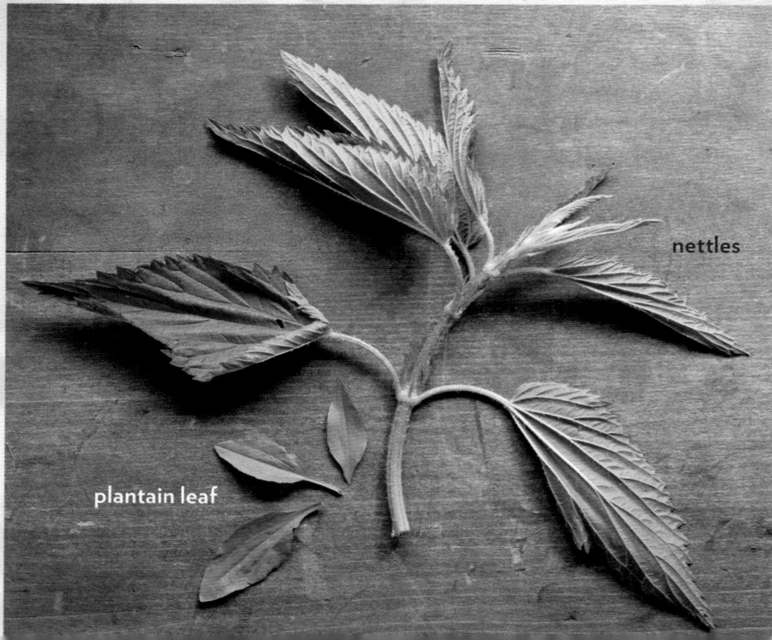

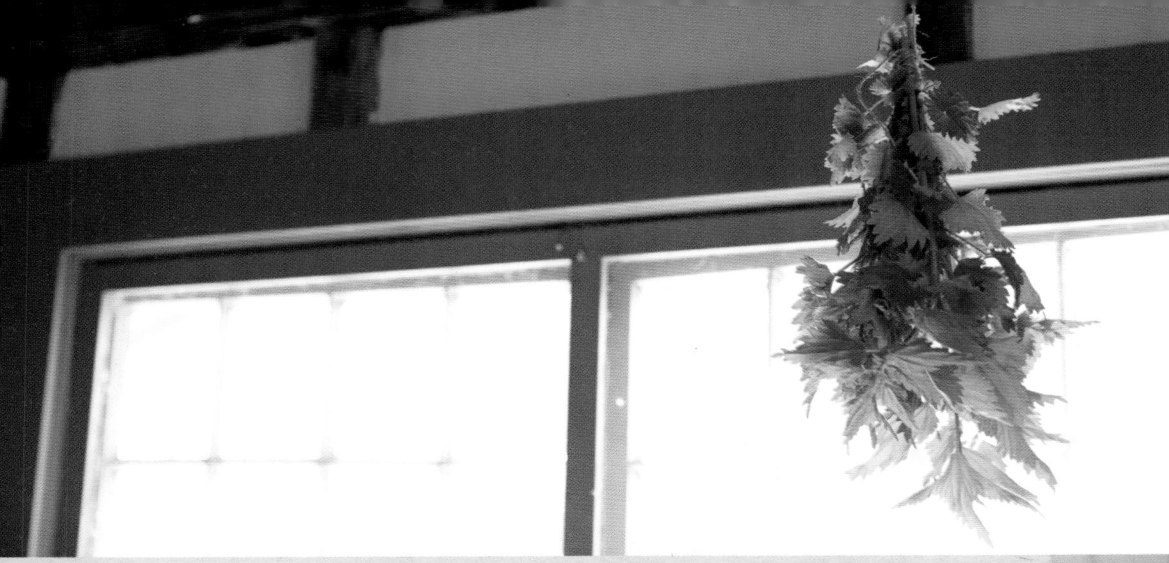

NETTLE MAGIC

FOR PROTECTION

There's no better "spell" for protection than simply carrying around the herb in question, or sprinkling it liberally throughout the house. According to folklore and practitioners who know such things, nettle is not your average protection charm. Oh, no. Nettles are adept at keeping evil away from your person and your home and sending it back from whence it came. That's right. *Evil.* That's some powerful mojo.

I like to carry a bit of nettles in a sachet if I'm traveling abroad or to a big city, to protect me from some of the crazy energy that is swirling around there. If, like me, you're susceptible to such chaos, then nettles will help protect and ground you. In the home, I like to hang bunches of nettles around the house to dry, both for magical and medicinal purposes. I also like to steep a nettle infusion, stick it in a spray bottle with some nice citrus essential oils, and spritz it around the house, especially when I'm doing a big spring or fall cleaning.

FOR RECOVERING FROM ILLNESS

Have you noticed how often an herb's medicinal and magical attributes work so well together? If so, it shouldn't surprise you that nettles are magically good for clearing illness, but what might surprise you is the method of its delivery. Head out to a nettle patch (wear your protection, of course) and cut a big handful of stalks. Place these in an open container (such as a plastic tub) and put them beneath the sickbed. As the nettles age and wither, they'll absorb the energy of the illness, helping the patient to recover. (Remember to thank the nettle patch before you harvest! Good karma!)

TEAS

Tea for allergy season. There's nothing quite like stinging nettles for allergy season. For a big brew, grab a quart jar and dump in 1 cup dried nettles (twice that for fresh; really, for fresh nettles, just cram as much in there as you can). Pour boiling water all the way to the top and stir. Cover and let steep. I usually let this cool, then put it in the fridge overnight. I strain it the next day and top it off with some filtered water so that I have a full quart. I like to drink a cup a day, adding a dash of lemon juice for extra hydration and vitamin C and a squeeze of liquid stevia for sweetness. You could also reheat your infusion and add a bit of local honey for extra-strong allergy relief and an immunity boost.

Note: If you're already on diuretics or have low blood pressure, take it easy with nettle tea. A cup per day would be just fine (2 to 3 teaspoons of dried herb per 8 ounces of water).

Tea to restore nutrient balance. Nettles are high in minerals, especially iron, and they help replenish and tone the kidneys and adrenals. For a great detox brew, grab a quart jar and mix ½ cup dried nettles, ¼ cup dried dandelion leaves, and ¼ cup dried alfalfa (double those amounts if you have fresh ingredients on hand). Boil up some filtered water and steep this brew overnight. Strain the next day, top off so you have a full quart, and drink cold or hot with a dash of lemon and sweetener. If drinking hot, add warm non-dairy milk, honey or maple syrup, and cinnamon.

Tea for digestive upset. When you find yourself suffering from overindulgence in rich foods like dairy and high-fat meats, reach for your nettles. Steep 1 tablespoon dried nettles in 10 ounces of water for 10 minutes. This tea will help reduce mucus and relieve bloating, and it moves wastes through the body while replenishing potassium supplies.

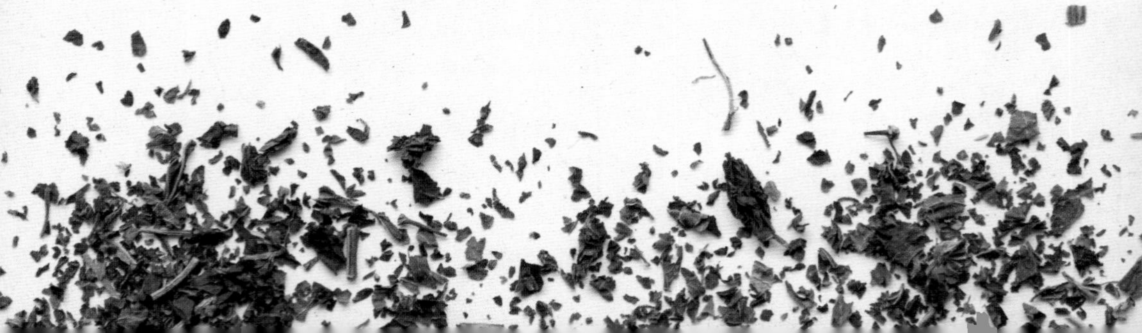

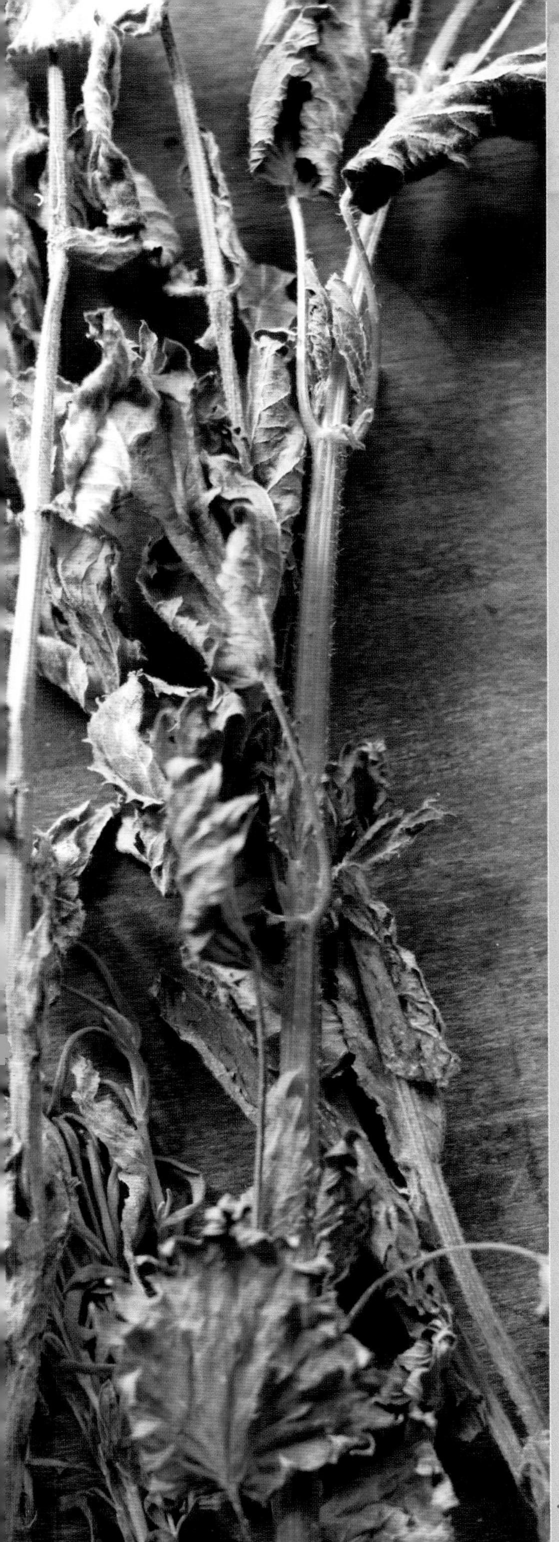

HOW TO "CURE" CAFFEINE ADDICTION

Caffeine, especially the high amounts found in coffee, can sap the body of minerals. If you're hooked and you want to un-hook yourself, then follow herbalist Susun Weed's advice and replenish your mineral supplies before you even look at a cup of decaf.

Give yourself six weeks to completely come off caffeine. Start each day with a cup of nettle tea (follow the tea for allergy season recipe on page 104) before you indulge in your caffeine. The nettles will help restore kidney and adrenal function and infuse the body with minerals. If you have some oat straw handy, you can add a tablespoon or two of this to your daily brew as well (for nervous-system health).

Then s-l-o-w-l-y cut back your caffeine intake. If you're trying to cut back on coffee, start with taking away one-quarter of your daily amount, substituting it with roasted dandelion root (this will help build the liver as you come off the addiction; see "coffee" box on page 65 for roasting instructions). Stay there for a few days, then take away the next quarter. Keep going until you're off all the way. If you experience detox symptoms (headaches, especially), back off more slowly.

If you're trying to come off caffeinated tea, follow the same formula, but substitute peppermint (or spearmint if, like me, you're not really a peppermint person) for one-quarter of your leaves. According to Susun Weed, this will help give you energy, but not "false energy."

recipes

BODY CARE

Nettle Hair and Scalp Stimulating Rinse

Nettles are wonderful for stimulating the hair follicles, resulting in more (and healthier) growth. Apple cider vinegar is invaluable for your hair and scalp. It balances the pH, removes product buildup, eases dandruff, combats hair loss by strengthening the follicle and stimulating growth, detangles, adds shine, reduces frizz, and prevents split ends. Plus, it's cheap. I mean, wicked cheap. What's not to love?

1 cup dried nettle leaves

4 tablespoons apple cider vinegar

1. Start by brewing your old friend, nettle tea, in a quart jar. Combine the leaves with 4 cups boiling water and steep for at least 15 minutes, or overnight. Strain and add the apple cider vinegar.
2. Pour this rinse over your head after you shampoo, and massage it into the scalp. Run your fingers (or a wide-toothed comb) from roots to ends to distribute it. Give your hair a quick rinse (optional) with cool water, and you're good to go. You can add this treatment to your daily regimen.

Makes 4 cups

Nettle Tonic for Burns and Rashes

Not only does apple cider vinegar do wonders for your noggin, but it's also amazing for treating rashes and burns — you know, those painful injuries that can't really be helped with a Band-Aid. Its antibacterial qualities will help keep the area germ-free while nettles provide anti-inflammatory and pain-relieving benefits.

½ cup dried nettles

1 cup apple cider vinegar

1. Combine the nettles and vinegar in a sterilized pint jar and shake. Keep in a dark cupboard for 2 weeks, shaking daily. Strain out the nettles.
2. Using a cotton pad or spray bottle (for extremely tender burns and rashes, dilute with a little water), apply liberally and as needed. Cover lightly with a clean cloth. You can even spray this cloth down and cover it with another clean, dry cloth, if you want to leave the cloth in place. Change the dressing daily.

Makes 1 cup

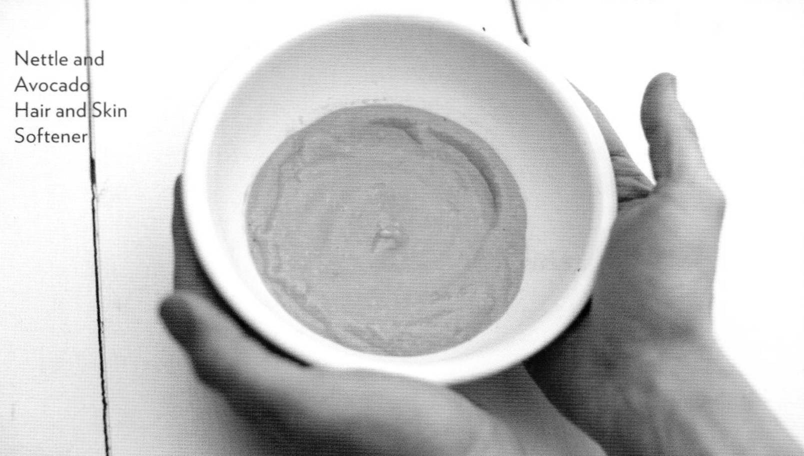
Nettle and Avocado Hair and Skin Softener

Nettle and Avocado Hair and Skin Softener

This is the easiest mask ever. It removes old skin cells, toxins, and impurities while leaving behind nutrients, hydration, healthy fats, minerals, and clear skin and hair.

1 ripe avocado

1 cup nettle tea

1. Slice open the avocado. (If you have some that have ripened behind your back and are too soft to eat, this is the perfect use for them.) Scoop out the green goodness and plop it into a bowl.
2. To begin, pour ½ cup cool-room-temperature nettle tea into the bowl and mash the avocado with a fork until you have a (mostly) lump-free paste (you could also do this in a food processor or blender). You should have a smooth consistency. If you don't, add more tea.
3. Stick your hands into the goo and spread it on your face or your still-wet hair (concentrating on the more fragile ends). Let the mask sit for 15 minutes, then rinse.

Makes 1 rinse

ARTHRITIS POULTICE

The easiest way to make a poultice is to simply mash up fresh or dried leaves with a bit of hot water. Since we're talking nettles here, and fresh, raw nettles sting, simmer a (gloved) handful in a bit of water for a few minutes. Then strain, cool, and apply the nettles directly to the painful joint. Cover with a warm, damp towel, and cover that with a dry, fluffy one. Keep the compress in place until it cools, then apply it again, if needed.

recipes

FOOD

Nettle Soup

If you've ever had a thick, warming kale-and-potato soup, then you know where I'm going with this recipe. Since nettles don't have the body that kale does, I use both in this recipe, but for a lighter soup, you could easily double the amount of nettles, up the liquid content, and leave out the kale.

- **4 cups (plus more as needed) vegetable stock, chicken stock, or water**
- **6 good-sized red potatoes (I leave the skin on), quartered**
- **1 super-ripe apple, chopped (optional)**
- **1 bunch kale (6–8 stalks), chopped**
- **2 cups chopped lightly blanched nettle leaves**
- **Salt and pepper to taste**

1. Pour the stock or water into a large pot, and bring to a boil over medium-high heat. Add the potatoes and apple, if using, and cook for 25 minutes, or until soft. Mash the potatoes and apple in the pot.
2. Add the kale, nettle leaves, and salt and pepper. Stir and let the soup simmer for 10 minutes.
3. Using a stick blender (or put in batches in a blender or food processor), blend the soup until creamy. If it's too thick, add more stock and reheat. Taste and add more salt and pepper if needed.

Serves 4

Garlicky Sautéed Nettles

Sometimes you just need a good, hearty green side dish. Enter a nettle dish with a good olive oil, lots of garlic, and shallots.

- **1 tablespoon extra-virgin olive oil, plus more if needed**
- **2 cloves garlic, chopped**
- **1 shallot, chopped**
- **2–3 cups lightly steamed nettle leaves**
- **Salt to taste**

1. In a large sauté pan, heat the olive oil over medium-low heat. Toss in the garlic and sauté until fragrant. Add the shallot and turn the heat to low (like, super-low) and cook about 10 minutes or until brown, sweet, and caramelized.
2. Add the nettles. If you need more oil, add a teaspoon at a time. Stir and sauté for 5 more minutes. Serve hot.

Serves 2

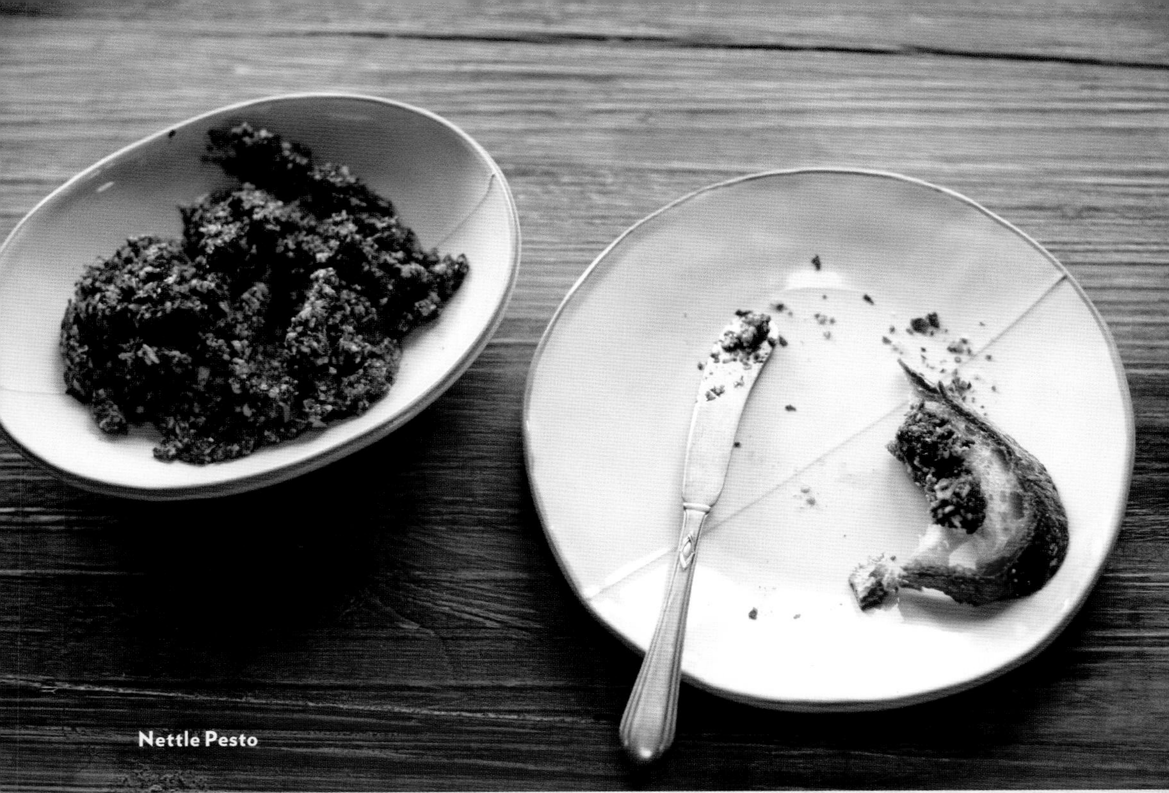
Nettle Pesto

Nettle Pesto

If you have nettles growing on your property, then you probably have more of them than you know what to do with. The solution? Make nettle leaf pesto. Lots of it. Make batches, and freeze them in plastic bags, pulling them out throughout the year. I love to spread this over firm tofu, then bake it.

- 3–4 **cloves garlic**
- ½ **cup extra-virgin olive oil**
- ¼–½ **cup pine nuts or walnuts (optional)**
- 2–3 **cups lightly steamed nettle leaves**
- ¼ **teaspoon salt**
- **Freshly ground black pepper to taste**
- ¾ **cup freshly grated Parmesan cheese (optional)**

1. Place the garlic, one at a time, into a food processor, and mince. With the blade spinning, slowly pour in the oil.
2. Add the nuts and pulse until chopped. Add the nettle leaves and pulse until well blended. Add the salt and pepper and the cheese, if using, and pulse again.

Makes 1 cup

NETTLE YOGA

Since nettles are useful for building strength in the body, easing joint pain, and protection, we're going to focus on spine, abdominal, liver/kidney, and digestive health and strength with Boat Pose (*Navasana*). Boat Pose stimulates the kidneys and liver, strengthens the abdominals and digestion, strengthens the hip flexors, and reduces stress. Wicked, right?

Starting position for Boat Pose. Let's start out easy. Take a seat on the floor. Bend your knees, plant your feet, and rest your hands behind you. Keep your spine straight, shoulders down, and belly drawn in.

Exhale, and, using your abdominals, pull your knees in toward your chest. You should feel this down the entire abdominal wall — just don't round your back. If this is too challenging, try one knee at a time.

Moving into Boat Pose. Easy enough? Let's step it up. If your knees were easily drawn in, try straightening your legs so that your shin and thigh create a 90-degree angle. Still easy? Stretch your arms out in front of you, straight out from your shoulders, running parallel to the ground. Still easy? Step it up once more and straighten those legs as much as you can. Breathe. *Breathe.* Don't hold your breath. This is Boat Pose.

Fine-tuning. Check in with your spine — is it rounding? If so, bring your legs back down or use your arms for support. This tones your belly, without stressing your back.

Check in with your belly — is it still drawn in? Try to draw the heads of your femurs (thigh bones) into your body. This will help take the weight off your spine and strengthen your hip flexors. Hang out there for 10 seconds, working up to 1 minute.

Finishing. Take a nice, long rest on your back (3 to 5 minutes — no skimping!) when you're done.

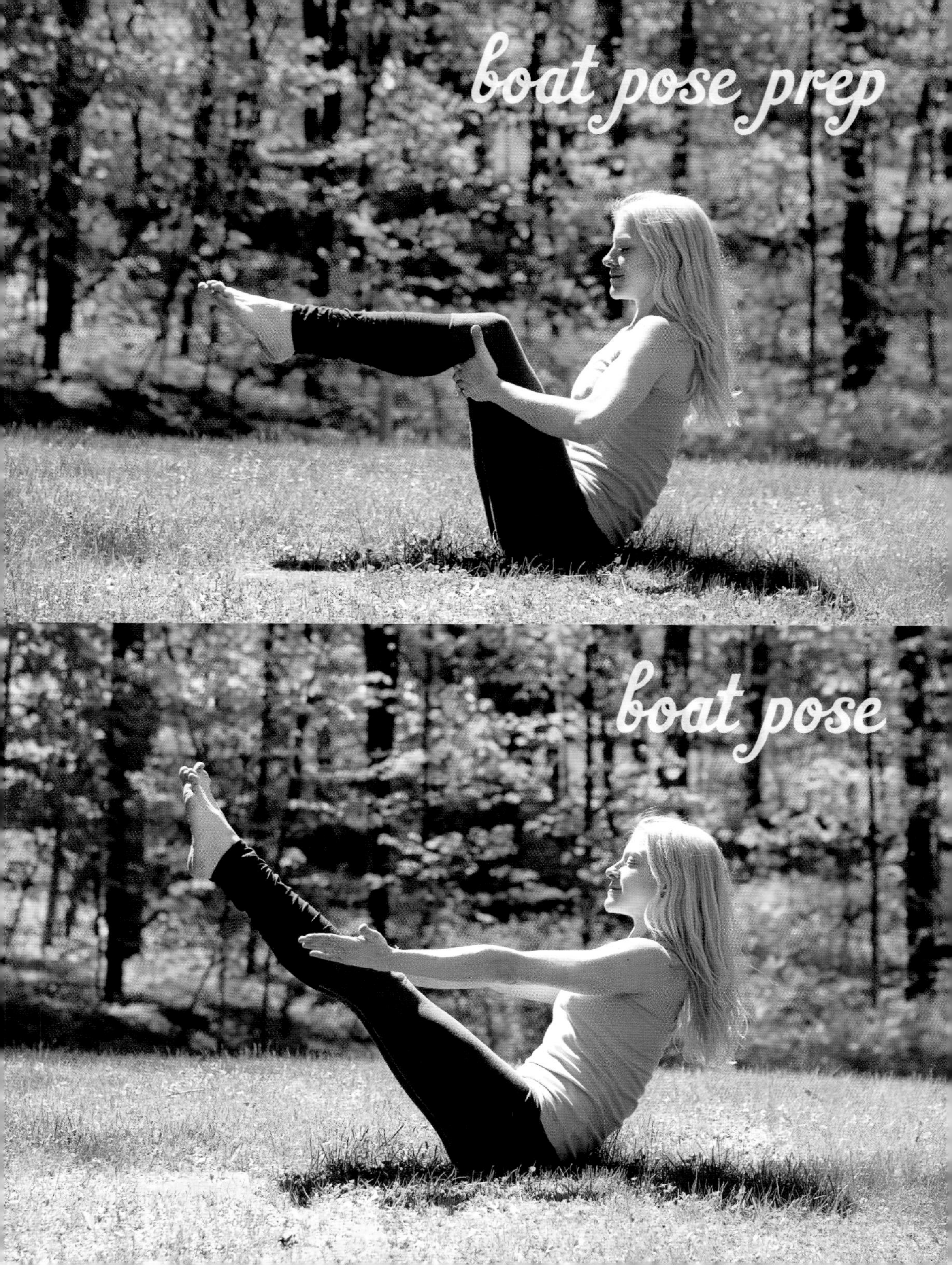
boat pose prep
boat pose

6 Healing with CALENDULA

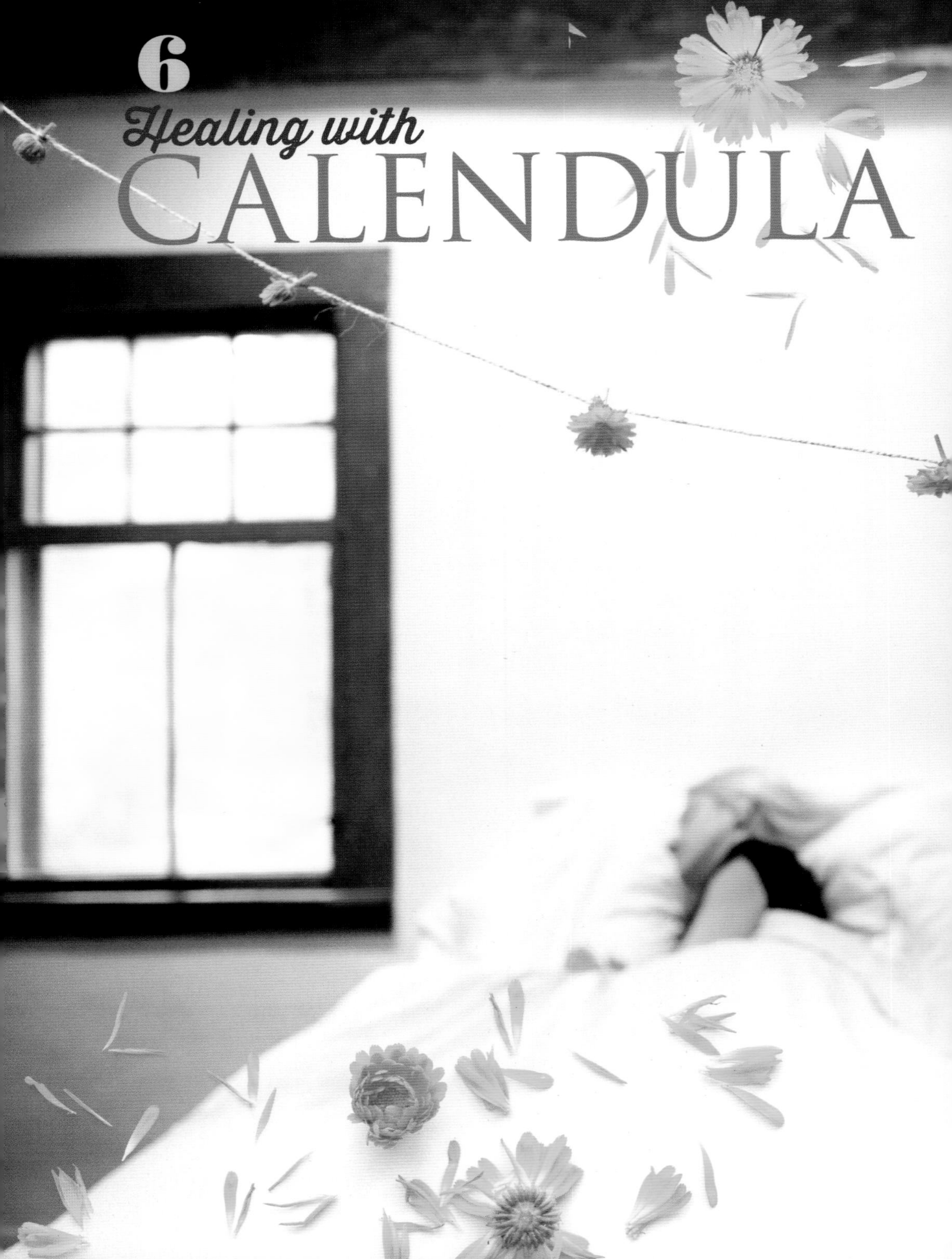

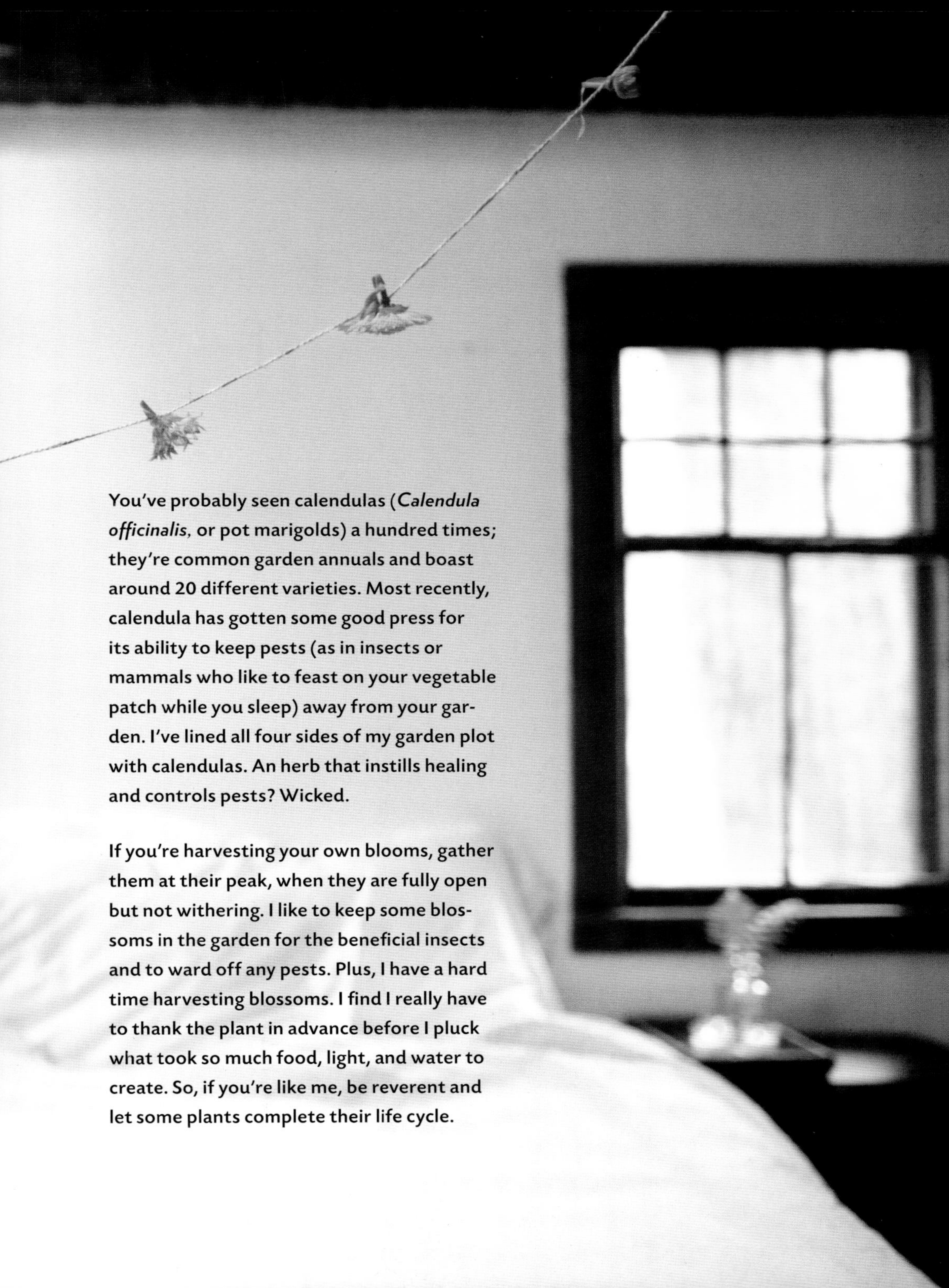

You've probably seen calendulas (*Calendula officinalis,* or pot marigolds) a hundred times; they're common garden annuals and boast around 20 different varieties. Most recently, calendula has gotten some good press for its ability to keep pests (as in insects or mammals who like to feast on your vegetable patch while you sleep) away from your garden. I've lined all four sides of my garden plot with calendulas. An herb that instills healing and controls pests? Wicked.

If you're harvesting your own blooms, gather them at their peak, when they are fully open but not withering. I like to keep some blossoms in the garden for the beneficial insects and to ward off any pests. Plus, I have a hard time harvesting blossoms. I find I really have to thank the plant in advance before I pluck what took so much food, light, and water to create. So, if you're like me, be reverent and let some plants complete their life cycle.

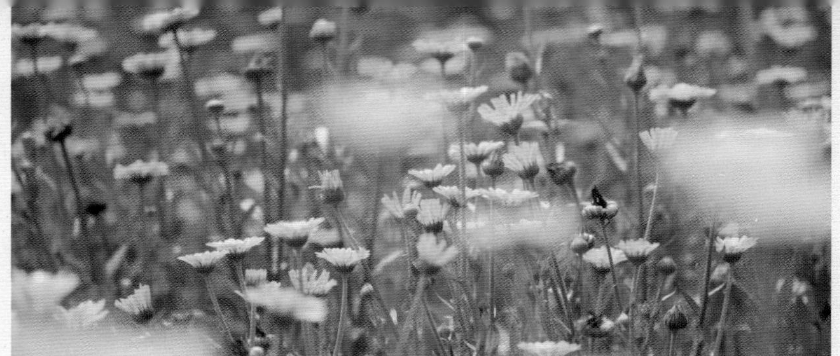

When you have your blossoms, remove the petals and compost the center (it's very bitter, so keep it only if you're using calendula solely to aid digestion). The petals can be dried and stored for use throughout the year. I have a gas stove, so I just spread them out on a baking sheet in the oven (turned off); the pilot light provides enough heat to dry them quickly. Alternatively, scatter the petals on a screen, and keep them in a dry place out of the sun until they're ready to store. Fresh or dried, the petals can be tossed in salads or added to veggie broth or the cooking water for your grains.

Note: Be sure to check the Latin name of your calendulas/pot marigolds and only ingest *Calendula officinalis*. Common marigolds are in a different genus from calendulas. Although there are no scary-poisonous marigolds, some do contain a mild toxin that can cause a skin reaction. No worries, though! If you accidentally ingest them, they won't have any dangerous effects on the body — but they won't have any medicinal ones, either. Just be sure and be safe before ingesting any wild plants. *Calendula officinalis* is safe for everyone.

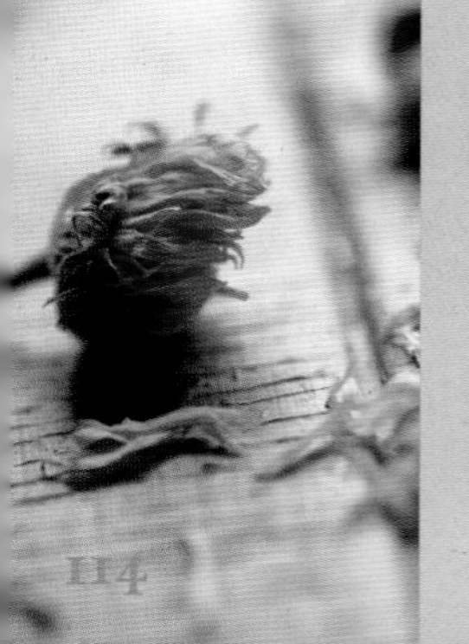

CALENDULA

Calendula officinalis

Parts used: Flower petals

How to harvest: Snip the flower heads from your calendula plants on a sunny morning, after the dew has dried, far from any roadsides or pesticide-dressed gardens

Effects on body: Nutrient-dense, antioxidant, antiseptic, healing, pain-relieving

Effects on mind and spirit: Warming, bravery-inducing, freeing, calming

Safety first: Be sure to check the Latin name of your plants before growing/harvesting them and only ingest *Calendula officinalis*; although no marigolds are truly dangerous, it's best to be sure of your plant before you ingest anything

for the Body

Despite my reservations about picking them, I really love it when flowers are used for healing and nutrition. I mean, how often does that happen, really? Most people are still unfamiliar with edible flowers, so it is so much fun to surprise my guests with a beautiful salad or veggie dish topped with these striking, golden, buttery (okay, and slightly bitter) flowers.

So, why eat them? Good question. The gold color that radiates from these little guys is a sign of high beta-carotene content (as in carrots and sweet potatoes). The body converts beta-carotene into vitamin A (or retinol), which is a superfood for the eyes (as well as the mucus membranes, immune system, and skin). Beta-carotene is also an antioxidant, which helps rid the body of free radicals (those nasty little things that stomp around our bodies, destroying cells through oxidation and aging us prematurely). Because calendula soothes and boosts mucus membranes, it is good for sore throats, digestive upset, ulcers (in the mouth or elsewhere in the digestive tract), internal swelling, lymph issues, infections, and pain relief.

So that's what it does to our bodies internally, but calendula really shines when used externally on the skin. I'm telling you — calendula is amazing, miraculous, and flipping fast when it comes to healing chapped skin, wounds, inflammation, diaper rash, fungal infections, bacterial infections, burns, stings, and bites of any kind. How can it do all this amazing stuff? It's antiseptic, antibacterial, and hemostatic (helps stanch bleeding). It's also an emollient (softens skin), so it makes a wonderful wound dressing that not only rids the body of infection but also prevents the skin from hardening into scar tissue. And, since it draws infection from a wound, it's also good for cleansing and drawing toxins from the lymph nodes (when taken internally).

Calendula is a heating herb, which means it is good at dispelling fever, moving infections out of the body, and warming you on bone-chilling, damp winter nights, so be sure you dry enough of this happy, sunny blossom to last you throughout the year. Not only does calendula keep you warm, but it will keep the lymph system flowing properly and the immune system ready to fight off any of those cold winter flus.

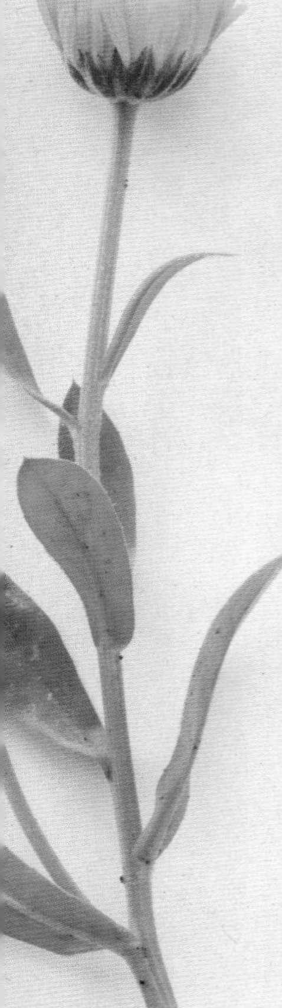

for the Mind

Warmth, warmth, warmth. That seems to be calendula's theme (not surprising, given its color and affinity for full sun). The calendula flower essence is no different. It has a special kinship with those who are good with the spoken word — poets, lawyers, teachers, singers, lecturers, and those who love to argue and debate. Healers and teachers should almost always experiment with the gentle warmth of this essence, especially when verbal communication is key to their practice, therapy, or message. Calendula also helps those who tend to be argumentative or who commonly suffer misunderstandings.

Think loving communication as the theme here. I once took this essence after a dear friend's mother passed away. While I tend to communicate well (I hope) via the written word, I'm often stumped when it comes to the spoken one. Calendula guided me toward the "right" thing to say (and to say it with warmth), and it helped me know when it was time simply to listen.

Also think of calendula if you're going through a particularly frustrating period. Frustration, miscommunication, and anger are all hot situations (think "heated argument," for example, or "hot under the collar"). Calendula helps you tap into the cool well of peace that does (I promise) reside deep within us all.

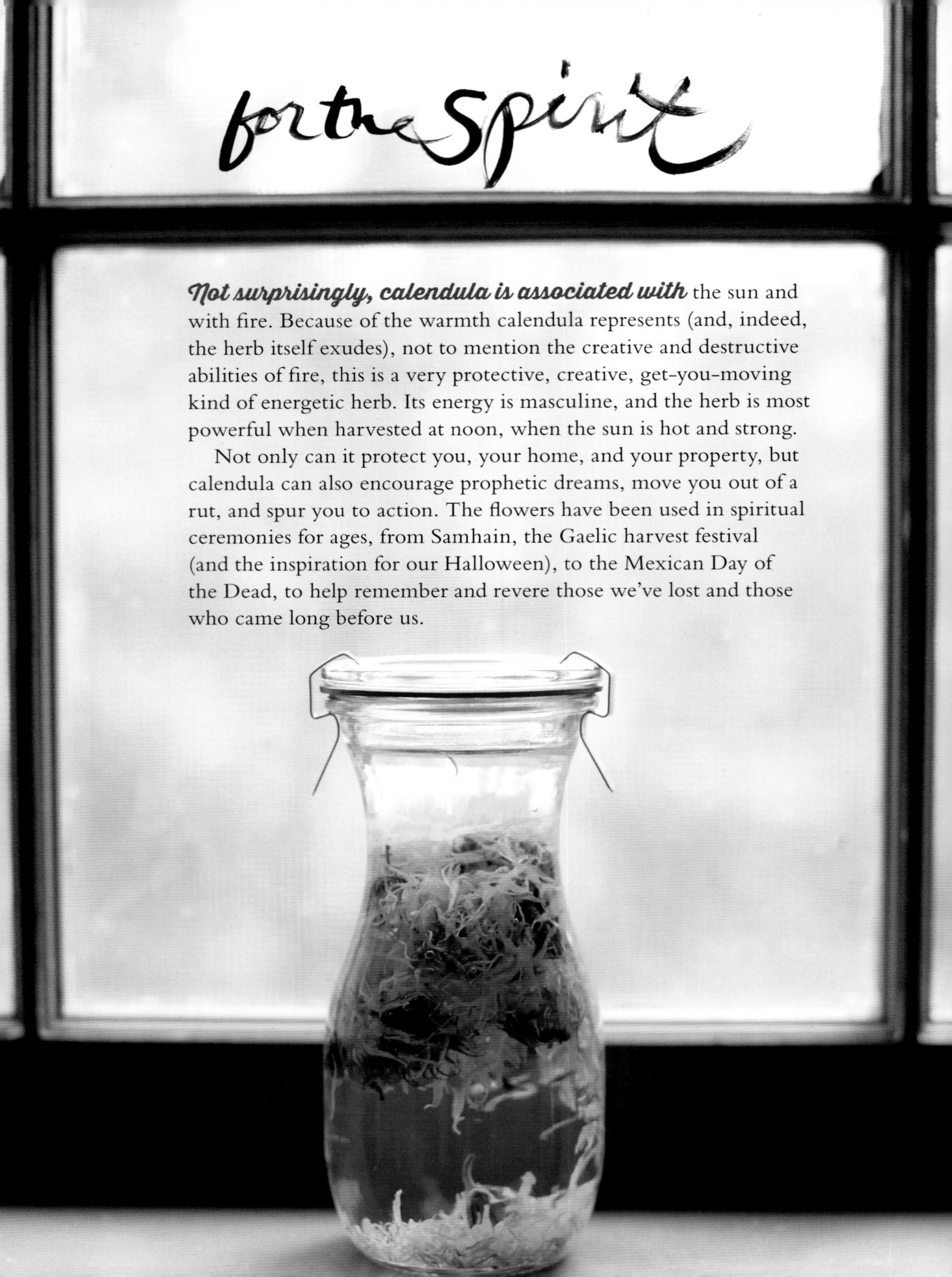

for the Spirit

Not surprisingly, calendula is associated with the sun and with fire. Because of the warmth calendula represents (and, indeed, the herb itself exudes), not to mention the creative and destructive abilities of fire, this is a very protective, creative, get-you-moving kind of energetic herb. Its energy is masculine, and the herb is most powerful when harvested at noon, when the sun is hot and strong.

Not only can it protect you, your home, and your property, but calendula can also encourage prophetic dreams, move you out of a rut, and spur you to action. The flowers have been used in spiritual ceremonies for ages, from Samhain, the Gaelic harvest festival (and the inspiration for our Halloween), to the Mexican Day of the Dead, to help remember and revere those we've lost and those who came long before us.

CALENDULA MAGIC

FOR RELEASING DEPRESSION

To get the most powerful, most uplifting magic from the calendula, gather the blossoms at noon. Why? This is when the sun is at its peak, and this is a sun plant (its other names include "bride of the sun" and "summer's bride") full of fiery, powerful magic.

Once you have gathered your blossoms, carry them close to your heart. Meditate on their color, scent, and feel, and the infinite variety of crenellations and patterns of their petals. Realize how complicated, yet beautiful, the marigold is; realize how briefly it blooms, yet how powerful its magic and its medicine. Realize, too, that your heart is just as complicated, just as lovely; and though this depression, this downturn, is powerful at the moment, it too is short-lived.

After the ritual, run a bath and offer your blossoms to the water. Soak there for 20 minutes or so, feeling fully whatever emotional state you are in, then as you let the water drain away, let it carry the darkness. Emerge cleansed from water and from the bride of the sun.

FOR INSPIRING PROPHETIC DREAMS

Pick your blossoms at noon(ish) and string them into a garland by using a long tapestry needle attached to kitchen twine or ribbon. Thread the needle through the center of the flower bud and lace it along the twine or ribbon. Make this garland as full or as spare as you like, and then drape the garland over your headboard or pin it above your bed (see the chapter opener photo).

Alternatively (or in addition), scatter blossoms beneath the bed, and sweep them up the next day.

FOR REMOVING STAGNATION

Again, gather your blossoms and string them into garlands (your color string of choice — whatever gets you going!). Drape the garlands over doors or windows — any exit or entry into your home. Because this is moving energy *through*, I like to drape windows or doors at either end of my house, creating a marigold tunnel of sorts.

Then open up the doors or windows and let the air do most of the work for you. This will move energy through and out, blowing that stagnation, boredom, dullness, and what-have-you out of your place. Gaze on the marigold's bright blossoms and feel that energy, that color, that *life* radiating in and through you.

TEAS

Base tea for internal healing. For internal injuries (ulcers, cuts, scrapes, inflammation, illness), I like calendula best as a tea. To brew up a pot, steep a few handfuls of dried flowers (about a scant cup of dried, twice that of fresh) in 4 cups freshly boiled water for 10 to 15 minutes. Strain and drink throughout the day. I really like this with nut milk and a touch of stevia or honey. Drink three cups per day, iced or hot.

Tea for soothing a sore throat. To 1 cup of your base tea, add 1 tablespoon antibacterial raw apple cider vinegar, a pinch of salt, and a spoonful of honey. You can gargle with this tea (gargling by the swig for 10 seconds at a time until the cup is gone), or go ahead and drink the concoction, vinegar and all.

Tea to aid digestion. Since calendula is a bitter herb, it's fantastic for stimulating the digestive organs. Brew a strong tea by steeping 1 tablespoon of the dried herb (or 2 tablespoons fresh) in 1 cup hot water for 15 minutes. For a digestive kick, add peppermint. Don't add sweetener or milk to this particular brew. It will be bitter, just a warning, but oh will it make digestion and assimilation *so* much better. Drink 20 minutes before a meal, or drink 30 minutes after a meal if you're feeling overly indulged, sluggish, bloated, or grumpy.

Tea for pain relief. Put a whole quart (4 cups) of water on the stove with about an inch of freshly sliced gingerroot (or a heaping tablespoon of the dried herb), and simmer, covered, for 10 minutes. Add ½ cup dried calendula flowers (twice that if fresh), and cover again, steeping for 10 minutes longer. The sweet spiciness of the ginger helps tone down the bitterness of the calendula, while the earthiness of the flower deepens the sweetness of the root. Drink straight or add honey for extra comfort and healing, along with a healthy dose of unsweetened nut milk.

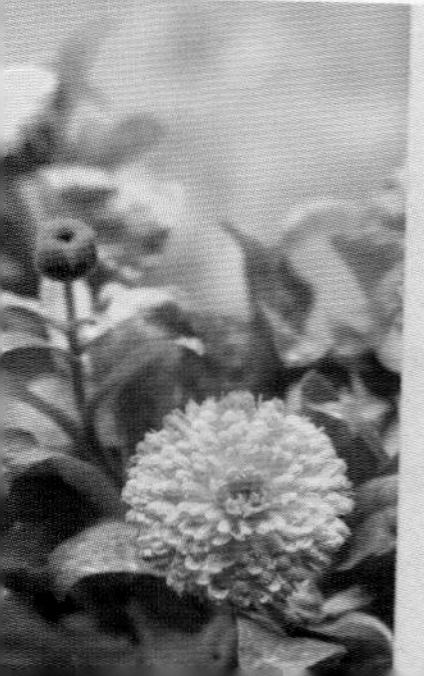

CALENDULA FOLK STORY

One of the most beautiful folk/magic stories about calendula I found was the following from *Cunningham's Encyclopedia of Magical Herbs* by Scott Cunningham: "If a girl touches the petals of the marigold with her bare feet, she will understand the language of birds." Now you want to plant some marigold, don't you? If not, be sure to ask your neighbor before you go tramping around in her marigold beds.

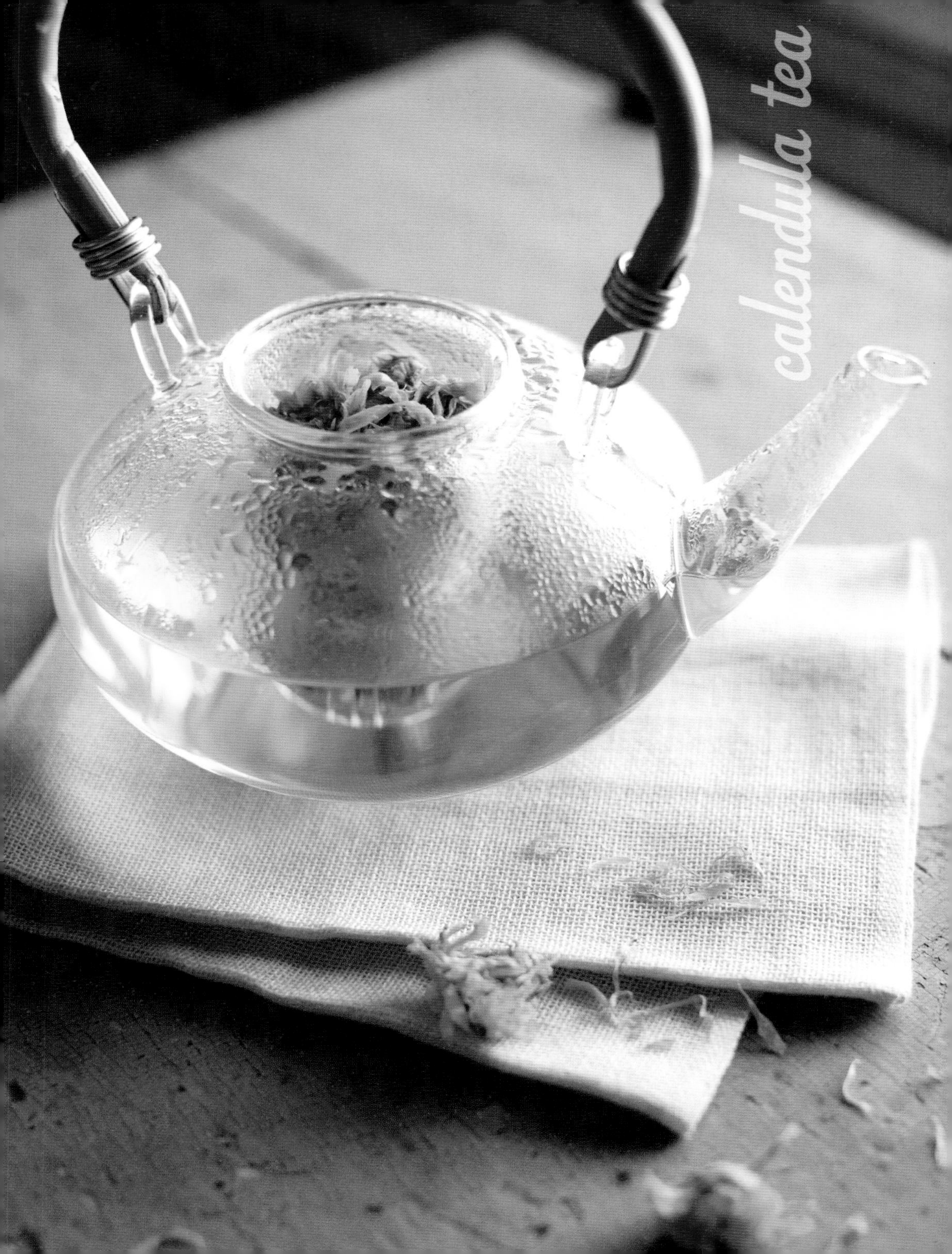
calendula tea

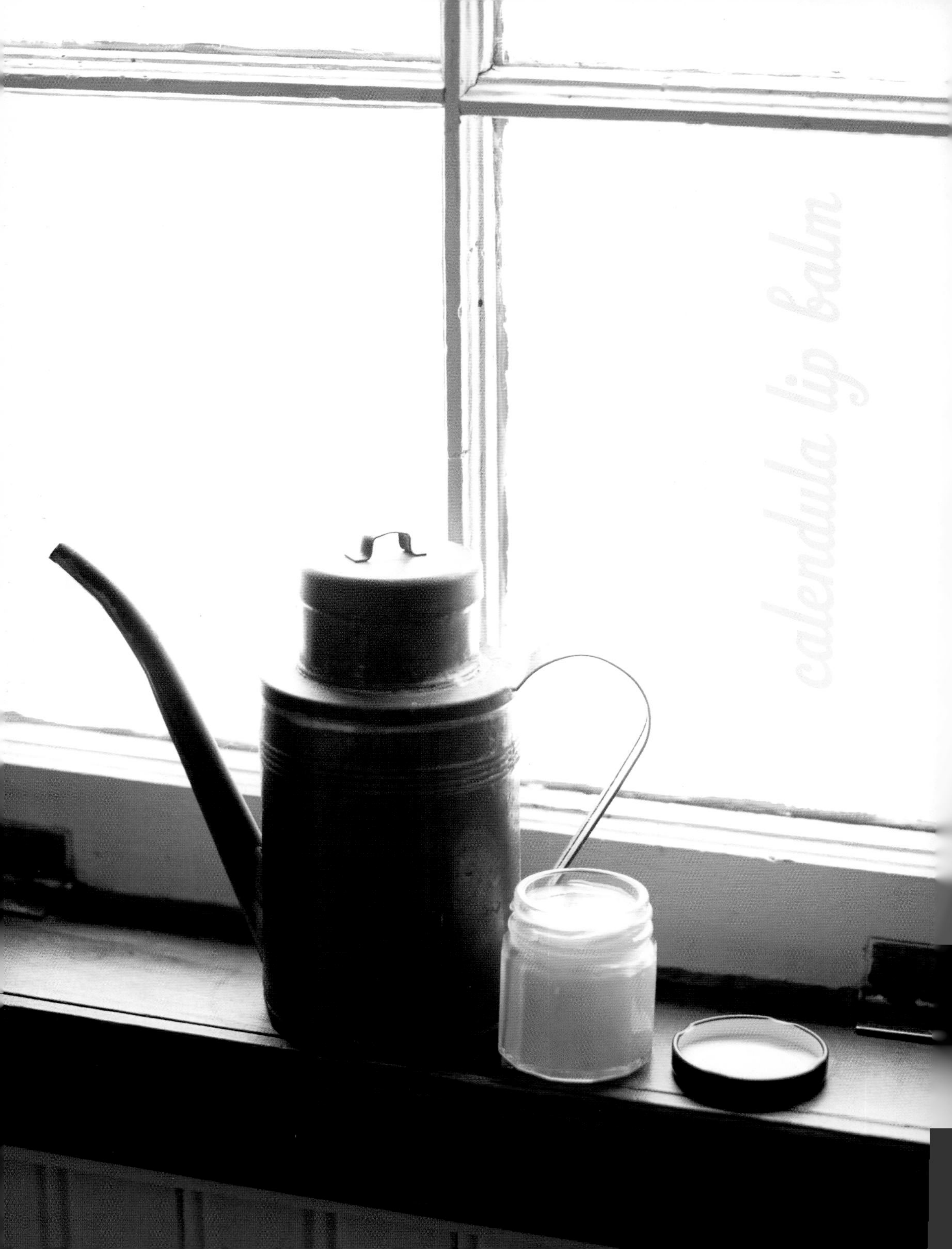
calendula lip balm

BODY CARE

Calendula Lip Balm

I am a lip balm addict. Dry skin haunts me no matter the season. I usually make a huge batch of lip balm right around Christmas, give away tons, and then keep a stash for myself. I like to experiment with flavors, colors, scents, and herb additives. It's not just the application of lip balm that is sweetly compelling, but the making of it, too.

This one is especially good for cold sores, cracked lips, or intensely dry skin (lips or elsewhere). It will last 1 year.

- **2 tablespoons calendula oil in a base of almond, coconut, or jojoba oil (or more to preference; see Appendix II)**
- **2 teaspoons grated beeswax**
- **5 drops calendula essential oil**
- **3–4 drops essential oil of your choice (vanilla, cinnamon, lavender, peppermint — go crazy!)**
- **1 teaspoon honey, for taste and extra demulcent action (optional)**
- **12 ¼-ounce tins or 20 tubes**

1. In a double boiler or your handy heat-proof bowl set over simmering water, warm your calendula oil over low heat for 5 minutes. I like my lip balm to be hard(ish), so I use 2 tablespoons oil. If you want a softer, more jelly-like consistency, add an extra teaspoon of oil.
2. Add the beeswax. When the wax has melted, stir the mixture and remove the pan from the heat. Let cool.
3. Add the essential oils and honey, if using, and stir (I like to use an eggbeater to really get it smooth).
4. Dip a spoon in the balm and stick it in the fridge for 5 minutes. Check the consistency. Too firm? Heat and add oil. Too soft? Ditto and add wax. Once you're happy, pour it into lip balm tins (see Resources) or recycled lip balm tubes/funky containers, label, and save or give away. Happy lip smacking!

Makes 3 ounces

Calendula Shampoo for Babies and Sensitive Scalps

I say babies and those with sensitive skin, but really, this shampoo is fantastic for anyone. It's healing and stimulating for the scalp, with no buildup or chemicals; a bottle of this shampoo makes a great gift for the person who has everything.

I like to use an all-natural liquid castile soap, and then add a touch of glycerin to

Recipe continues on next page

keep the soap from becoming too drying. As a demulcent, glycerin helps attract and retain moisture without weighing down the hair follicles or blocking pores.

- **¼ cup dried calendula blossoms**
- **¼ cup castile soap**
- **2 tablespoons vegetable glycerin**
- **7 drops lavender, chamomile, or rosemary essential oil (optional — use one, none, or any combination; chamomile is good for itchy or sensitive scalps; lavender for soothing and gentle cleansing; rosemary for stimulating hair growth)**

1. In a small saucepan, heat 2 cups distilled water over low heat and bring to a simmer. Turn off the heat and add the calendula blossoms. Steep for 10 minutes, strain, and let cool.
2. Add the soap, glycerin, and essential oil, if using, to the calendula tea and blend. Decant the mixture into a clean plastic bottle. You can keep this right in the shower, but replace after a month or so if you haven't used it all. Follow up with an apple cider vinegar rinse or your usual conditioning regimen.

Makes approximately 12 ounces

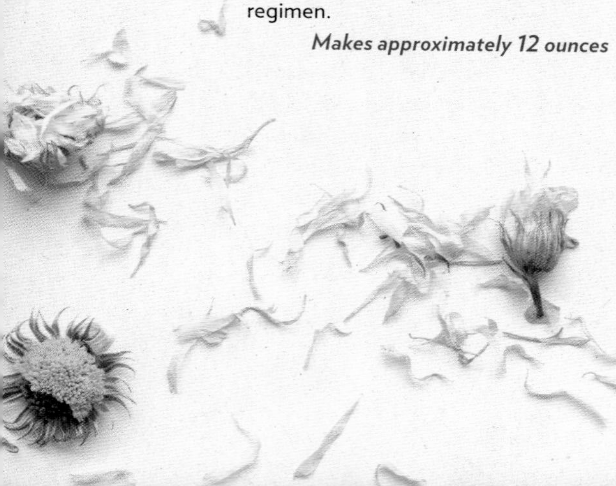

Calendula Salve for Injured and Infected Skin

Salves are a wonderful way to carry herbs around with you, since they're not as messy as oils. Just place a lip-balm-sized tin of calendula salve in your first-aid kit, glove compartment, or purse, and take it with you anywhere.

- **1 cup calendula oil (see Appendix II for herbal oil recipe; for added healing, especially in summer, you can make lavender calendula oil instead)**
- **¼ cup grated or shaved beeswax (or, if you're like me and you're too lazy to grate it, just put a block in a plastic bag and sort of beat it about with a hammer; noisy, but it gets the job done)**
- **1 tablespoon lavender flowers (optional)**
- **16 ½-ounce salve tins**

1. In a double boiler or a heat-proof bowl sitting over simmering water, gently heat the oil over low heat.
2. Add the beeswax to the oil. When it melts, turn off the burner and remove the pot from the heat.
3. Dip a spoon into your salve and stick this in the freezer for a few minutes. If it's too hard for your liking, reheat and add more oil. Too mushy? Add more beeswax. Test a teaspoon at a time so you don't have to backtrack. Keep notes!
4. Pour the mixture into individual salve tins (see Resources), and carry them around with you.

Makes 8 ounces

FOOD

recipes

Calendula Blossom Springtime Salad

You can use whatever greens and fresh veggies are in season, but I find this particular combination works well in this salad. The mustard in the French vinaigrette helps cut the slight bitterness of the calendula. You'll have a lot of leftover dressing, so store it in the refrigerator.

For the salad:

- **3 cups mixed spring greens (baby lettuces, young dandelion leaves, arugula, watercress, mâche)**
- **3 asparagus spears, cooked and chopped**
- **3 young carrots, chopped**
- **2 early tomatoes, chopped**
- **6 radishes, chopped**
- **3–4 fresh, rinsed calendula blossoms**

For the dressing:

- **¾ cup olive oil**
- **¼ cup red wine vinegar**
- **2 tablespoons Dijon mustard**
- **1 teaspoon salt (optional)**
- **¼ teaspoon pepper**
- **1 clove garlic, crushed**

1. In a large bowl, combine the greens, asparagus, carrots, tomatoes, radishes, and calendula blossoms.
2. In a blender, mix together the olive oil, vinegar, mustard, salt, pepper, and garlic. Add 2 tablespoons water and blend until smooth.
3. Dress the salad, toss, and serve immediately.

Calendula Cornbread

One of my favorite childhood memories is of weekend mornings spent at my grandparents' enormous house in Rhode Island. I'd wake up to Grandpa's cornbread, cooked in a cast-iron skillet and smothered in butter. These days, it's more of an occasional treat.

- **⅓ cup vegan shortening, regular shortening, or butter**
- **1½ cups plain cornmeal**
- **¾ cup all-purpose flour**
- **3 teaspoons baking powder**
- **½ teaspoon baking soda**
- **½ teaspoon salt**
- **2 tablespoons dried calendula flowers, chopped in a coffee grinder**
- **1 cup buttermilk or vegan alternative (see box on next page)**
- **2 eggs, well beaten or vegan substitute**

Recipe continues on next page

1. Preheat the oven to 425°F/220°C.
2. Put the shortening or butter in a 10-inch cast-iron skillet, and place in the oven to melt.
3. In a large bowl, combine the cornmeal, flour, baking powder, baking soda, salt, and calendula flowers. Add the buttermilk and eggs and stir until well blended. Add the melted shortening or butter and stir to mix.
4. Pour the batter into the cast-iron skillet, and bake for 20 to 25 minutes or until golden brown on top.

Serves 4

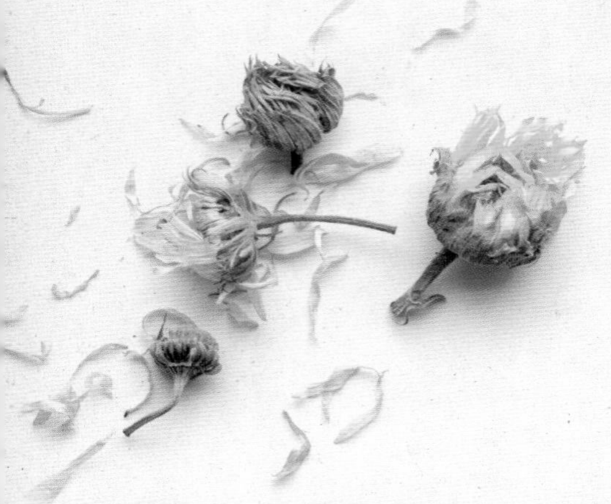

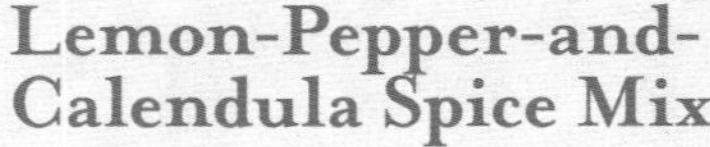

Lemon-Pepper-and-Calendula Spice Mix

I love spice mixes. I use them to dress salads, potatoes, and rice dishes. I like to make all kinds of different varieties so that I can indulge wherever my taste leads.

- **¼ cup salt**
- **2 tablespoons ground calendula flowers**
- **1½ tablespoons onion powder**
- **2 tablespoons garlic powder**
- **2 tablespoons black pepper**
- **2 tablespoons white pepper**
- **1 tablespoon dried lemon rind**
- **¼ teaspoon ground mustard**

Combine the salt, ground calendula flowers, onion and garlic powder, pepper, lemon rind, and mustard in a small jar, and shake everything up. The mix can be kept in a tightly covered glass jar in a cool, dry place out of direct light for up to 4 months.

Makes 2 ounces

VEGAN BUTTERMILK

To make vegan buttermilk, you can do one of two things: Add 1 tablespoon white vinegar or lemon juice to 1 cup soy milk and blend well, or blend together ½ cup vegan sour cream and ½ cup non-dairy milk. The former isn't as thick as buttermilk but has a similar flavor, while the latter is thicker but not quite as sweet.

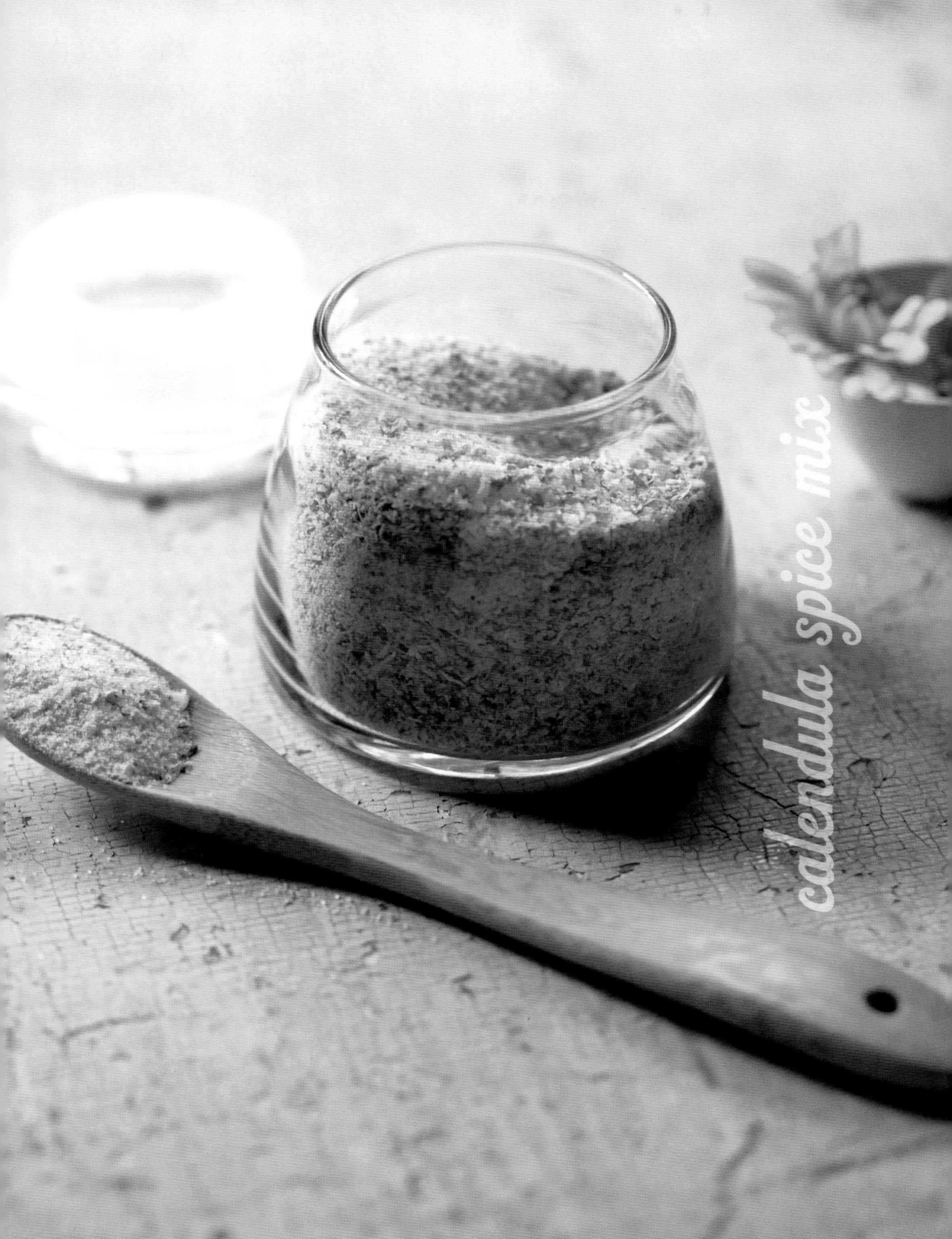
calendula spice mix

CALENDULA YOGA

Sun and heat are the themes of calendula. When we apply these concepts to the body, we come up with the solar plexus (*Manipura* chakra, or the yogic concept of energy centers in the body; *Manipura* is the third chakra). The solar plexus, or navel center of the body (the abdominals), is all about fire — digestive fire, courage, will, and discipline. If the solar plexus is weak, then you might suffer from fatigue, back pain (because the abdominals are weak), poor digestion and elimination, weak will and discipline, and general listlessness.

We're going to explore Bow Pose ("bow" as in archer's bow and also called *Dhanurasana*) to help strengthen the back and massage the abdominals and digestive organs — we're talking every muscle from the chest all the way down to the pelvis. Fiery intensity, people! (With modifications if needed, of course.)

Warming up for Bow Pose. Make a few simple twists or spinal extensions/contractions, such as Cat and Cow poses.

Moving into Bow Pose. Lie facedown on your mat. As you exhale, bring the heels of your feet as close to your bum as you can. Reach back with your hands and grab your ankles. As you inhale, draw your heels away from your hips. Because you're holding on to your ankles, this action is going to lift your chest and shoulders off the floor. Try to keep your knees hip distance apart, but if you're a little wider (and it doesn't cause you pain), then you're okay.

If this is pretty simple for you, intensify it. Try lifting your thighs off the floor and raising your chest higher, dropping your shoulder blades down your back. This not only further strengthens the muscles of your back (which you're trying to keep soft; if you clench them too much, you might cramp), but it also increases pressure on your belly. Try to breathe into the back-space of your body. This is the full Bow Pose.

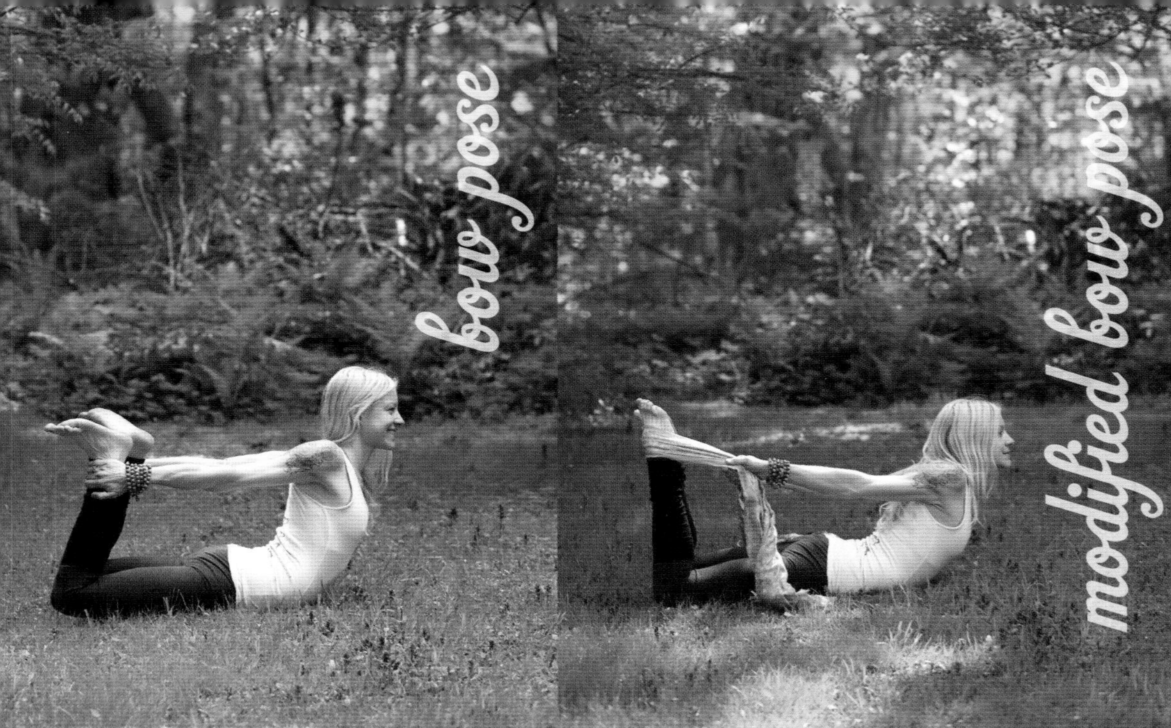

Finishing. After your last Bow Pose, on the exhale, lie down and turn one ear to the mat. Allow your arms to rest at your sides and bring your big toes together to touch (to relieve any tension in your low back). Take a few breaths here, then turn your head to the other side. Feel free to take Child's Pose at any time.

Bow Pose Variation

Can't reach your feet? No worries. Grab a yoga strap, cloth belt, tie, or scarf and wrap it around your ankles. Grab the ends of the strap with your hands and practice the same actions as above. You might have to adjust your grip — you want your arms to be extended here. Keep working; you can inch your way up the strap, bringing those hands closer and closer to your ankles, as time passes.

Can't lift your thighs off the floor? Again, no worries. Either just leave them and do your best, or prop your thighs on a rolled-up blanket or towel so you can get the feel of the full pose. If you can't yet get your chest off the floor, that's okay too. You'll have a nice stretch through your shoulders nonetheless.

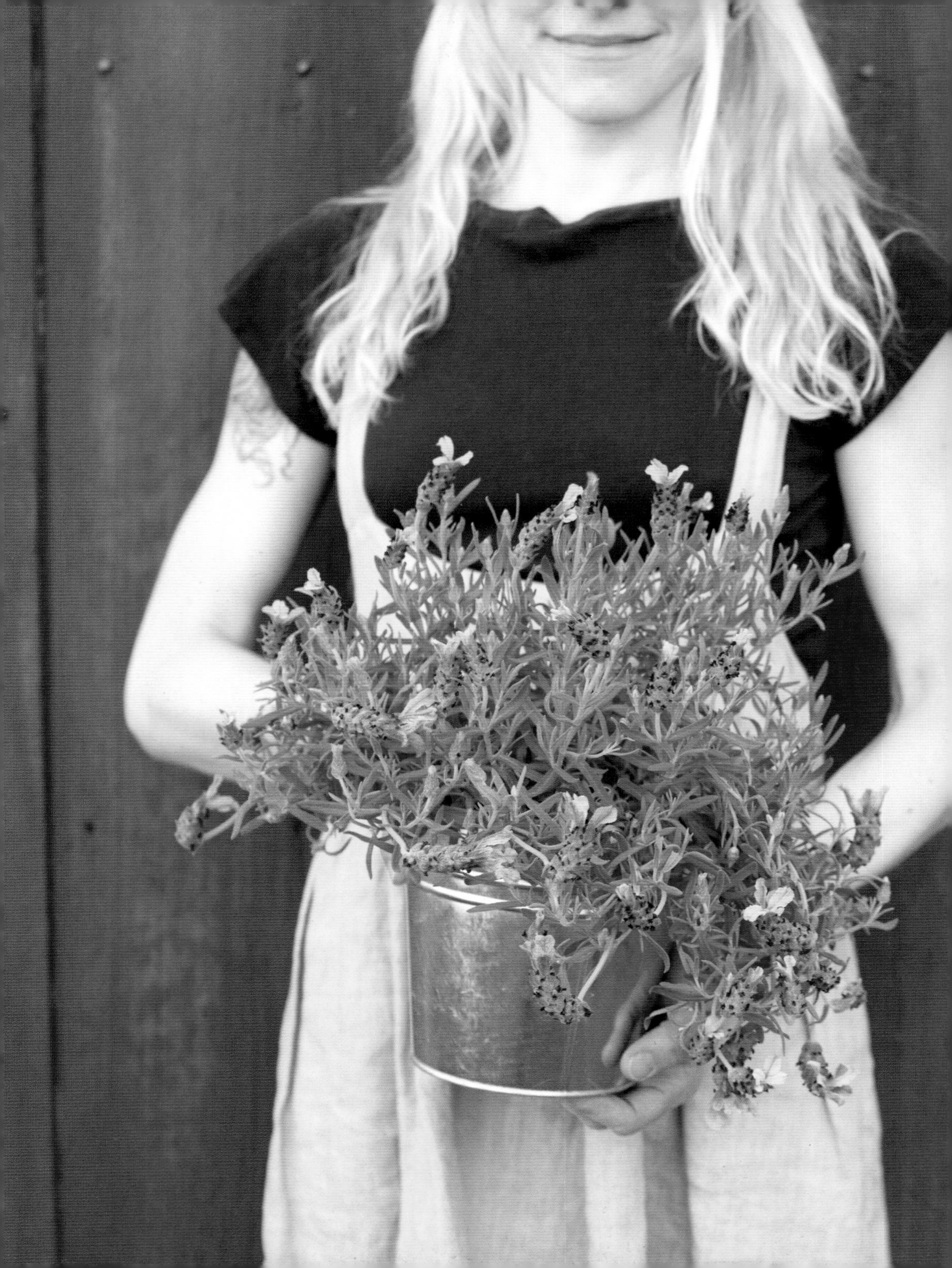

7

Having a Lie-Down with LAVENDER

Lavender (*Lavandula angustifolia*) is a member of the mint family, which always surprises me. It shouldn't, since mint is a very extended, welcoming family that includes most of the herbs you can think of. There's lots to think about and explore with lavender. I have a feeling (unless you really, *really* don't like the scent of lavender) that this is going to become a lifelong friendship.

While lavender is known for being relaxing, it can, in some cases, be stimulating, so be sure to check in with your mind, your mood, and your energy level after each recipe. Perhaps you find that the lavender in skin care is stimulating, while lavender tea is relaxing. Or, perhaps the scent is such a sedative for you that you should avoid the herb altogether until later in the day. And when you buy an essential oil, be sure to take a sniff, wait a few moments, and see how you feel. Remember: Herbs affect each of us differently, so it's important to carefully observe your own experience. You're the expert when it comes to your own, individual life.

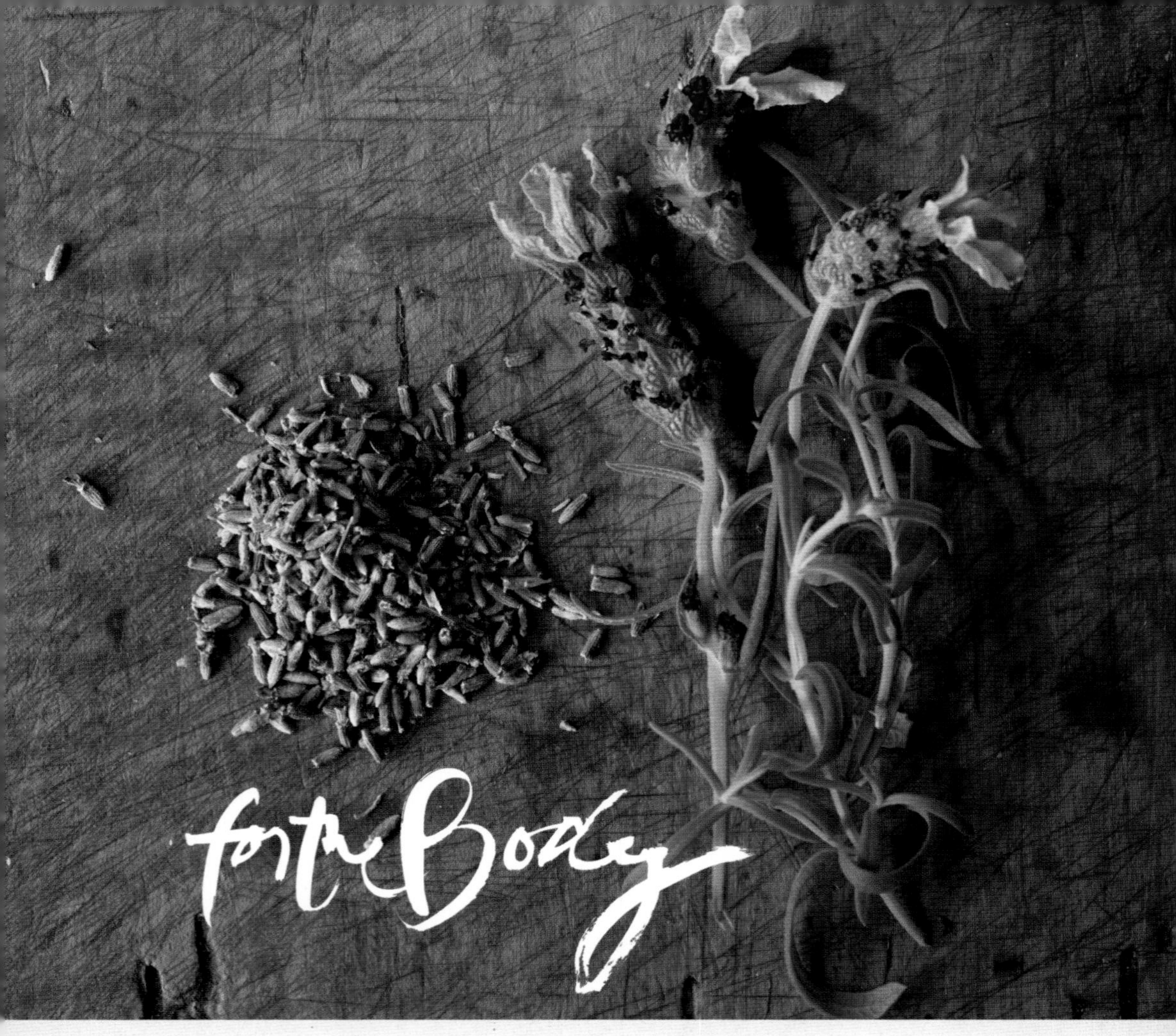

for the Body

Like most mints, lavender is a cooling herb, but most varieties are not stimulating (a notable exception is Spanish lavender or *Lavandula stoechas*). This is where lavender is different and also what makes it super-groovy. Lavender is singular for calming the mind when it's anxious (cooling hot heads, if you will), which is what makes it a wonderful remedy for easing into sleep.

Here's the fine print: Lavender is antiseptic, antibacterial, antifungal, anti-inflammatory, and analgesic (pain relieving); it's a nervine and an antidepressant. More often than not, the essential oil, rather than the herb itself, is used medicinally. However, you can brew quite an exquisite floral tea with dried lavender flowers (never take the essential oil internally). I like to brew the tea for insomnia, anxiety, nausea (although avoid this if you're pregnant), indigestion, flatulence, and headache relief. Inhaling from a bottle of essential oil or putting a few drops of the essential oil on a pillow or in a tablespoon of carrier oil (like almond oil) and rubbing it on your temples will work well, too.

One thing that makes herbs a lot of fun is getting to know the stories that trail along behind them. For example, the pain relief characteristics of lavender (especially for burns) were discovered by accident, or so the story goes according to herbalist James Duke. After burning his hand, a perfume chemist by the name of René-Maurice Gattefossé plunged it in the nearest vat of cool liquid. Luckily, it was a tub of lavender oil.

The lesson? Keep lavender near at hand in the kitchen. Conveniently, unlike most essential oils, lavender can be applied directly to the skin without a carrier oil (although, if you have sensitive skin, you may want to err on the side of caution and use a carrier oil; even lavender can sting in some cases). I usually carry a small bottle of it with me in my bag and use it on all manner of cuts, scrapes, bites, stings, and burns. Not only does it relieve pain (almost immediately, may I add), but its antibacterial properties will keep the cut germ-free in the absence of a handy soap dispenser.

LAVENDER

Lavandula angustifolia

Parts used: Flowers

How to harvest: Harvest your blooms on a dry, sunny day, after the dew has evaporated but before the heat of the day sets in

Effects on the body: Antiseptic, anti-inflammatory, pain-relieving

Effects on the mind and spirit: Calming, soothing, cooling, uplifting

Safety first: When using lavender, check the Latin name; *Lavandula stoechas* can be stimulating, while the much more common lavender, *Lavandula angustifolia*, is soothing and calming

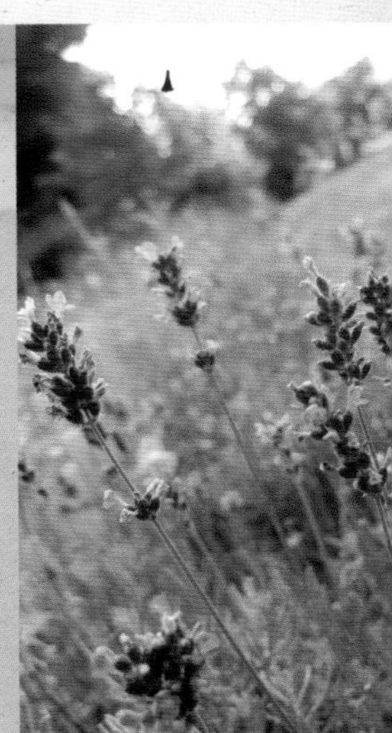

for the Mind

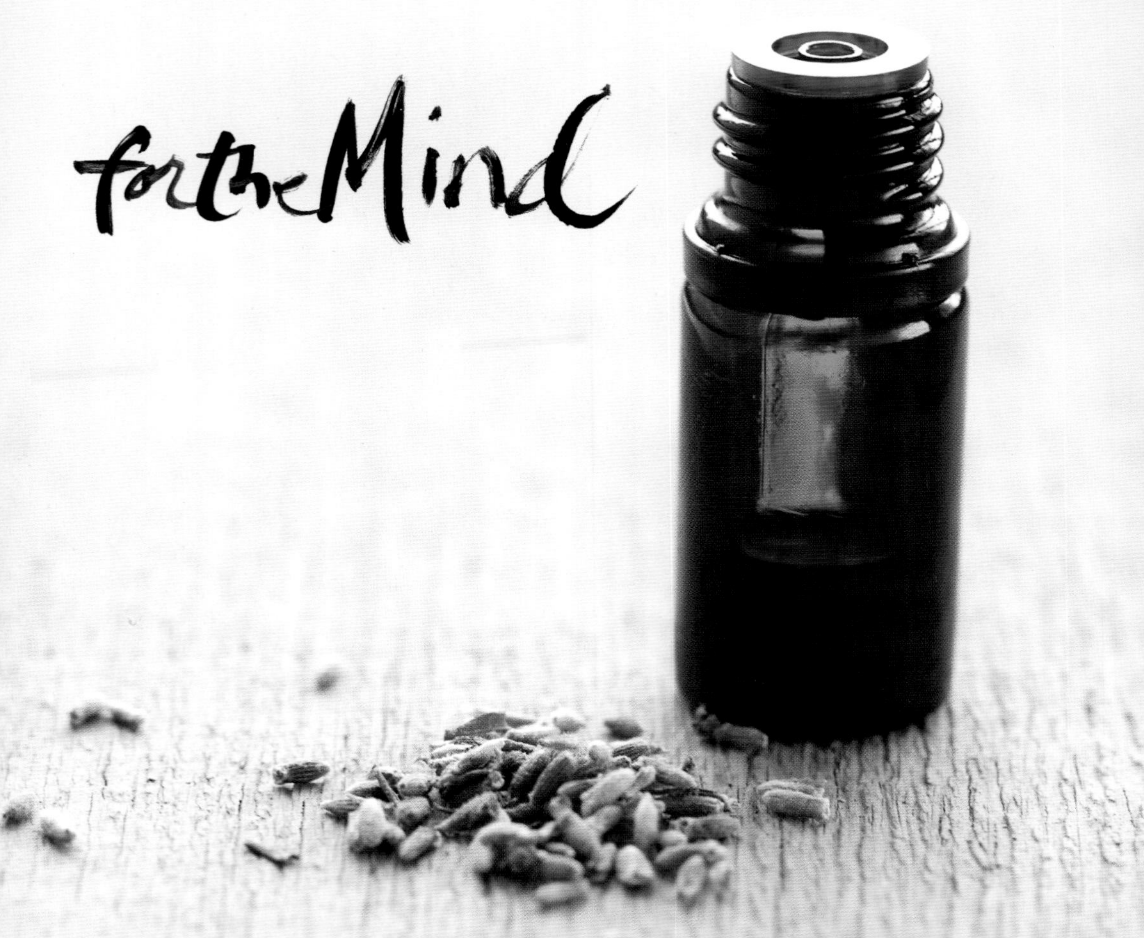

The aromatherapy aspect of lavender makes it a wonderful stress-reliever and antidepressant. You know the saying, "My bed is a magical place where I suddenly remember everything I was supposed to do"? I live that saying, which is why I keep a small bottle of lavender essential oil by my bed. Every time my mind gears up, I inhale deeply from the bottle until my mind calms down enough to sleep. (Note: Don't hyperventilate and get light-headed as you do this; seriously, I've done that to myself and it doesn't help the situation. . . .) Let the scent of lavender work double- and triple-time as it lifts you from depression, stress, worry, and anxiety and places you in a pool of tranquility reflected in the cool, calming blue and purple blossoms of its name.

Primarily, lavender has a cooling, calming, and uplifting effect on the mind, so it follows that a person who is nervous, easily startled, exhausted, or overly stimulated would benefit from this essence. Oftentimes, overstimulation is the result of having (and we're going to get into some yoga terminology here) an energy distortion in the third-eye chakra (or energy center, also called the *Ajna* chakra, whose color is, not surprisingly, indigo or lavender). Many of you have probably heard of the third eye; it's the spiritual, instinctual, and intuitive center of the body. When this is very open, you can feel others' emotions quite easily. Symptoms of energy center distortion include vagueness, forgetfulness, or agitation for no known (or good) reason. Lavender helps get this energy center under control, creating a kind of shield, or barrier, for those sensitive souls.

The flower essence works on multiple levels. It first soothes the stimulation; then, over time, teaches the body, mind, and spirit (or soul, intuition, sixth sense, what-have-you) to work together, regulating all three into better balance.

The flower essence is also helpful for those who wish to have a deeper spiritual or meditative practice but find that their minds just won't be quiet long enough, no matter how hard they try. The same goes for those who have insomnia due to an overactive mind. The lavender essence has the ability to ground the mind while, at the same time, elevating it and opening it safely, slowly, and carefully.

This is interesting because if you think of a lavender stalk itself, its roots take time to grow and establish themselves. Once rooted, the plant sends up slender stalks topped with a riot of purple flowers. Roots and crown — these are the key aspects of the lavender plant. Lavender also likes to be pruned or pinched back, allowing new growth to have a chance and letting old growth go. When you think of it that way, it's kind of a metaphor for life.

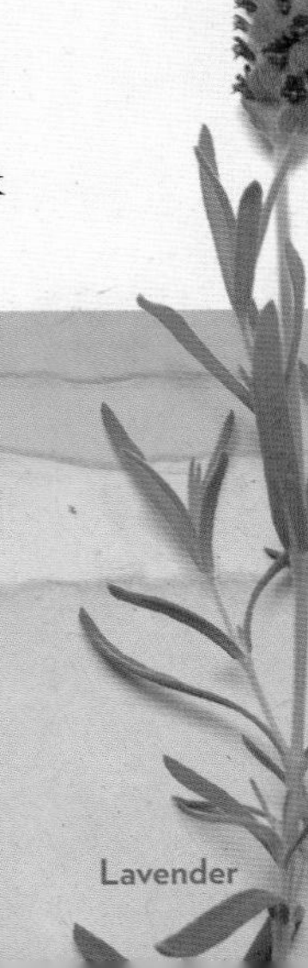

LAVENDER OIL FOR SOOTHING BURNS

This one is super-simple. Keep a bottle of lavender essential oil in your kitchen. Burn yourself? Uncap it, sprinkle a few drops into whatever oil you have handy, and rub it on. Pain? What pain? Done.

for the Spirit

Lavender's flower essence qualities closely align to its magical properties, namely: purifying the mind (and body) for a spiritual practice. Bathing or scenting yourself with lavender will ready you for steady, continuous spiritual or taxing work.

Intriguingly, lavender is also included in love spells. Now, this isn't just the romantic love of the rose, although there's definitely an aspect of that here. We're really talking about deeply spiritual and, yes, sexual, love. Lavender is good for attracting love, but it also protects against false love, fleeting infatuation, and cruelty by the potential beloved.

As for magical associations, lavender is masculine and its planet is Mercury. Mercury is the planet associated with communication, as well as creativity, resourcefulness, and swiftness, which is perhaps why lavender is such a good love charm; after all, true love can only accompany clear and honest communication.

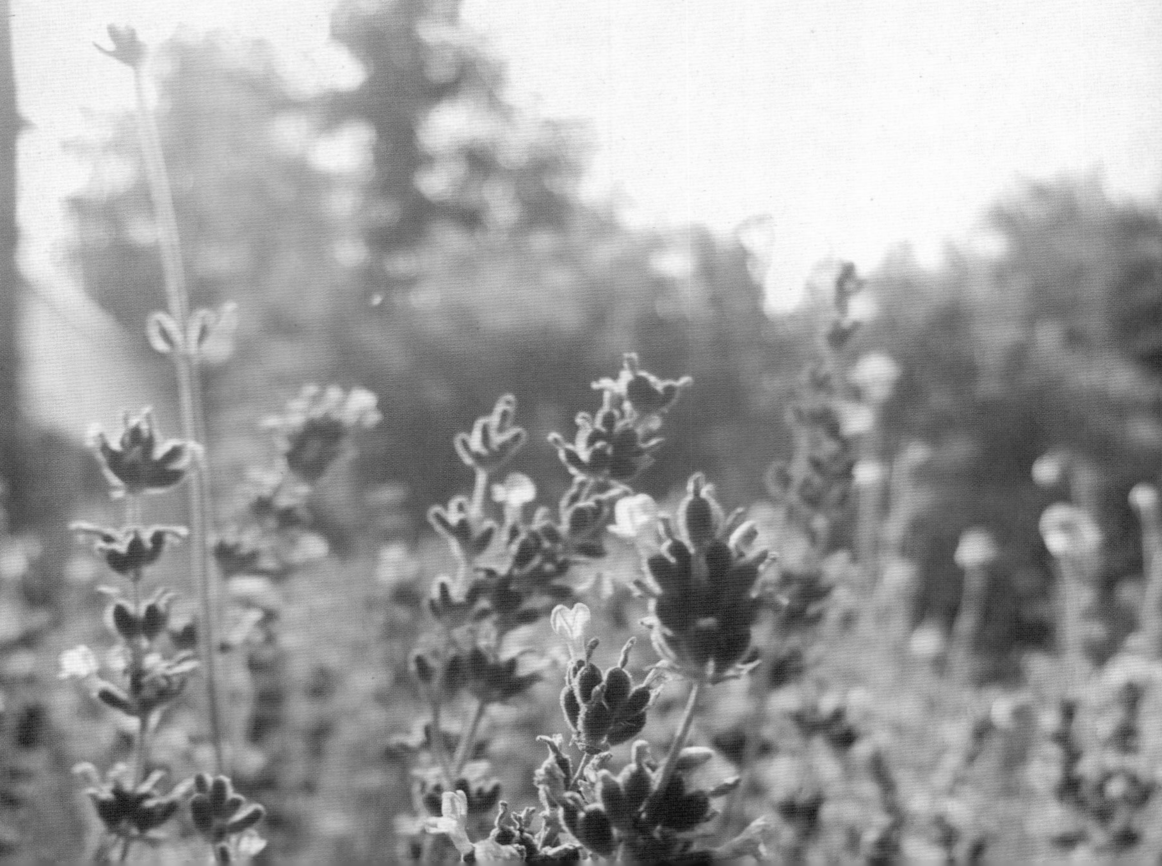

LAVENDER MAGIC

FOR LOVE

You can do pretty much anything with lavender to attract love. Bathe in it, sugar-scrub with it, wear the essential oil as perfume, add a few drops of essential oil to a washcloth and toss into the dryer with your laundry, sprinkle a few drops on your sheets . . . you get the picture. For some reason, love and lavender just can't keep their (astral) hands off each other. Just be careful what you wish for; lavender is strong love juju. Rest assured, though; while lavender attracts love, it also repels violence and ill intentions.

FOR LONG LIFE

As we now know, the scent of lavender is incredibly uplifting. It induces sleep and relaxation, allowing the body time to rejuvenate and repair. The tea is an antioxidant and keeps the body young and thriving from the inside out.

Burn lavender flowers as incense (or if you have a woodstove, as I do, toss a handful of flowers into the fire on a cold night). Burn lavender candles to promote harmony throughout your home, inviting joy into even the darkest corners.

FOR PURIFICATION

Carrying lavender on your person or wearing it as a scent (especially when dabbed at the third eye and at the center of the throat chakra — right in the front center of the neck) helps shield your entire energy field (or aura) from outside influences. Lavender protects your sense of self, your self-confidence, and your faith in your intuition. It strengthens resolve and repels those who wish to do you harm. I always wear lavender scent when traveling — especially in airports, bus or train terminals, and large or unfamiliar cities.

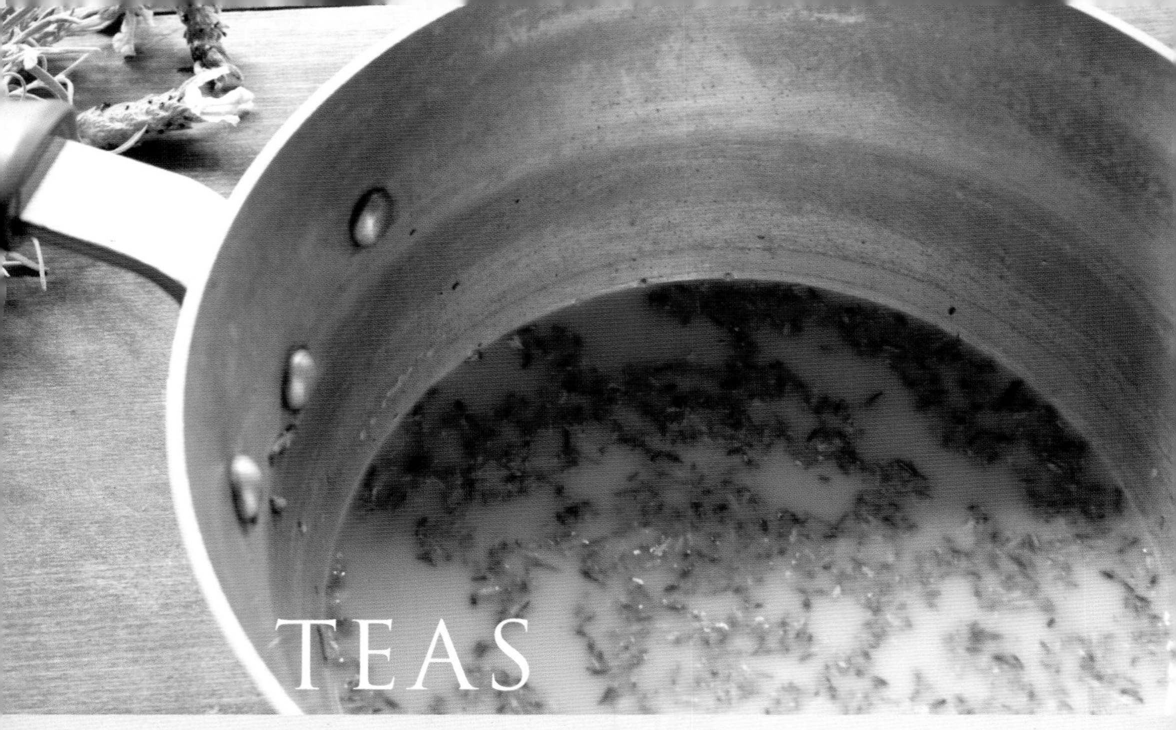

TEAS

Tea for anxiety and nervous stomach. As we've learned, lavender is marvelous for that pesky, tight state of anxiety. Bring 1 cup water to a boil and pour into a mug. Add 1 teaspoon dried lavender and steep for 10 minutes. If the flavor and/or scent are too much for you, add 1 teaspoon dried lemon balm. Lemon balm is especially talented at treating a nervous stomach, plus the subtle lemon and mint flavors of the balm blend beautifully with the lavender. Add honey and nut milk, if your tum will take it.

Tea and aromatherapy for insomnia. When you're trying to sleep, the aromatherapy power of lavender flowers steeped in tea is awesome. In a small saucepan, heat 1½ cups almond milk until steaming. Remove from the heat and add 1 to 2 teaspoons dried lavender and a sprinkle of cinnamon, if you like. Cover and steep for 10 minutes. Strain and add honey or stevia for sweetness. Reheat if necessary. Relax. Sleep well.

Tea to ease headaches. Lavender is a talented and gentle pain reliever. I like to add peppermint (if I'm cold) or spearmint (if I'm hot) for added pain relief and stomach-settling. Steep 1 teaspoon lavender and 1 teaspoon mint in 12 ounces hot water for 10 minutes, and doctor per your taste.

BODY CARE

recipes

Lavender Hair Rinse for Distressed Scalps

Remember our old friend apple cider vinegar? Remember all those fabulous hair and scalp nourishing qualities? Mix that good madness with lavender, and you have unstoppable soothing relief for itchy, dry, irritated, or sunburned scalps.

- **1 tablespoon dried lavender**
- **1–2 tablespoons apple cider vinegar**

1. In a small saucepan, boil 2 cups water. Remove from the heat, add the lavender, and let steep for 10 minutes, covered. Strain and let cool, then pour into a bottle.
2. Add the apple cider vinegar to the bottle and shake. After shampooing, pour this rinse over the scalp and work it in with your fingers. There's no real need to rinse this out. The vinegar scent will dissipate, but if it bothers you, just rinse with cool water.

Makes 16 ounces

Lavender Candles

I love beeswax candles for their scent, their color, and their texture, not to mention their air-cleaning properties. Beeswax burns longer and cleaner than any other type of wax, and it is smokeless and basically drip-free. Not only does beeswax do all of that, but it is also the only fuel that releases negative ions into the air that cling to positively charged allergens, dust, dander, and viruses, and basically bear-hug them until they disappear. (This is science talking, by the way. . . .) The flames also burn up any positive ions that dare to enter within range of the flame. Have asthma? Burn beeswax.

- **Enough beeswax to fill your containers (2 tablespoons per tea light; ½ cup per votive candle)**
- **10 drops lavender essential oil (more if making candles larger than votives)**
- **Pure cotton, beeswax-coated wicks**

1. In a small saucepan or double boiler, melt the beeswax over low heat. When it's completely melted, remove it from the heat and let cool.
2. Add the essential oil and stir, adding more oil if necessary. Let your nose be the judge. The scent will fade a bit as the wax hardens but should activate again as the candle is burned.
3. If you are pouring your beeswax into a candle mold, grease the mold with a little almond or apricot oil (or any

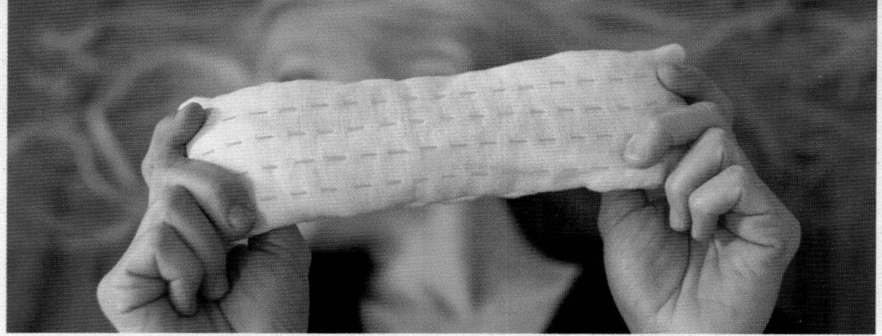

other non-scented oil). Fasten your wick to the bottom of your container with a bit of melted wax, wrapping the end of your wax around a pencil or chopstick and placing this across the opening of the container.

4. Carefully pour your wax into your container. You might need to straighten the wick, but don't tug too hard (I've made plenty of messes by pulling my wick out of the candle). Keep an eye on the wax as it cools. Sometimes a small hollow appears where the wick is. Fill this in with a bit of melted wax to allow the candle to burn evenly.

5. If you're unmolding your candle, stick your mold in the freezer for an hour or so; this should shrink the wax enough to allow it to slide out. Pop out your candle and decorate with a pretty ribbon if you want. I don't recommend dyeing beeswax candles; they're such a beautiful, natural color already.

Makes 1 votive or 4 tea-light candles

Soothing Lavender Eye Pillows

I love eye pillows. I give them away as gifts every year, usually in the company of soaps, lip balms, teas, or what-have-you. One of my favorite things to do is go to the fabric store and pick out fun, lovely, and/or crazy flannel fabrics. Flannel makes divinely soft eye pillows, and fun colors and patterns inspire people to use their eye pillows.

If you're going to use your pillow a lot, you can make a few slipcovers for it. That way, you can wash those and not worry about how to wash your actual eye pillow. I always make a bunch of covers in different fabrics and alternate them depending on my mood.

- 3/8 **yard fabric of your choice (double if you're making a slipcover)**
- ½ **cup rice (uncooked)**
- ½ **cup dried lavender flowers**
- 3 **drops lavender essential oil (optional)**

1. Cut two panels that are each 4½ by 10 inches.

2. Put the right (patterned) sides together, and stitch a ½-inch seam around the rectangle, leaving a 4-inch opening on one of the long sides. Backstitch around the opening. Turn the pillow right-side out.

3. Using a funnel or a measuring cup with a spout, fill your eye pillow with the rice and lavender flowers and add the essential oil, if using. At the opening, fold a ½-inch seam allowance toward the inside of the pillow and pin

it closed. Make nice, small stitches (by machine or hand) ⅛ inch from the outside of the pillow to seal the hole closed.

4. If you're making a slipcover, cut two rectangles that are 5 inches wide by 10½ inches long. Lay one of the rectangles right-side down. Fold back the right short side ½ inch and stitch in place. Do the same thing to the other rectangle. This gives your slipcover a nice, finished end.

5. Match right sides together, hemmed sides together. Stitch a ½-inch seam around the unfinished three sides of the slipcover. Turn right-side out and tuck your pillow inside. Voilà! Beautiful relaxation awaits.

Makes 1 eye pillow

Lavender Sugar Scrub

Sugar scrubs are a magical bathtime ritual. They feel indulgent, spa-worthy, and divine, leaving your skin whisper-soft and your soul just as cozy.

Just a note: Be sure to wash out the tub if it gets slick. The oil can make for some dangerous showering. Also be sure to avoid broken skin when exfoliating; while lavender is wonderful for bruises and wounds, sugar and friction may not be so welcome.

- **2 cups sugar (any kind)**
- **1 cup almond, apricot, or coconut oil**
- **½ teaspoon vitamin E oil, or two little capsules**
- **15–20 drops lavender essential oil**
- **1 teaspoon real vanilla extract**
- **1 tablespoon lavender flowers (optional)**

1. In a large bowl, mix together the sugar, oil, vitamin E oil, essential oil, vanilla extract, and lavender flowers. If you find that your sugar scrub is too crumbly, add more oil. Too oily? Add more sugar. You want a consistency that you can spread and rub easily onto the skin. Pour into a clean pint jar (or divide into smaller jars if you're giving this away as gifts). This should be good for a few months, so cut the recipe in half if you need to.

2. To use, wet your skin and massage in the scrub. You can leave it on your skin for a few moments or wash it off immediately. There's no need to use soap, unless you're feeling uncomfortably oily. And there's definitely no need to moisturize afterwards! Use as often as you like; once a week is a good exfoliating schedule.

Makes 16 ounces

AROMATHERAPY *for* HEADACHES

If you have a headache and don't feel like drinking tea, try a few drops of lavender and mint essential oils. Mix them with a teaspoon of carrier oil and rub on your temples and/or pulse points. Alternatively, simply mix the two together and sniff every few minutes or as the spirit moves you.

recipes

FOOD

"Four Thieves" Healing Vinegar

As the French folklore goes, during the seventeenth century this concoction of herbs and vinegar kept four thieves from falling to the dreaded black plague. Apparently these thieves (grave robbers, actually) doused face masks with this brew and were able to rob graves and houses willy-nilly, without falling ill.

I believe it — these herbs are potent antivirals, anti-inflammatories, and immune boosters. When you feel colds, flu, or (heaven forbid) the plague approaching, douse your salads and veggies in this, actually quite tasty, vinegar. You can also take it by the tablespoonful in warm water with a dash of honey and lemon.

- **2 tablespoons dried rosemary**
- **2 tablespoons dried sage**
- **2 tablespoons dried lavender**
- **2 tablespoons dried wormwood**
- **2 tablespoons dried peppermint**
- **1 quart raw, organic apple cider vinegar**
- **2 tablespoons fresh garlic, chopped**

1. In a clean quart-size glass jar, combine the rosemary, sage, lavender, wormwood, peppermint, and apple cider vinegar. Cover and steep in a cool, dark place for 2 weeks or so, shaking daily.
2. Strain out the herbs and return the vinegar to the jar. Add the garlic and cover. Let this steep for a few days and strain again. Since this is vinegar, it should keep for a long time, but store it in the fridge if you're not at the height of cold and flu season.

Makes 16 ounces

Lavender Rum Balls

This is another recipe from my Great-Aunt Lois. What can I tell you? The woman knew how to live.

- **2 cups crushed vanilla wafers (store-bought or homemade)**
- **½ cup nuts of choice, crushed**
- **¼ cup brandy**
- **¼ cup rum**
- **½ cup lavender-infused honey (see recipe on page 32; substitute lavender for chamomile)**
- **Lavender-infused sugar for rolling (see recipe on page 32; substitute lavender for chamomile)**

In a large bowl, mix together the vanilla wafers, nuts, brandy, rum, and honey. If the dough is too wet to roll into balls, add more crushed cookies. If it's too dry, add more honey. Roll balls in sugar and serve.

Makes approximately 2 dozen balls

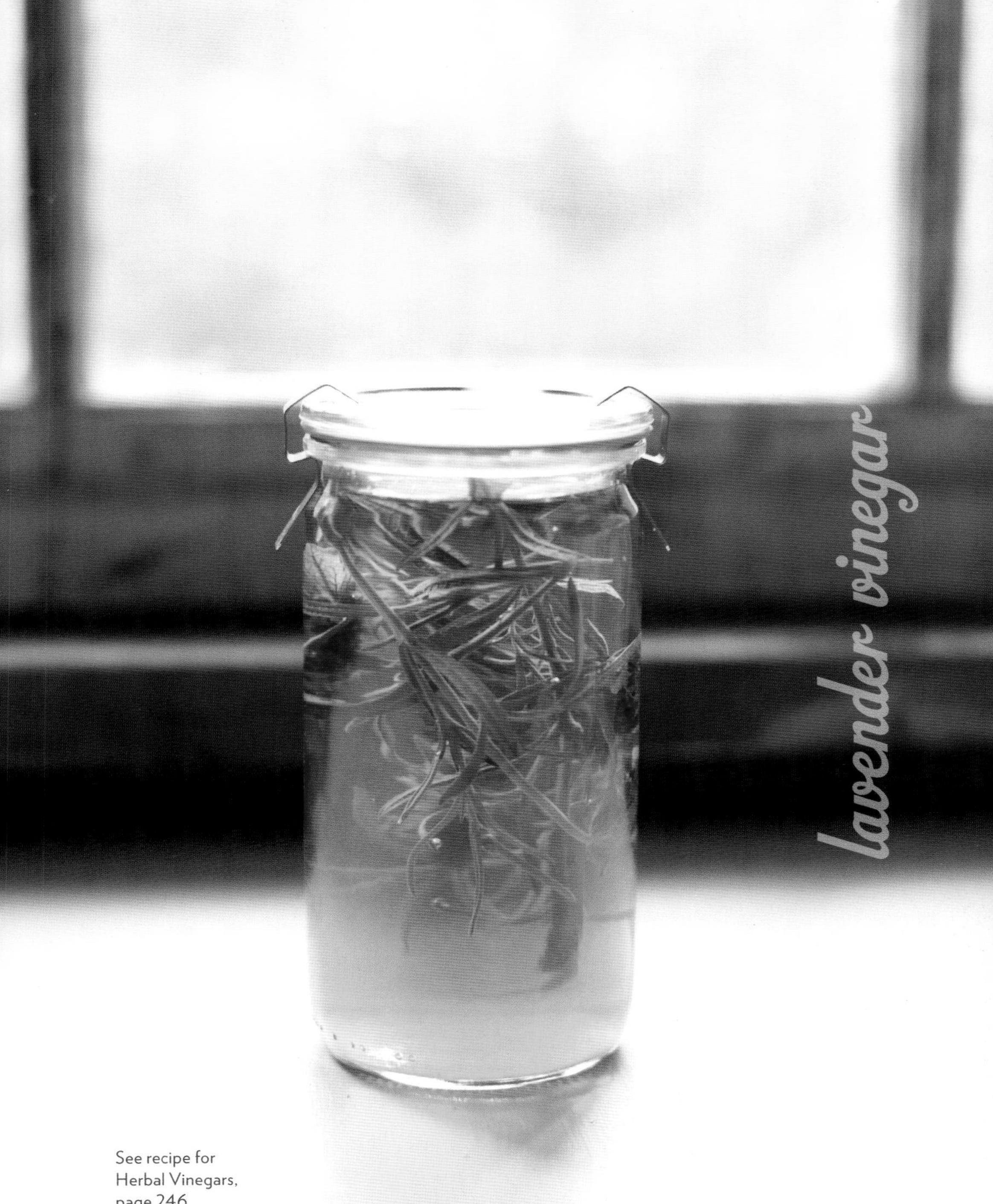

See recipe for Herbal Vinegars, page 246

Lavender-Lemon Bread

I love dessert breads — pumpkin, lemon, zucchini, whatever. You can combine many different flavors in these breads, but lemon and lavender? Heaven. And in this case, it's okay to take lavender essential oil internally because we're using such a small amount as a flavor additive, not in medicinal quantity. It's totally safe at this level. Promise.

- **6 tablespoons vegan shortening**
- **1 cup lavender-infused sugar**
- **2 eggs, beaten, or vegan alternative**
- **¼ teaspoon orange extract/flavoring**
- **⅛ teaspoon lemon extract/flavoring**
- **2 drops lavender essential oil**
- **1½ cups plus 1 tablespoon flour**
- **1½ teaspoons baking powder**
- **½ teaspoon salt**
- **Pinch of powdered cloves**
- **½ cup milk of choice**
- **Grated rind from 1 lemon**
- **2 tablespoons lemon juice**
- **¼ cup lavender-infused sugar (see recipe on page 32; substitute lavender for chamomile)**

1. Preheat the oven to 350°F/180°C. Grease and flour a 5×9-inch loaf pan.
2. In a large bowl, cream together shortening and sugar.
3. In a small bowl, whisk together the eggs, orange extract, lemon extract, lemon rind, and lavender essential oil. Add to the shortening and sugar mixture.
4. In a medium bowl, sift together the flour and baking powder. Add the salt and cloves and mix well. Add the dry mixture to the wet mixture and beat well. Add the milk and mix again.
5. Pour the batter into the greased loaf pan and bake for 1 hour, or until a toothpick inserted in the center comes out clean. Let the bread stand in the pan for 5 minutes before adding the sauce.
6. To make the glaze, combine the lemon juice and lavender-infused sugar in a small bowl and mix together. Slowly pour it over the loaf. Let the bread stay in the pan until all of the glaze is absorbed (trust me — it's much cleaner this way). When it's cool, de-pan the loaf and wrap it in parchment and a clean dishcloth. Let it age at room temp for 24 to 36 hours before cutting. Served with cinnamon tea, this is truly magical.

Makes 1 loaf

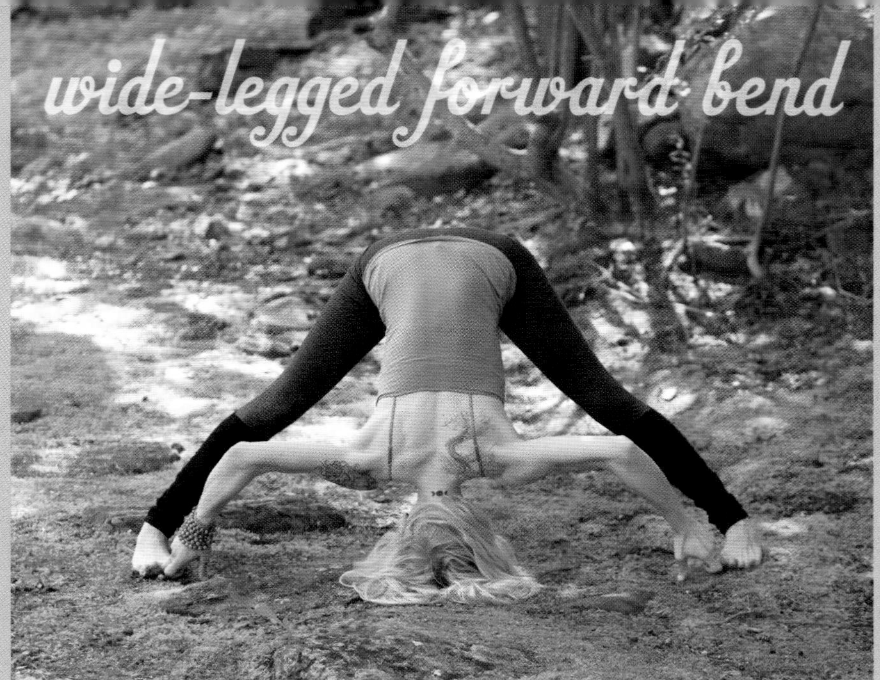

LAVENDER YOGA

Since lavender is so focused on calming the mind and stimulating the sixth chakra (*Ajna* chakra, or the pituitary gland if we're speaking anatomically), we're going to focus on the Wide-Legged Forward Bend (*Prasarita Padottanasana*), which puts the head below the heart, allowing the neck and shoulders to decompress while also allowing the blood to draw to the pituitary gland. I think of the pituitary as the "master gland." It's located in the middle of your brain, behind the bridge of the nose (the area of the third eye, funnily enough). Since it regulates all other glandular activity in the body, it's definitely a good idea to treat it well.

Starting position. Stand nice and tall, shoulders down, feet hip-distance apart. Now, step your feet wide (3 to 4 feet or more, depending on your comfort level). I like to pigeon-toe my feet a bit,

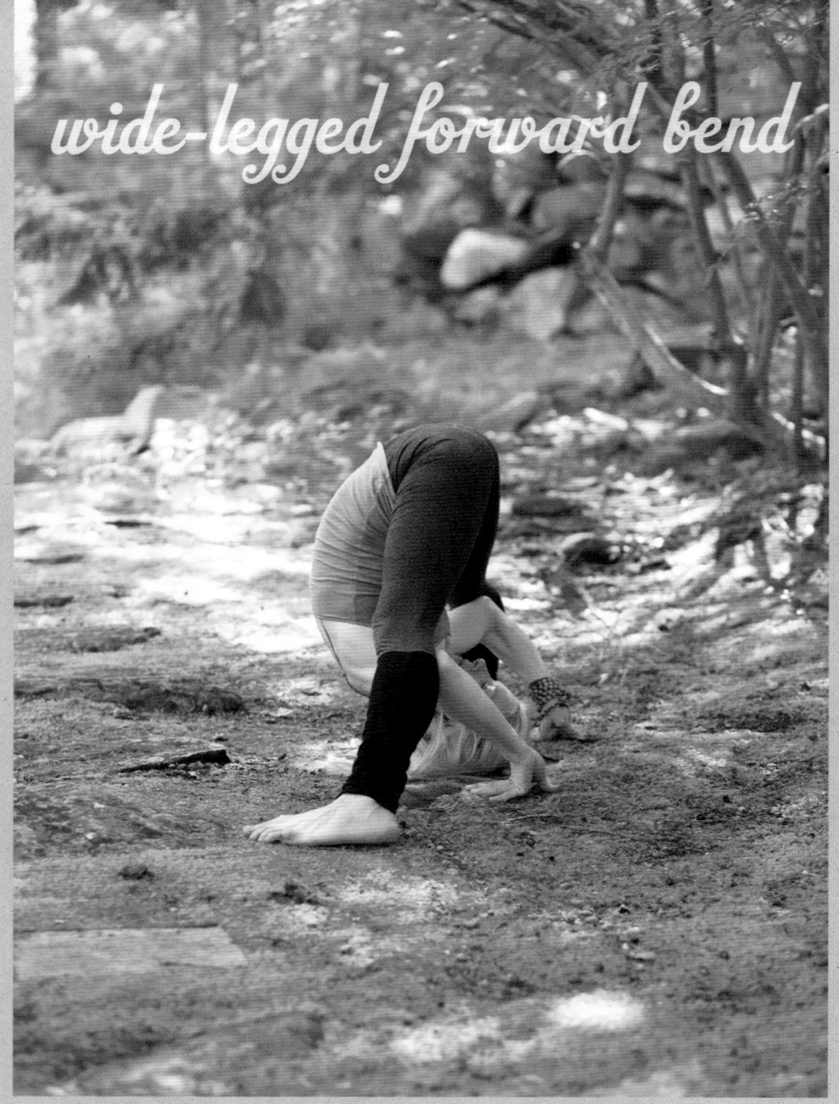

bringing my toes ever-so-slightly toward each other. I feel this gives me an easier stance, but you may find this is too stressful on your knees. Try the traditional, parallel, foot posture first and go from there.

Moving into Wide-Legged Forward Bend. From the wide stance, inhale and bring your hands to your hips, lift through your heart, and drop those shoulder blades down your back. Exhale and fold forward at your hips, keeping that nice, long torso for as long as you can. When you've gone as far as you can go, either let your arms dangle or bring your palms to the floor.

If you reach the floor easily, you can either narrow your stance or start to walk your torso through your legs; however, be careful to keep length in your spine. We don't want to compromise your back just to get closer to the ground.

Fine-tuning. Feel all four corners of your feet on the floor. Lift gently through your arches and spread your toes. Don't lock your knees; keep them firm, kneecaps drawn up into your quadriceps, legs active. Belly is drawn in and up slightly; doing this will give you greater length in your back (try it; you'll be amazed). Even though you're hanging upside-down, you still want those shoulder blades sliding down your back; don't hunch them toward your ears just to get a little closer to the ground. That will happen on its own. Technically, we want the crown of your head to rest on the floor.

Finishing. Stay in this pose 30 seconds to 1 minute. Inhale, bend your knees slightly, press your feet into the floor, and bring your hands to your hips. Rise on an exhale. Many teachers will instruct you to rise on an inhale. However, I tend to get dizzy if I come up from a forward bend that way, so I use the exhale, which usually takes care of the problem. Try it both ways and see what feels right for you. If you *do* feel dizzy, go back down and come up more slowly, bringing your head up last.

Modifications

If your head or hands won't reach the ground, you can rest them on a chair, a stack of blankets, or a bolster. If that still doesn't work, just keep hanging out and eventually you'll get there. Remember to keep your torso nice and long; it takes longer to get to the floor with the proper alignment (in other words, no cheating). You can also try widening your stance to see if it gets a little easier. Just be careful of your knees; we don't want too much pressure there.

If you have tight hamstrings, bend your knees. If your hamstrings *really* don't like this pose, take a seat in a chair, legs together or wide apart, and just drape forward over your legs. Place blankets or a bolster or a couple of pillows in your lap if it helps. Hang out there.

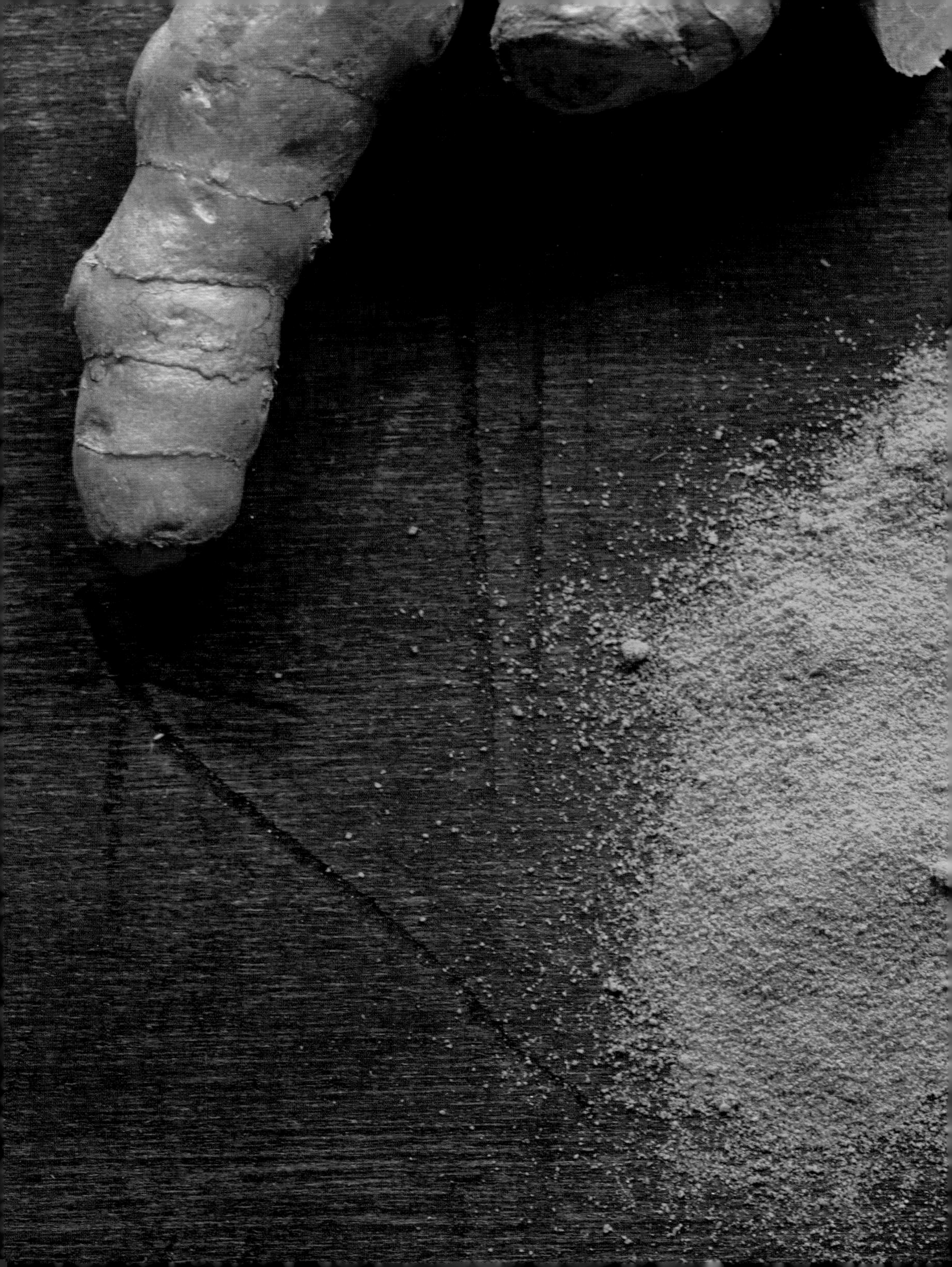

8

Treating It All with TURMERIC

I thought about putting this chapter off for last. Why? Because turmeric (*Curcuma longa*) does *so much* for the body that this chapter could be inexhaustible and easily take over the book. But I decided to take it one step at a time and boil it down to its essentials.

The root is the only part of the herb that is used in traditional medicinal preparations, while the flower is used for creating flower essences. Most turmeric you find for herbal use is dried and ground, but you can find fresh roots in natural food and ethnic grocery stores. You can try to dry the fresh roots yourself, but it's pretty tough, unless you have a really good dehydrator. Instead, I prefer to juice my fresh root or just slice it finely and either cook with it or simmer it into a tea. Just remember that the fresh herb is much stronger and more pungent than the dried and powdered variety.

for the Body

You could basically run through the alphabet and find a disease or malady that turmeric will help with (arthritis, Alzheimer's, bloating, colds, diabetes). I could go through every last one of them (we'll touch on some, never fear!), but there is one common denominator that links all of them together: inflammation.

There are some health experts — both in the allopathic and holistic world — who believe that inflammation is at the source of almost every disease. Once inflammation sets in, no matter what organ or muscle or vessel it chooses to inhabit, the body part can no longer play its proper role. Once *that* body part fails, the domino effect happens: one after another, each system fails. The blood supply is hindered, and health deteriorates. Most pain, too (and asthma, incidentally), is caused by inflammation. Take away the inflammation and, voilà! Pain-free and mobile.

Turmeric contains a particular constituent called curcumin (which is what gives it its bright yellow color, in case you're ever playing Trivial Pursuit and that question shows up). Curcumin is antibacterial and anti-inflammatory. The beauty of this powerhouse combo is that if there's a bug in the system (bacteria, that is; not a design flaw), then turmeric has it covered. Inflammation? Got that, too.

Because of these properties, turmeric can be used internally or externally. Internally, it is used for bleeding, infection, viruses, asthma, arthritis, and pain in general. Externally, it is used on cuts, wounds, scratches, and burns. Because turmeric is such an incredible medicinal herb for easing inflammation and preventing all kinds of disease, it would not hurt to take turmeric when you need a little extra help in the health department. I'd even recommend applying this flower essence externally on painful joints and areas of inflammation, just to see what would happen.

Now to the big stuff. Studies have shown that turmeric may be able to treat cancer. While we know that, as an antioxidant, turmeric protects the body against free-radical damage, herbalists and doctors have found that turmeric also seems to trigger the destruction of cancer cells. According to a phase-1 study by the UK's Cancer Research Center, "[it] seemed to show that curcumin could stop the precancerous changes becoming cancer." And, "A number of laboratory studies on cancer cells have shown that curcumin does have anticancer effects. It seems to be able to kill cancer cells and prevent more from growing."

Cautionary notes: More lab studies are being done. If this is a therapy you are interested in trying, please do so with the guidance of a professional practitioner. You need to take large doses of turmeric to get enough curcumin into your system, and while turmeric is widely considered to be completely safe, those who are on blood thinners or prone to kidney stones or gallstones may have trouble. Also, if you find yourself experiencing stomach distress, dehydration, or constipation, dial it back.

TURMERIC

Curcuma longa

Parts used: Rhizome, flower (for flower essences)

How to harvest: Wait until the plant has died back for its dormant season, then gently dig up the rhizome, gather what you need, and return a small portion back into the soil for regeneration and a new harvest the following year

Effects on the body: Anti-inflammatory, healing, immune-boosting, detoxifying, cleansing, nutrient-dense

Effects on mind and spirit: Groundedness, willpower, determination, grants a sense of safety and induces courage

Safety first: Use turmeric in moderation. In very large quantities, it can cause stomach distress. While this isn't likely to happen when using the amounts we're talking about here, go slowly if you have a history of stomach disorders. Also, turmeric temporarily dyes your skin, so depending on your complexion, you may not like the shade. See the box on page 161 for more details.

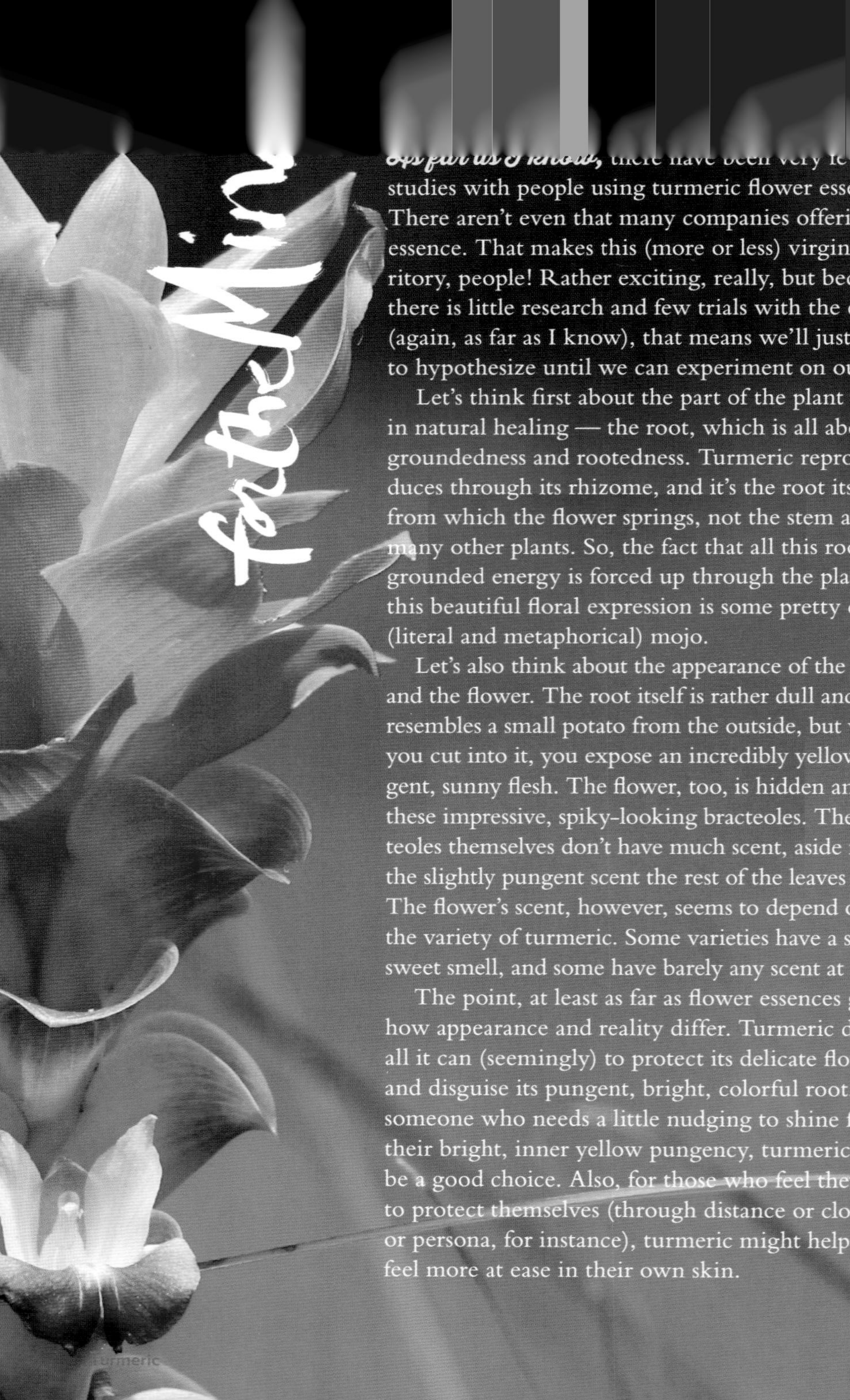

Turmeric

As far as I know, there have been very few case studies with people using turmeric flower essence. There aren't even that many companies offering the essence. That makes this (more or less) virgin territory, people! Rather exciting, really, but because there is little research and few trials with the essence (again, as far as I know), that means we'll just have to hypothesize until we can experiment on our own.

Let's think first about the part of the plant we use in natural healing — the root, which is all about groundedness and rootedness. Turmeric reproduces through its rhizome, and it's the root itself from which the flower springs, not the stem as in so many other plants. So, the fact that all this rooted, grounded energy is forced up through the plant into this beautiful floral expression is some pretty deep (literal and metaphorical) mojo.

Let's also think about the appearance of the root and the flower. The root itself is rather dull and resembles a small potato from the outside, but when you cut into it, you expose an incredibly yellow, pungent, sunny flesh. The flower, too, is hidden amongst these impressive, spiky-looking bracteoles. The bracteoles themselves don't have much scent, aside from the slightly pungent scent the rest of the leaves have. The flower's scent, however, seems to depend on the variety of turmeric. Some varieties have a strong sweet smell, and some have barely any scent at all.

The point, at least as far as flower essences go, is how appearance and reality differ. Turmeric does all it can (seemingly) to protect its delicate flowers and disguise its pungent, bright, colorful root. So for someone who needs a little nudging to shine forth their bright, inner yellow pungency, turmeric would be a good choice. Also, for those who feel they need to protect themselves (through distance or clothing or persona, for instance), turmeric might help them feel more at ease in their own skin.

for the Spirit

In my research, I've found turmeric associated with the sun and with fire. However, I've also found turmeric associated with Mars, which is fiery and masculine; with the moon, which is feminine; and also with a water element. Why the discrepancy? Magic is not a well-documented science; at least, it doesn't have money for research behind it. All we really have to go on is the experience, practice, and information from our own workings.

Let's take the first association with fire, Mars and the sun, and masculine energy. Turmeric is yellow. It tastes and feels fiery. In the ancient Indian healing system of Ayurveda, turmeric is associated with Pitta (the fire element), digestion (again, fire), and it induces sweating. This makes a good case for association A.

But! Turmeric was traditionally used mostly by women and in the kitchen. It had cosmetic use (the yellow pigment on the skin) and was very often prepared and served in milk (also an obviously feminine association). It was used as an offering to Lakshmi, the goddess of wealth and prosperity. The Sanskrit name for turmeric is *Kanchani*, which translates to "golden goddess."

So, which association is it? There's no definitive answer, but I feel turmeric has a healing, feminine quality. I have nothing but instinct to back that up, but hey, that's magic for you.

Despite its associations, everyone seems to agree on turmeric's magical uses: protection, sensuality, love, and prosperity; and the ability to uplift emotions, uncover hidden beauty, heal, and even (in one bit of research) ward off crocodiles. I mean, come on! Crocodiles? You just can't beat that.

WHY ISN'T TURMERIC A COMMON FLOWER ESSENCE?

I imagine one reason why I can't find many outlets carrying turmeric flower essence is because turmeric takes so long, and is rather tricky, to grow. The flowers, too, are nestled inside spiky-looking protective bracteoles and are not the easiest thing to harvest. Or maybe because its flowers don't produce seeds (that's right — flowers, but no seeds), no one has thought of adapting turmeric for this purpose. I don't know. But it's a beautiful flower that is very exotic and ginger-looking.

TURMERIC MAGIC

TO INSPIRE DESIRE

Sensual, warm vanilla meets hot, sunny, and passionate turmeric. For this desire-stoking magic, mix ½ teaspoon turmeric powder with ½ teaspoon vanilla extract and 2 teaspoons almond oil. Apply to the pulse points. Vanilla invites warmth, love, attraction, and passion. Turmeric adds a desirable glow to your body, aura, speech, and presence.

Not only that, but turmeric sprinkled in food or in small dishes set around the bedchamber (a passion spell just calls for a word like "bedchamber," no?) invites desire, warmth, truth, and true soul connections. Invite your loved one in for a sensual curry or spicy Indian-themed meal. Burn yellow candles anointed with the vanilla-turmeric scented oil.

TO CALL ON COURAGE

Invoke some fiery courage by ingesting turmeric — especially in spicy curries and other Indian cuisine; the spices add to the bravery-stoking fires. You can also anoint yourself with a special, sunny, courage-inspiring oil. Combine ½ teaspoon turmeric powder, 1 teaspoon almond oil, and 2 drops cinnamon essential oil. Mix up and apply to the pulse points. If you have extra-sensitive skin, skip the pulse points and combine the ingredients in a little vial, inhaling when you find yourself in need of courage.

FOR HEALING

Magical spells aren't just incantations and intentions (although that's a part of magic, surely). Often, most of the magic comes from ingesting, bathing, or wearing the herb.

If your loved one is sick, keep a turmeric plant or fresh root in their room, allowing all that energy to seep where it's needed. Alternatively, take turmeric baths (1 tablespoon turmeric powder in a nice, warm bath), or sip on turmeric milk (1 cup nut or dairy milk with 2 teaspoons turmeric powder). Heat, blend with a teaspoon (or more) of honey, and sip with intention. Anoint the body with turmeric powder, either on the pulse points (extra power) or anywhere with pain. (Worried about staining? See the box on page 161).

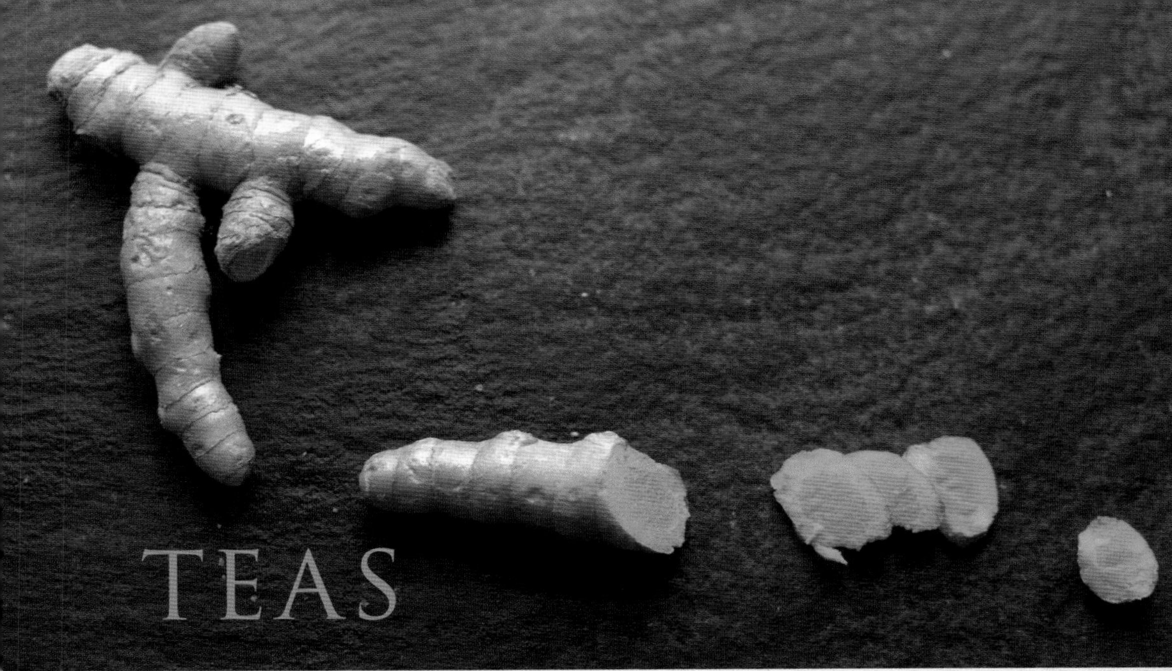

Basic teas/decoctions. You must boil turmeric root and can't steep it like a regular tea, so technically, these are decoctions and not teas. To decoct the root, you can do two things: You can buy (or grow) turmeric fresh and slice thinly or grate it, then simmer the root for 10 to 15 minutes. Or you can buy the herb already dried and powdered, add water to it, simmer for 5 to 10 minutes, then blend it up and drink (blending it gives it a highly recommended fluffiness, not to mention that it distributes the turmeric particles so you ingest as much as possible, leaving less sediment on the bottom of the cup). For the fresh herb, I'd recommend a scant tablespoon of grated turmeric per cup; for dried, try a heaping teaspoon.

Tea for inflammation. To fight inflammation, I recommend using the basic powdered herb decoction (see above). The powdered herb has the most surface area, so its medicinal qualities are more easily extracted. Since turmeric is best absorbed by the body when taken with a bit of fat, add 1 teaspoon cold-pressed coconut oil to your tea, then blend. Avoid dairy and nut milks; dairy milk aggravates inflammatory conditions, and commercial nut milks have preservatives that can cause inflammation. Blending it up (I use a nifty stick blender, but you can also use a standard blender) allows you to drink the actual herb itself, getting all kinds of the bonus nutrients and anti-inflammatory action.

Tea to heal the stomach. If you're a longtime sufferer of acid reflux or acid conditions, then you must heal the lining of the stomach. Marshmallow (sadly, I'm talking about the herb, not the fluffy, sugary, gooey goodness of campfire and hot chocolate fame) has been shown to heal and protect the stomach lining as well as the esophagus, fixing any damage an overly acidic condition has wrought. And the antibacterial qualities of the turmeric and the coconut oil will keep those sore spots clean and healthy while they heal. ***Note:*** Marshmallow root likes to soak up everything around it and hustle it through the body, so don't take any medicines or supplements 30 minutes before or after you drink this tea.

Brew the powdered turmeric base decoction, but add the contents of 2 marshmallow capsules when you add the turmeric. Then add 1 teaspoon cold-pressed coconut oil when you blend up the drink. Drink three cups a day (or more, if you really, really like it).

Tea for sweetening sleep. Turmeric, as an anti-inflammatory, eases pain and stiffness that can keep you awake at night. For a nighttime tea, gently heat 1½ cups milk in a small saucepan. Add a sprinkle of cinnamon, ¼ teaspoon fennel powder, 1 licorice capsule (opened, the powder sprinkled into the brew), ½ teaspoon turmeric powder, and, if you have some, the contents of 1 (or 2, if you're especially agitated) kava-kava capsule. Simmer for 10 minutes. Add a good dollop of honey or stevia to taste, then blend until foamy. Pour into a preheated mug and sip until sleepy.

Note: If you have low blood pressure, you might want to limit using licorice to only once in a while.

Tea for joint and bone health. Combine a chunk of fresh turmeric root (or 1 teaspoon powder), 1 tablespoon dried dandelion root, a ½-inch piece of fresh chopped gingerroot (or 1 teaspoon dried), and 2 cups water in a small saucepan. Dandelion contains calcium, silicon, and boron — all essential for bone health. Simmer this for 10 minutes, then strain. Sweeten and add non-dairy milk, if you like.

Tea to ease depression. Turmeric has the ability to lighten the mood while, at the same time, bringing us out of our heads (where most of our troubles begin) with its earthy qualities. Add to this a good dose of licorice (which, you may not know, is an MAO inhibitor; see note on previous page if you have low blood pressure) and Saint-John's-wort, which is famed for its antidepressant qualities, and you pack a powerful wallop against depression.

In a small saucepan, combine 1½ cups milk or water (I prefer milk), 1 teaspoon turmeric powder, 1 teaspoon licorice powder (or a couple of capsules opened and dumped in), and the contents of two Saint-John's-wort capsules. Simmer for 5 minutes. You can also add a touch of vanilla extract along with sweetener for sweetness and comfort. Blend up and sip as often as you like.

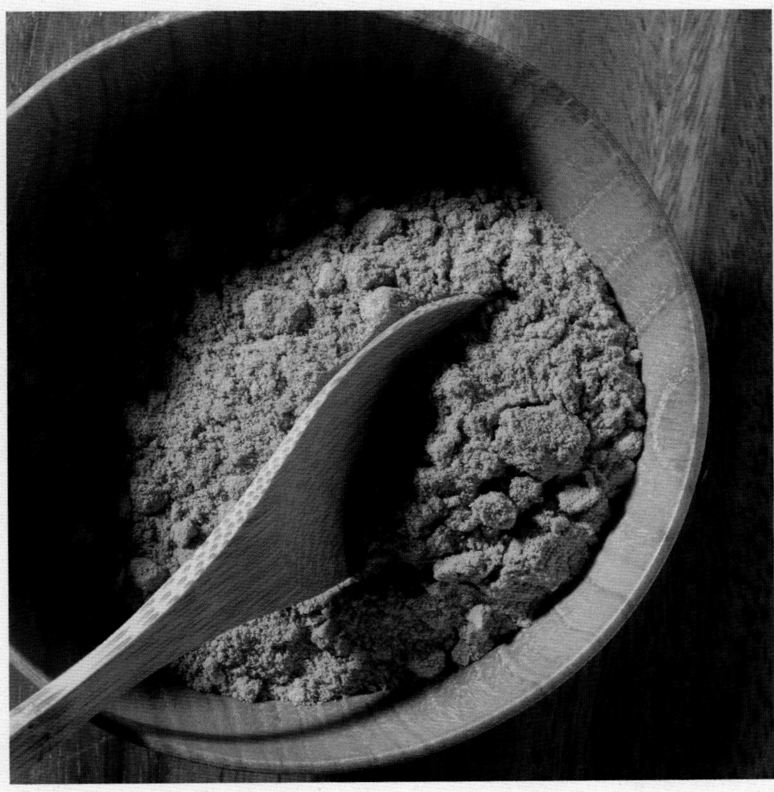

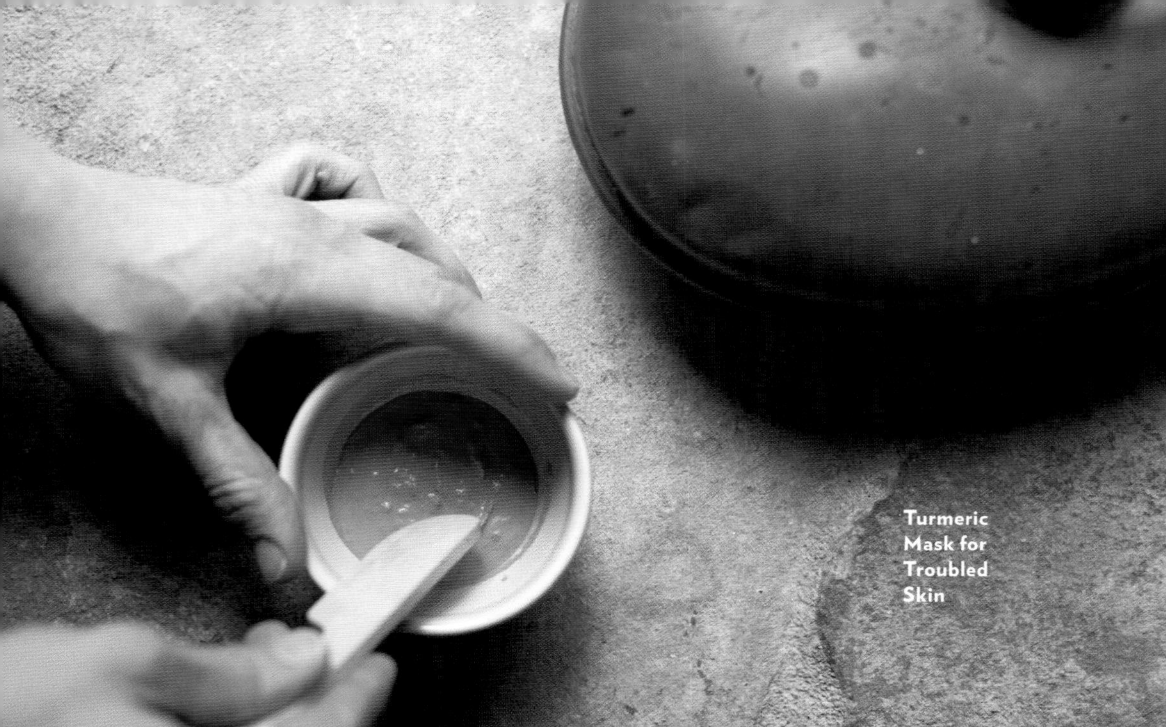

Turmeric Mask for Troubled Skin

recipes

BODY CARE

Turmeric Mask for Troubled Skin

Turmeric is wonderful for drawing blood to the surface of the skin, flushing out dirt, oils, impurities, and any infection — virus or bacteria — that may be lurking just under the skin (but do test for discoloration first; see box on page 161). This paste should keep for about a week, but make less if you don't think you'll use it all.

- **½ cup French green clay, bentonite clay, or white cosmetic clay**
- **2 tablespoons powdered turmeric**
- **1 tablespoon apple cider vinegar**
- **2 tablespoons witch hazel**

In a small bowl, mix together the clay, turmeric, apple cider vinegar, witch hazel, and as much water as you need for a paste consistency. Apply the mask to your face, and then sit and relax for 10 minutes. Rinse off with warm water.

Makes 2 applications

Sore Throat Gargle

Sore throats are caused by many things: voice overuse, inhalation of smoke or other pollutants, illness, dry air, allergies, and irritation. I like to hit all causes of sore throat pain in this one-stop-shop gargle. And slippery elm is as awesome as it sounds — lots of mucilaginous, slippery, soothing coating all over your poor sore throat. You can also make a nice slippery elm and turmeric tea; use the same ratios as below, but leave out the salt.

- **¼ teaspoon good-quality sea salt**
- **1 teaspoon powdered turmeric**
- **1 teaspoon slippery elm bark powder, or the contents of 2 capsules**

In a small saucepan, heat 1 cup water until hot (but not boiling). Pour it into a mug and add the sea salt, powdered turmeric, and slippery elm bark powder. Mix this all together and throw back a glug. Gargle for 30 seconds and repeat until all of it is gone. Repeat as often as necessary.

Makes 1 cup

Ache-Relieving Turmeric Bath

There's nothing like a bright yellow bath to convince you that you're not at home and in pain, but actually basking in a sulfur hot spring somewhere where people in organic cotton lounge pants bring you healing drinks and warm towels. (Worried about staining? See the box on page 161.)

- **½ cup Epsom salts (good for inflammation and restoring the body's mineral balance)**
- **⅛ cup powdered turmeric**
- **Essential oils of choice (just stay away from strong, minty scents, as they can burn sensitive skin)**

Start by running a nice warm bath. To this, add the Epsom salts, powdered turmeric, and essential oils. Soak in the tub for at least 20 minutes, then rinse in a warm shower and bundle up. As a follow-up, you can sprinkle a bit of turmeric in a carrier oil (I like castor oil, since it penetrates the skin into the muscle or joint) and rub it into the affected area.

Makes enough for 1 bath

BLACK DRAWING SALVE

I like to purchase my black drawing salve (see Resources) instead of making it. Its key ingredient, pine tar, is hard to source and even more challenging to work with. However, if you're really gung-ho on making it, you can find how-to's online (see Resources).

Turmeric Paste for Cancer Prevention

Black drawing salve is a pretty incredible substance. A lot has been written about it, but basically, it contains one key ingredient: pine tar (from the pine tree). Yes, pine tar makes it black and weird-looking, but it also has this amazing, magnetic, and almost magical ability to draw impurities, including (some think) cancer-causing constituents. Mix this with turmeric (whose cancer-fighting actions we've already discussed), and you've got some potentially powerful purifying action.

This paste is especially good for melanoma or troublesome skin conditions, but also try it for any infected or inflamed skin areas, including stubborn splinters that just won't emerge from the skin.

1–2 teaspoons black drawing salve (see box, page 159)

2 teaspoons powdered turmeric

In a small bowl, mix together the salve, turmeric, and 2 tablespoons water to form a paste (add a bit more water if the mixture is too thick). Spread the paste on the affected area and cover with a bandage. Let it stay there for 24 hours. Now, here's the freaky part: You may find that the drawing salve is, well, actually drawing something out of the skin. Don't be alarmed. Just wash the area, reapply the salve, and bandage. Continue these steps until the salve stops drawing.

Makes 1 application

Turmeric Poultice to Ease Pain

Turmeric meets ginger in this spicy, anti-inflammatory, paste-y goodness. For a bonus, sip on anti-inflammatory turmeric tea while the paste is setting.

2 tablespoons turmeric powder

2 tablespoon ginger powder

Castor oil

In a small bowl, mix together turmeric powder, ginger powder, and enough warm castor oil to make a paste. Apply the mixture to the area of pain, avoiding any broken or infected skin. Cover this with a clean towel and then a hot water bottle or heating pad. Keep the area warm for 15 minutes, then remove the paste with cool water. Repeat throughout the day as needed.

Makes 1 poultice

Turmeric Paste for Eczema

Eczema sufferers know how irritating, itchy, and inconvenient an outbreak is. Luckily, we have an ally in turmeric, especially when coupled with our old friend calendula.

1 tablespoon turmeric powder

1 tablespoon ground dried calendula flowers (grind them yourself with a coffee grinder)

Almond oil (for dry conditions)

Witch hazel (for wet conditions)

In a small bowl, mix together the turmeric powder and ground calendula, then add enough almond oil or witch hazel to make a paste. Apply to the skin and let it sit for 20 minutes. If it's irritating, rinse it off and try again, using less herb and allowing it to sit for less time. Rinse off with cool water, pat dry, and let the air circulate on the skin. Repeat as necessary.

Makes 1 application

Turmeric Rinse for Blond Locks

I'm a blondie (which may or may not be a gift naturally given to me . . . I'll never tell), but whether you're a natural blond or not, turmeric is fabulous for bringing out bright highlights. If you're white-blond, however, you might want to skip this treatment; it could temporarily give you a yellow glow.

- **1 cup cool chamomile tea (see recipe on page 25)**
- **1 tablespoon apple cider vinegar**
- **1 teaspoon lemon juice**
- **1 teaspoon powdered turmeric or ½ cup turmeric tea (see recipe on page 155) if powder in your hair doesn't sound all that pleasant**

In a bottle, combine the chamomile tea, apple cider vinegar, lemon juice, and turmeric powder or turmeric tea. Pour the rinse on your hair after shampooing but before conditioning. Let it sit on your hair and scalp for a few minutes, then rub your scalp vigorously and rinse it out. Condition as usual. Use this rinse once a week.

Makes 8 ounces

DON'T WANT TO GLOW? TEST FIRST

Turmeric temporarily dyes your skin, and depending on your complexion, you may not like the shade (although, if you mix it with milk or yogurt, as in these recipes, staining isn't usually a problem). If you're concerned, rub a little of the turmeric mask/rinse/paste on the inside of your elbow. If you don't like the color, simply use it at bedtime or try a different herbal treatment that doesn't include turmeric.

If your skin *does* get stained, just mix a bit of granulated white sugar with enough water to form a paste and rub this into the stain. Rinse with warm water and repeat if necessary.

Wash the turmeric off of your skin before handling fabric, and use old towels and clothing, just to be safe. If your fabric does become stained, try spot-washing the stain by hand, using cool water and laundry detergent. Pour the detergent right onto the stain and work it in. Place the soapy fabric in cool water, and let soak for 30 minutes or so, then rinse. If the stain is still too visible for your taste, rub a cut lemon on the stain and let that sit for 30 minutes more, then launder as usual.

recipes

FOOD & DRINK

Turmeric Hot Chocolate

Can you tell I like cold weather? Or maybe I just like to cook when it's cold out. Adding turmeric counters the sweetness of the traditional hot chocolate, lending depth and an earthy taste.

- **4 cups non-dairy milk**
- **4 tablespoons good-quality cocoa powder**
- **4 cinnamon sticks**
- **Dash of nutmeg**
- **½ teaspoon ground turmeric**
- **Dash of ground cloves**
- **1½ teaspoons vanilla extract**
- **Marshmallows (optional, but awesome)**
- **4 3-inch cinnamon sticks or candy canes for garnish (optional)**

In a medium saucepan, combine the non-dairy milk, cocoa powder, 4 cinnamon sticks, nutmeg, turmeric, and cloves, and stir with a wire whisk. Cook over low heat until thoroughly heated (but not boiling). Remove from the heat and discard cinnamon sticks. Stir in the vanilla extract; then pour into individual mugs and top each mug with marshmallows. If you like, garnish with a fresh cinnamon stick (or a candy cane if it's the holidays).

Serves 4

Oven-Fried Tofu

Here's another one of my dad's decadent gems. It used to be oven-fried chicken, but just because I left meat behind didn't mean I had to leave behind things like this. I added turmeric for a little extra kick.

- **½ cup sour cream (vegan or dairy)**
- **1 tablespoon lemon juice**
- **1 teaspoon Worcestershire sauce**
- **1 teaspoon celery salt**
- **2 cloves garlic, chopped**
- **½ tablespoon paprika**
- **2 teaspoons turmeric**
- **Pinch of salt, and freshly ground black pepper to taste**
- **2 pounds firm tofu, cubed**
- **1 cup breadcrumbs**

1. Preheat the oven to 350°F/180°C and grease a baking pan.
2. In a large mixing bowl, mix together the sour cream, lemon

Recipe continues on page 165

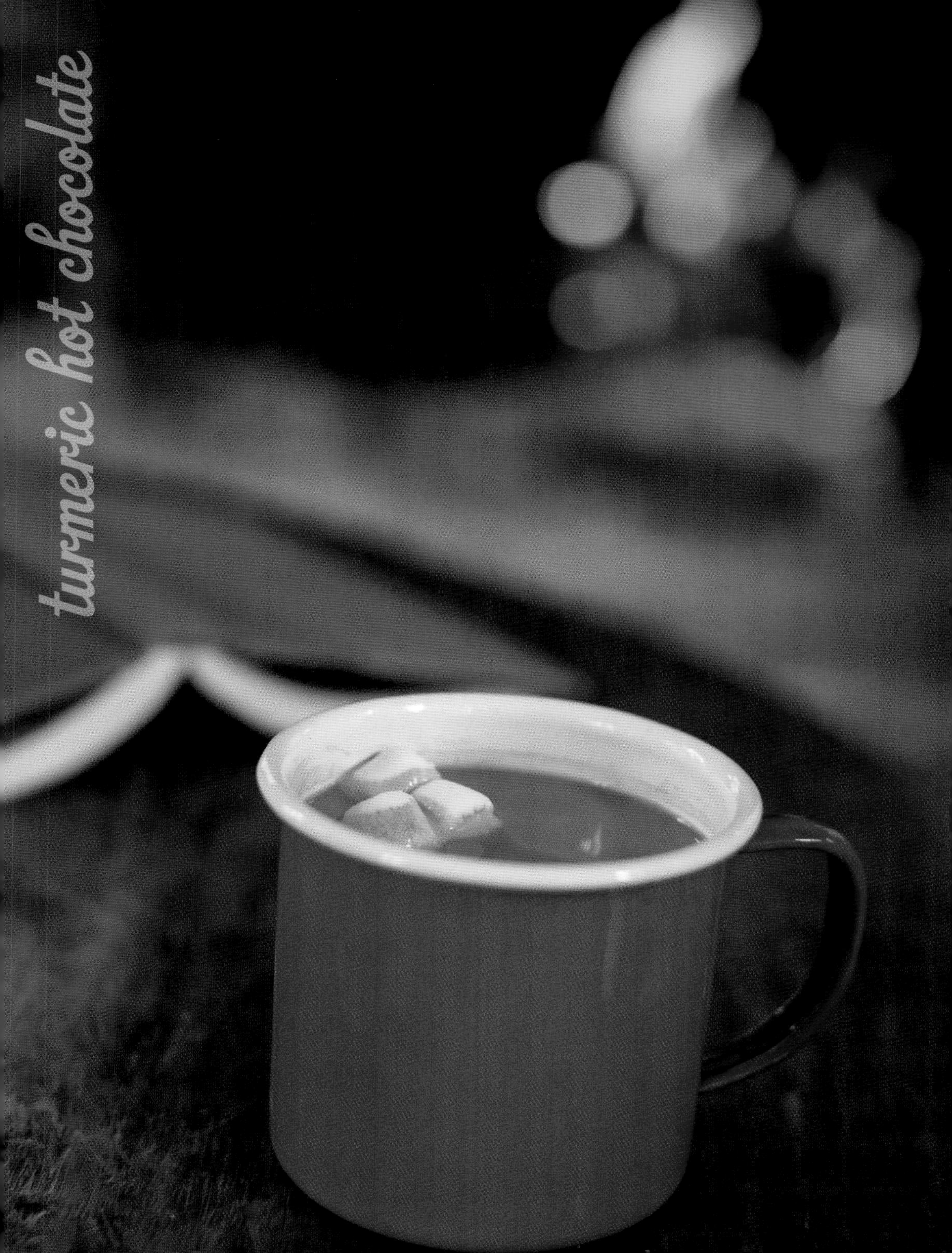
turmeric hot chocolate

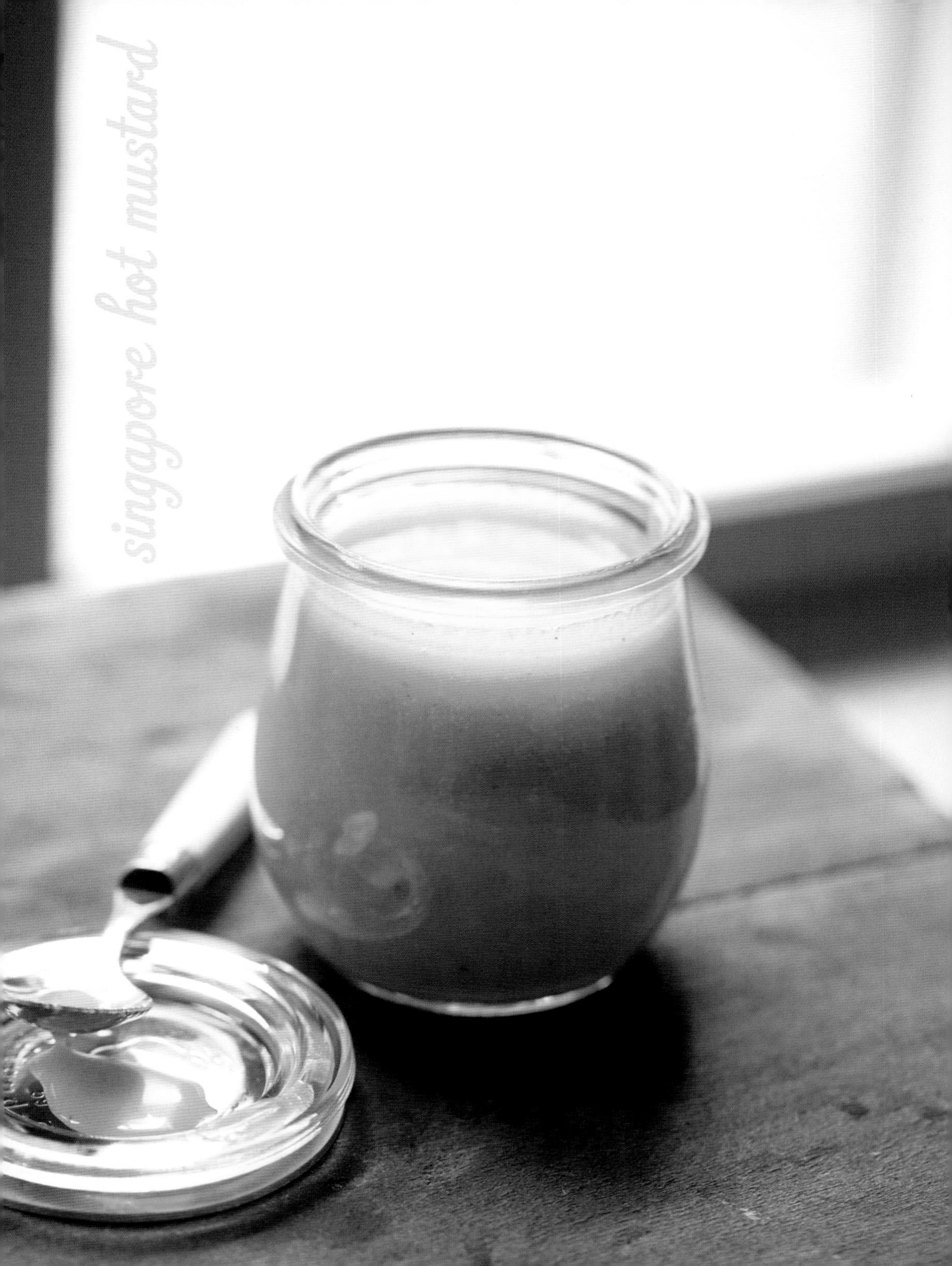
singapore hot mustard

juice, Worcestershire sauce, celery salt, chopped garlic, paprika, turmeric, salt, and pepper. Add the cubed tofu and mix well. I like to use my hands so that I don't break the tofu. ***Note:*** If you wear contacts or don't want your hands stained yellow, wear gloves or use a rubber spatula to fold in the tofu.

3. Add the breadcrumbs to the bowl and coat the tofu well. Pour the tofu mixture into the baking pan and bake, uncovered, for 45 to 60 minutes (check often toward the end). Serve over rice or greens.

Serves 4

Singapore Hot Mustard

This recipe came from my maternal grandmother. My parents made it all the time, and now my sister and her husband make it to give away as gifts each Christmas. Yes, it is that awesome.

- 6 ounces dry mustard
- 2 cups sugar
- 1½ cups apple cider vinegar
- 1 teaspoon salt
- ½ teaspoon turmeric
- ½ teaspoon black pepper
- ¼ teaspoon white pepper
- ⅛ pound butter (vegan or dairy), softened at room temperature
- 3 well-beaten eggs or vegan substitute

1. In a medium saucepan, mix the mustard with enough water to make a paste. Add the sugar, vinegar, salt, turmeric, and black and white pepper. Mix well and put on the stove to cook (if you need more water, go ahead and add it) over medium-low heat.

2. When this starts to heat up, after 5 minutes or so, add the butter and eggs. Stir constantly. When you see the first bubble that precedes boiling, take the pan off of the heat and stir until thickened (5 minutes or so). Then pour the mixture into a blender (or use a stick blender). Blend until smooth.

3. Pour the hot mustard into four sterilized 4-ounce canning jars and lid them. (Sterilize the jars either by running them through the dishwasher or by submerging them in boiling water for 10 minutes. Add the lids to the boiling water at the last minute.) Store the jars in the fridge to let the mustard thicken. The lids should suck down to make a seal as the mustard cools. If they do, then you can store it for a year. If any don't seal, keep the jar in the fridge and use it within a month or two.

Makes 16 ounces

Turmeric-Spiced Sweet Potato Soup

I love, love, love thick veggie soups in the winter. Being a New England girl raised on chowder and stew, I associate a good soup with the coziness of a warm house on cold, dark winter evenings.

- 1 tablespoon butter (vegan or dairy)
- 2 cups coarsely chopped onions
- 2 pounds sweet potatoes, peeled and cut in small cubes (about 5 cups)
- 2 large Granny Smith apples, cut into small pieces (I like to leave the peel on)
- 3 cups veggie broth
- 1¾ cups unsweetened apple juice
- 1 teaspoon thyme
- 1 teaspoon powdered ginger
- 1 teaspoon powdered turmeric
- Salt to taste
- ¼ teaspoon ground black pepper

1. Heat the butter in a large stockpot or Dutch oven over moderate-high heat until hot. Add the onions and sauté, stirring frequently, until they start to brown, about 5 minutes.
2. Add the sweet potatoes, apples, broth, 1 cup apple juice, thyme, ginger, turmeric, salt, and pepper. Cover and simmer 25 minutes or until the sweet potatoes are soft. Remove from the heat and let stand until cool enough to handle.
3. Use a stick blender (or purée in batches in a food processor or blender), blending until the texture is coarse. Return the soup to the pot, add the remaining ¾ cup apple juice, and heat thoroughly. For a thinner soup, add more juice.

Serves 4

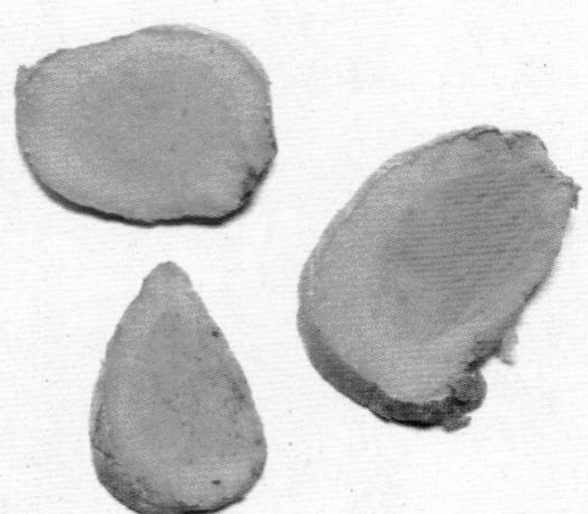

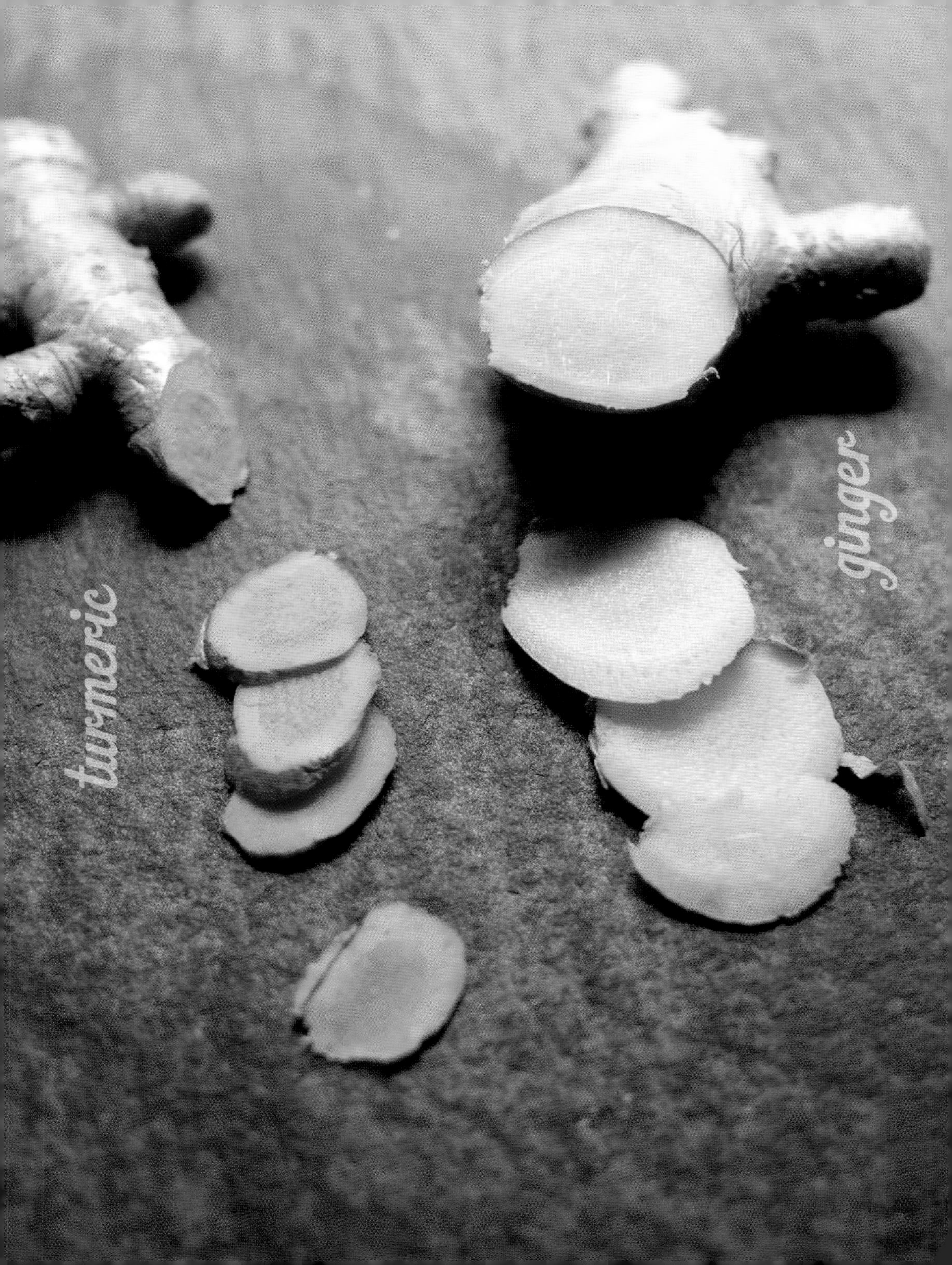

turmeric

ginger

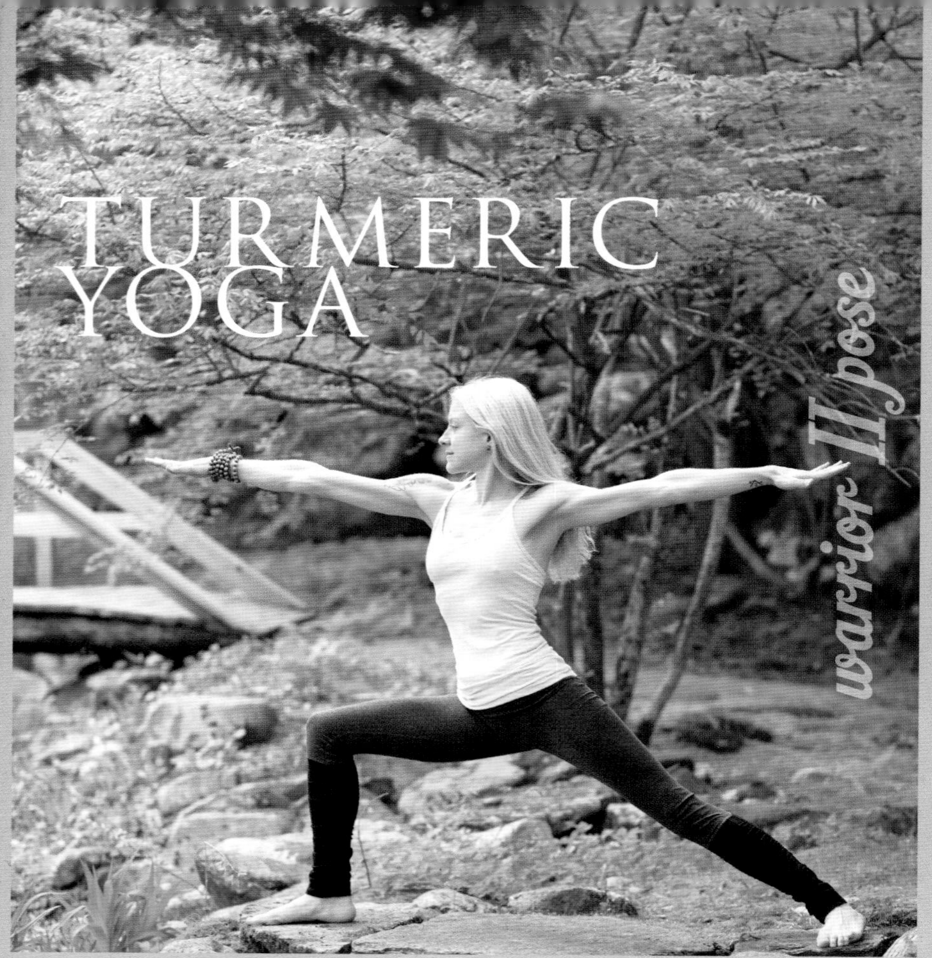

Here, we'll focus on the more spiritual aspect of turmeric. We've already explored how turmeric boosts courage, offers protection, strengthens resolve, and offers grounding. The yoga pose that offers these same supports is Warrior II (*Virabhadrasana II*).

Virabhadrasana translates as "fierce warrior" and is associated with the Hindu deity Shiva, the god of destruction and rebirth known as "Śiva the Destroyer" and "Śiva the Regenerator." If we want to get *really* deep (and, heck, I've got time if you do), then we can look at Shiva himself. Shiva is often described as having a thousand feet. If *that* won't ground you, well, I don't know what will. Furthermore, Hindu and Buddhist monks traditionally wear saffron-colored robes, which were originally dyed with turmeric.

Starting position. Begin in Mountain Pose (*Tadasana*). Stand on your mat with your feet together or hip-distance apart — your choice — facing the long side of the mat. Breathe. With all four corners of your feet, feel the earth beneath your feet. Inhale and step or lightly jump your feet about 3 feet apart.

Moving into Warrior II. Turn your right foot toward the short side of your mat, keeping your left foot facing the long side of your mat. Your body itself will keep facing the long side of your mat. Inhale and raise your arms out, stopping when they reach shoulder height. Turn your head to look out over your right arm, and as you exhale, bend your right knee to 90 degrees (or thereabouts). Make sure that your knee is over your ankle; if it's pushing forward over your toes, wiggle that foot out farther so you're lined up correctly.

Fine-tuning. Make sure those shoulder blades are gliding down your back — don't scrunch them up by your ears. Keep your navel drawn in toward your spine and your entire spine lifting upward, out of your pelvis (in other words, good posture!).

Lift through the arches of your feet. We want grounding, not slumping through the arches; not only will this hurt your feet and ankles, but it will cause your knee to round in a weird and painful way. On that note, glance down at that bent knee. You should see your big toe; if so, draw that knee (and thigh, from the hip) toward your baby toe. You'll feel your outer thigh being activated when you do this. That's good; that's what we want. We don't want your knee to collapse.

Take a break if you need to — those arms are heavy, I know. Then, keep drawing that tailbone down toward the earth. Grounding. Remember grounding. We want a nice long spine — no bunching or pinching in your low back. Keeping your belly drawn in will help, too.

Finishing. After 30 seconds to 1 minute, inhale, straighten your right leg, and drop your arms. As you exhale, turn your left foot to the short side, your right foot to the long side, and repeat everything, this time with your left knee leading.

Modifications

If it's hard for you to support yourself on that 90-degree leg, then feel free to support that bent leg with the seat of a chair. Place the seat under the leg that's bending and lower into it; the seat should be under your thigh. If you're graced with height, you may need to stack a few blankets or towels on the seat of the chair to make this modification work for you.

If you're finding it hard to keep your spine straight (in other words, not stick out your bum), then you can try this pose with your back against a wall. Do everything the same way, but try to keep your shoulder blades and both sides of your bum against the wall. Try to stretch your arms out along the wall as well.

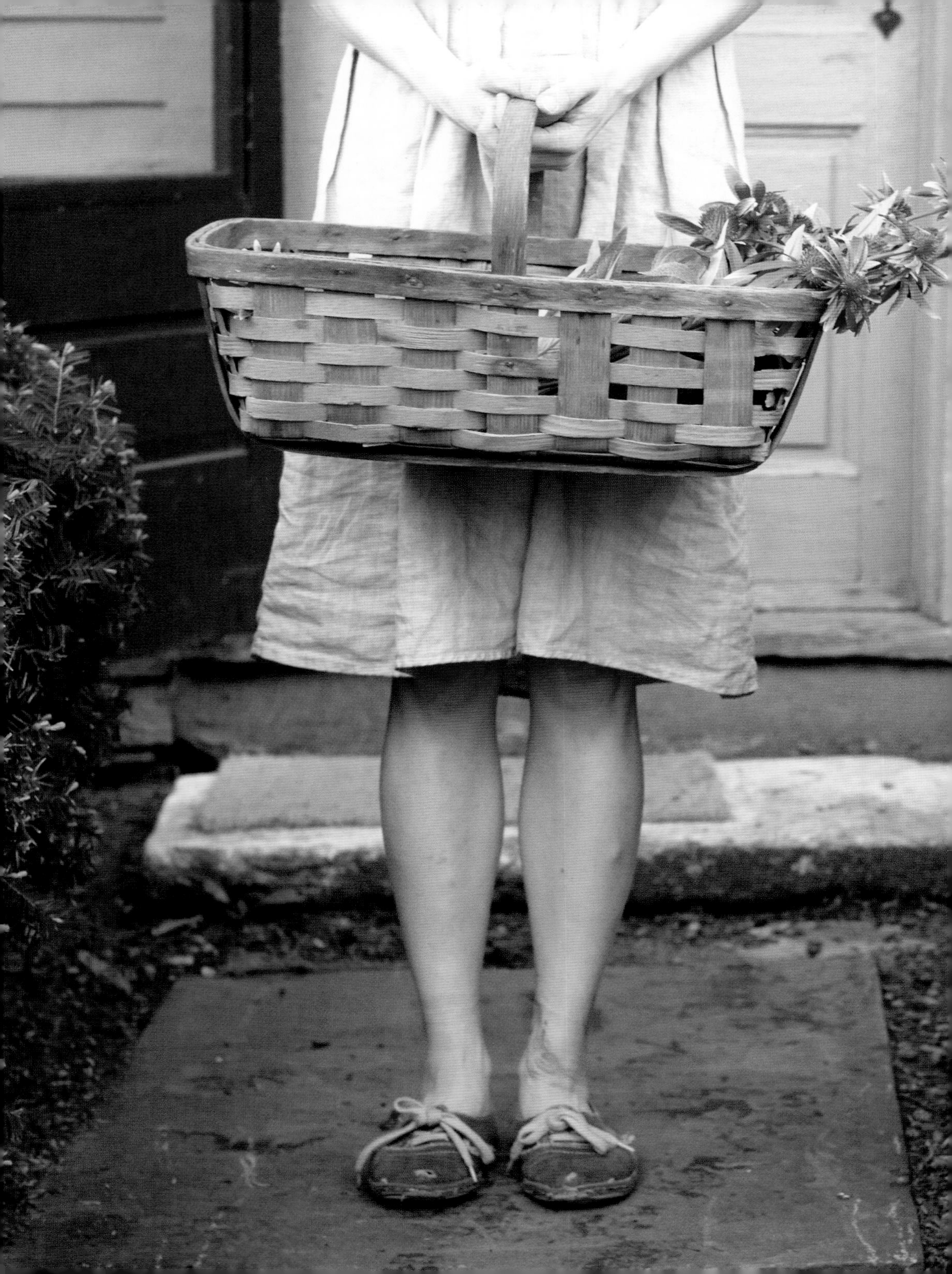

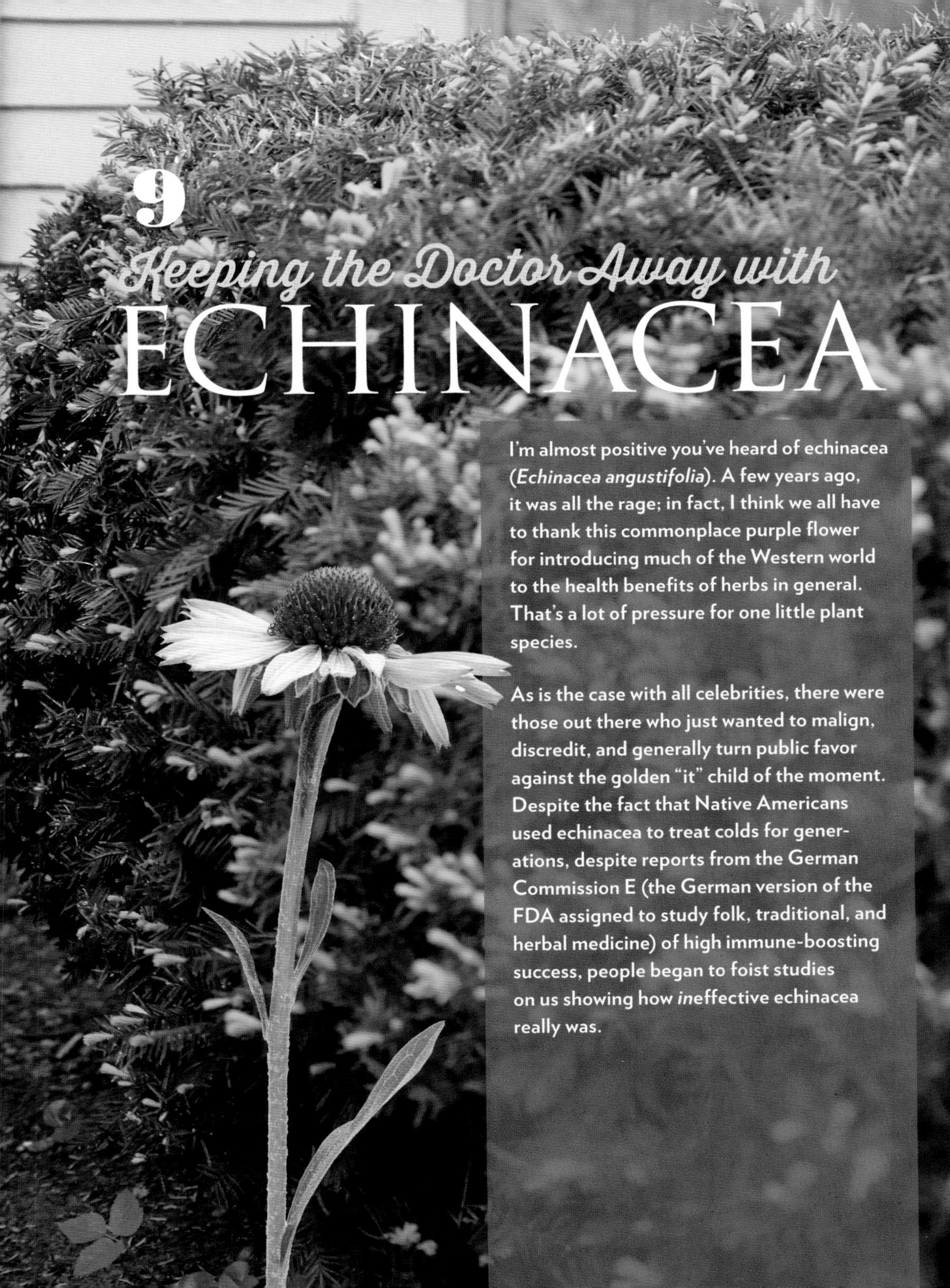

9

Keeping the Doctor Away with ECHINACEA

I'm almost positive you've heard of echinacea (*Echinacea angustifolia*). A few years ago, it was all the rage; in fact, I think we all have to thank this commonplace purple flower for introducing much of the Western world to the health benefits of herbs in general. That's a lot of pressure for one little plant species.

As is the case with all celebrities, there were those out there who just wanted to malign, discredit, and generally turn public favor against the golden "it" child of the moment. Despite the fact that Native Americans used echinacea to treat colds for generations, despite reports from the German Commission E (the German version of the FDA assigned to study folk, traditional, and herbal medicine) of high immune-boosting success, people began to foist studies on us showing how *in*effective echinacea really was.

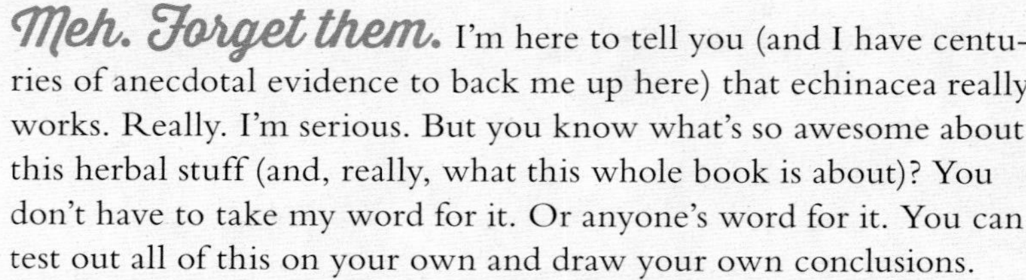

Meh. Forget them. I'm here to tell you (and I have centuries of anecdotal evidence to back me up here) that echinacea really works. Really. I'm serious. But you know what's so awesome about this herbal stuff (and, really, what this whole book is about)? You don't have to take my word for it. Or anyone's word for it. You can test out all of this on your own and draw your own conclusions.

Echinacea is a hardy perennial that will do well in soil beds or in pots. If you live in the Central Plains, then you've probably seen echinacea growing wild. Feel free (after making a positive identification, of course) to forage for your immune-boosting herb.

When it comes time to harvest, the roots are the part of the plant you'll use. You can make a tea or tincture out of the flowers and leaves, but the root is where the mojo lies. It's best to let your echinacea live two years before harvesting anything, but if you're impatient (like me), you can carefully harvest leaves and flowers during the first year.

If you're harvesting the flowers or leaves, do so right after they bloom, in the morning, after the dew has dried but before the heat of the day (be sure to leave some flowers for the bees). You can dry the flowers or leaves for a few days if you want to store them, or brew up a tea with fresh plant material.

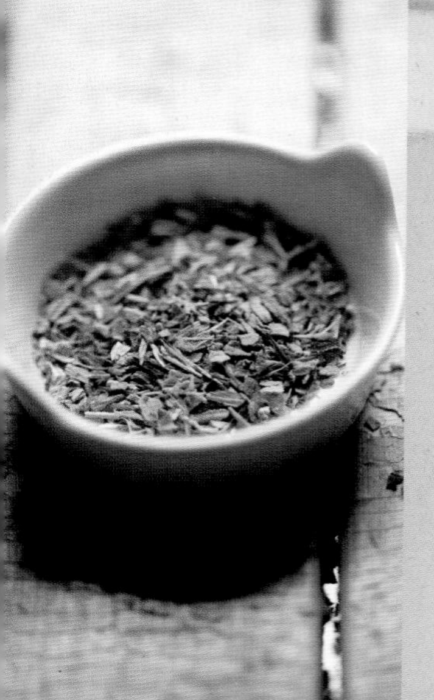

ECHINACEA

Echinacea angustifolia

Parts used: Leaves, flowers, roots
How to harvest: Dig up roots after the first frost of the season, when the plant is two years old; leaves and flowers can be harvested in the first year on a sunny day after the dew has dried
Effects on the body: Immune-boosting, antiviral
Effects on the mind and spirit: Reconnects you to your absolute core of self — what makes you happy, dance, sing, spin around, and live with excitement
Safety first: Use with caution if you have a ragweed allergy

When harvesting roots, wait until after the first frost of the second year, when the plant itself has browned and died back. This is when all of the plant's life energy has moved to the root to be stored for the winter. Carefully dig around your plant with a trowel, being cautious not to gouge or damage the root system. Find roots that are far from the central body of the plant and have no dependent rootlets growing off of them. Carefully cut these with scissors or a sharp knife. Clean them and, if you like, chop them up for easier brewing. Let them dry on a screen in a cool, dry part of your house or, if you have a gas stove, in an unlit oven (using just the pilot light) for a few days. You can also use a dehydrator or a barely warm oven (you don't want it to exceed 110°F/40°C).

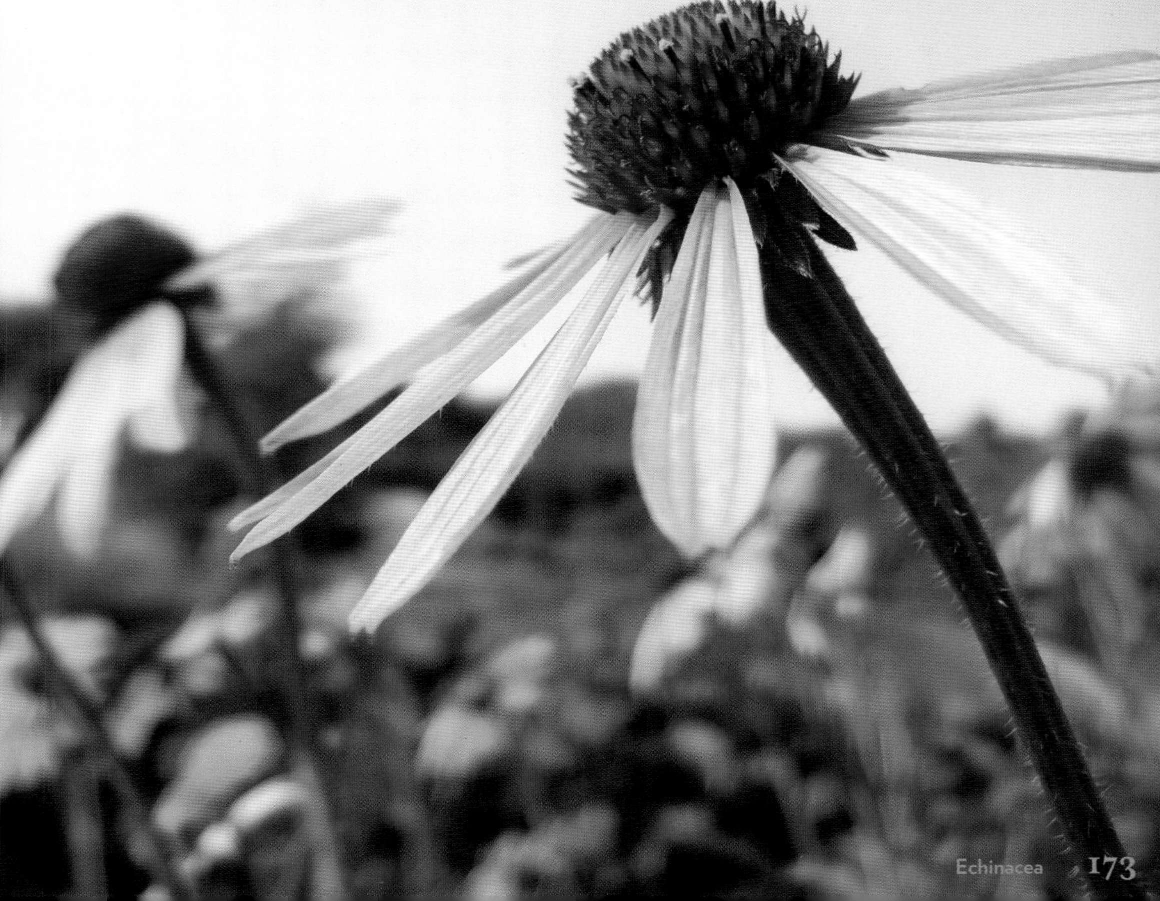

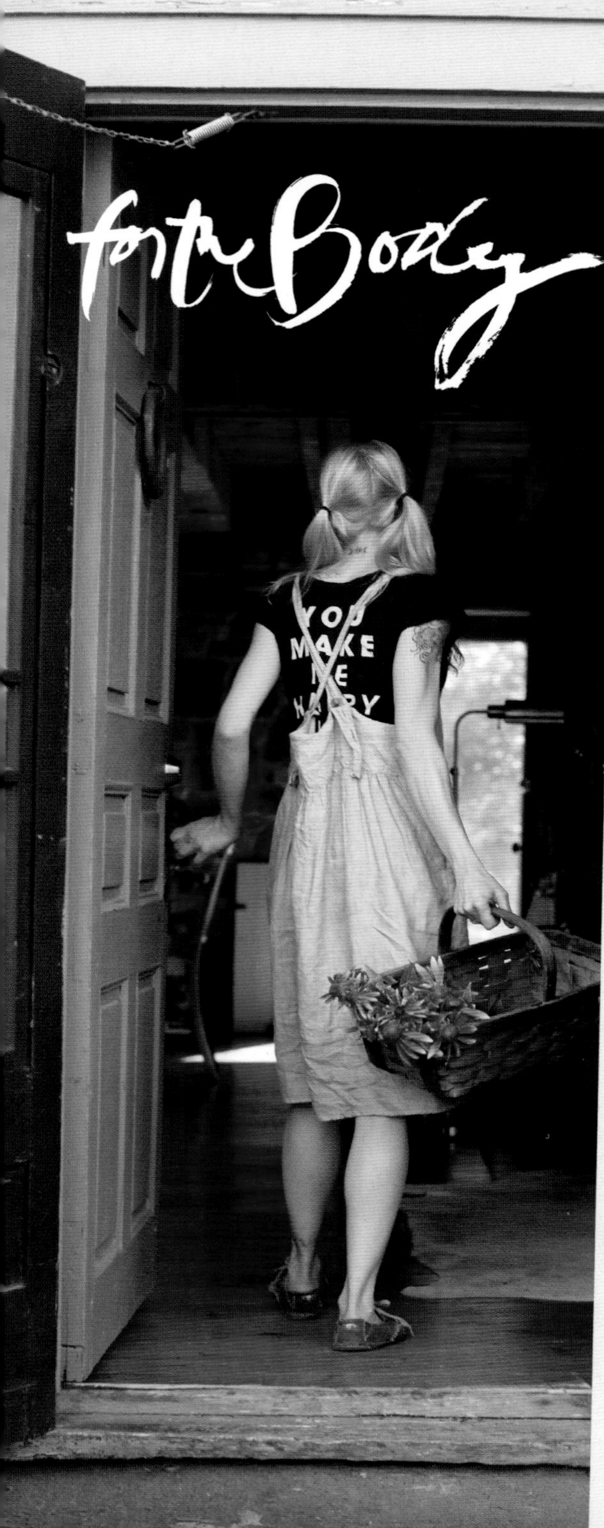

for the Body

So, the question you are asking yourself now, the answer you are just *dying* to know, is why echinacea works in the first place. Am I right? (See? We know each other so well by now.) Well, I'll tell you (but no worries — there won't be a quiz later, unless you're planning on writing one yourself). Your body has a protein found in the blood serum called properdin. This protein, when triggered, signals to the immune system to hurry up and arm itself because there's been a slew of viruses and bacteria reported in the system and it's time to get serious. Echinacea increases the levels of properdin in the body, making your body all the more efficient, organized, and all-around dangerous to invading organisms. As an antiviral, echinacea is also good at fighting off cold, flu, and even herpes viruses (in that case, apply echinacea tea or poultice topically — preferably before an outbreak erupts).

Good god (you're thinking); how do I get some of this mad, antiviral action for myself? The trick with echinacea is that you have to take it at *the first sign* of cold or flu or viral outbreak. That means you need to take it at the *first* unusual sneeze, cough, sniffle, or itch, or take it before then if anyone in your general day-to-day vicinity is ill. You can take it a few days into a full-blown illness, but it's *much, much* more effective if you take it at the first signs. Try 900 mg per day in tincture or tea. You know you have a really stellar echinacea product if your tongue goes numb and tingly for a bit after you take it (no worries; this is temporary).

Besides being antiviral and antibacterial, echinacea is also anti-inflammatory and antifungal. So, no matter *what's* wrong with you — from sore or scratchy throats to stomachaches to urinary or kidney infections to cuts and scrapes (internal or external application) — echinacea is a good way to go. Of course, I'd be remiss if I didn't add that if you have an autoimmune condition, consult a physician before going forward with echinacea. Otherwise, this herb is totally safe — even if you're allergic to daisies, of which it's a family member.

If you're the kind of person who succumbs to perennial illness — like bronchitis or pneumonia *every* winter — or if your body (like mine) is just naturally slow to heal, then echinacea will transform your life. For some of my clients who deal with chronic illness, I just have them take echinacea daily for maintenance (two weeks on, one week off seems to be the best plan; it keeps the body fighting off illness on its own while also boosting immunity). Then, once the first sign of a cold comes on, I have them up the dose until they're symptom-free.

Echinacea is also great for stubborn cuts, scrapes, bites, or stings. I like to make a paste to apply topically. To do this, just open a few echinacea capsules into a small dish and stir in a bit of water. Many of the chronically sick have issues with candidiasis (yeast overgrowth) as well, which can be treated with tea or tincture internally. You need to make a lot of lifestyle changes in order to really beat a *Candida* overgrowth (such as a whole-food diet that's devoid of refined sugars and simple carbohydrates and that includes lots of fresh fruits and veggies), but you can do a lot with herbs (of course!). When taken daily, echinacea will help cull the yeast herd and get your body back to being a good home for friendly bacteria.

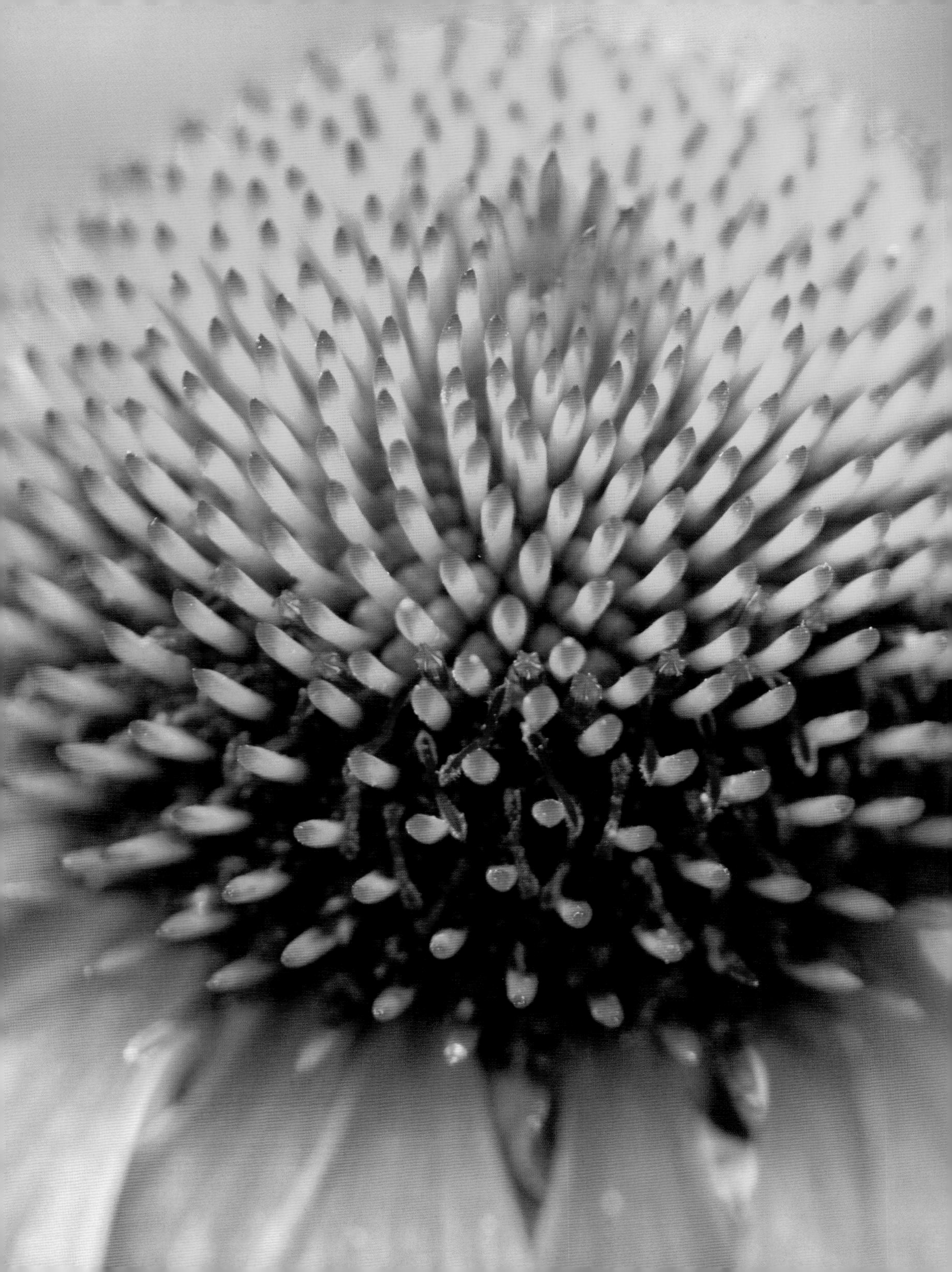

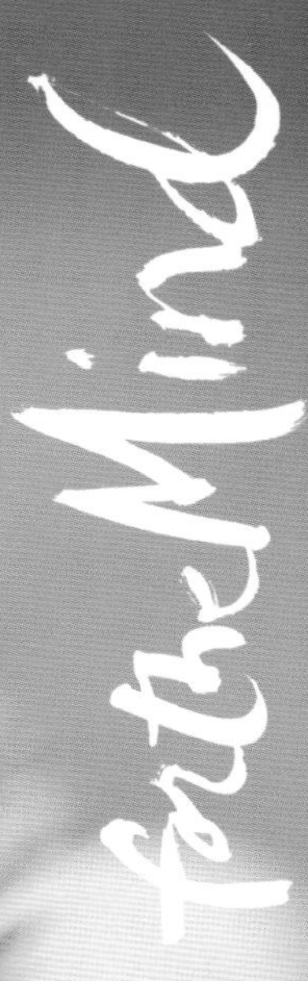

If you've explored the natural health field at all, you've probably come across the idea that the mind has a lot to do with the body and disease. Through my own experience and in counseling clients, I've come to believe that this is true for many of us (of course, lots of illness is just illness, but we've all seen how a positive attitude can benefit healing).

One of the causes of illness, according to those smarties in the flower essence field, is a lack of connection to our true minds, our true selves — knowing what makes us truly happy. We're so bombarded by images of what we *should* be and how we *should* look that we forget to get to know the person we really are. The body, mind, and soul into which we were born disappears, and we morph into some strange and uncomfortable version of ourselves. Without our vital, energetic connection to our own happiness, to knowing our own minds, we lose our ability to fight off everyday invading organisms.

Enter echinacea flower essence. The essence awakens that connection, reminds us of who we were before we were told who we should be, and brings our interests and our passions back into our day-to-day lives. You see, when you're not connected to what makes you truly happy, truly inspired, and truly passionate, the mind doesn't know what to do with all of that spare energy. So we become anxious, depressed, nervous, and withdrawn. All of that constriction saps our body of energy — energy that is vital for fighting disease and boosting the immune system.

So what makes the mind happy? Think of it this way: You know when you're wandering through a place (a field, forest, bookstore — whatever gets you going) and you suddenly become overwhelmingly excited and optimistic because you see something you connect to and love, and feel deeply in your soul that you were meant to understand, have, or do it? That feeling, right there, is true happiness. That's how we want to feel as often as humanly possible (and, yes, it is possible).

The benefits of this ongoing happiness are more than just a healthy body and mind. Suddenly your entire outlook changes; you have direction, passion, knowledge, and ability. I mean, think about what you could do with that kind of energy. Heck, you wouldn't have time to get sick.

So, if you're prone to chronic illness, chronic fatigue, or are fighting such long, debilitating illnesses as cancer, autoimmune syndromes (the flower essence is totally safe in this case, unlike the herb), or depression, then this essence is worth a try.

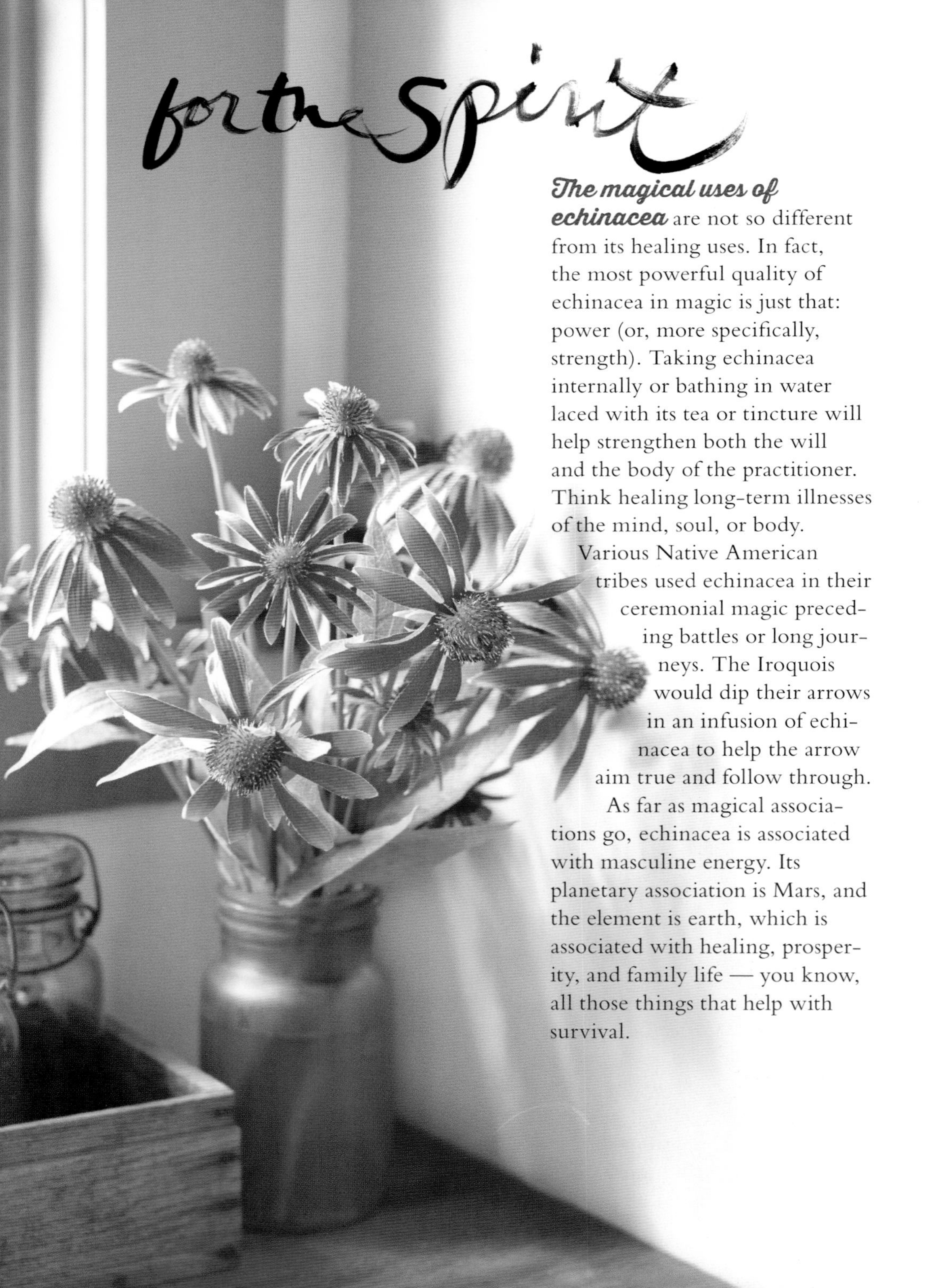

for the Spirit

The magical uses of echinacea are not so different from its healing uses. In fact, the most powerful quality of echinacea in magic is just that: power (or, more specifically, strength). Taking echinacea internally or bathing in water laced with its tea or tincture will help strengthen both the will and the body of the practitioner. Think healing long-term illnesses of the mind, soul, or body.

Various Native American tribes used echinacea in their ceremonial magic preceding battles or long journeys. The Iroquois would dip their arrows in an infusion of echinacea to help the arrow aim true and follow through.

As far as magical associations go, echinacea is associated with masculine energy. Its planetary association is Mars, and the element is earth, which is associated with healing, prosperity, and family life — you know, all those things that help with survival.

ECHINACEA MAGIC

AS SPELL STRENGTHENER

I'm not exactly sure why echinacea is a spell-strengthener, but I can guess. To me, echinacea signifies strength and resiliency in a (somewhat) hostile environment. Growing wild in the Great Plains — in poor, sandy, or loose soil; frequent droughts; hot sun; cold winters; and unforgiving wind — takes a heck of a lot of moxie. Not only that, but when we think about what echinacea does for the body, strengthening the immune system against invaders of all kinds, well, that's a pretty good calling card. I definitely want echinacea at my back.

When I'm setting intentions, meditating, or doing a little home brewing, I like to ask permission for and gather a few stalks of echinacea flowers. I set them in a big vase near my workstation and enjoy their quiet, sturdy presence. Next time you need a little grounding or a little encouragement, cut some echinacea flowers or carry a few dried blossoms in your pocket, your wallet, or a small parcel. Hang on to them when you need strength; use their innate dependability to enhance and echo your intent to the world around you.

FOR INCREASING VIRILITY

As far as I know, the herb itself has no medicinal effect on virility, but magically, it's been used to this end here and there within the annals of folklore (just think about its physical presence — the *coneflower* — and the way its winter stalk stands straight up against the flat grasses of the winter plains; you get the idea). Sprinkle a few coneflower petals on your food or the food of the person in question (be sure you have his permission, however). Cut stalks and place them under the bed for a little encouragement. Keep bouquets of the sturdy plant here and there around the house. Brew a strong cup of echinacea flower tea and offer the brew to the earth. Ask for strength, health, virility, and vitality — especially on a full moon. These nights are especially good when asking for fulfillment or increase of any kind.

FOR HEALING AND PREVENTING ILLNESS

As we've already discovered, the divine and the mundane uses of plants often go hand in hand. Naturally, an herb that is so physically powerful when introduced into the body must (logically speaking) have some magical effect as well.

Echinacea flowers, when picked (with blessing, after requesting permission) in full sun at the height of their bloom, are wonderful instillers of, and inspiration for, good health. Place an arrangement in a sunny window of the sickroom. Feed the patient a few echinacea petals or a sweet, mild echinacea brew. Dose it with honey and warm milk, offering comfort, well-being, and security through the sweet and earthy taste.

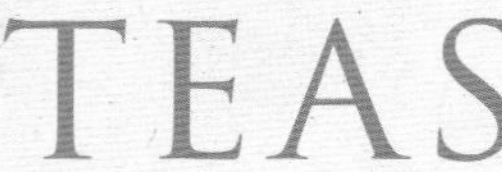

TEAS

Tea for boosting immunity. This tea is for short-term use (two or three weeks at a time is fine; just take off a week or two after that so that your system gets stronger and is able to fight colds and flu on its own). ***Note:*** Avoid sarsaparilla if you are pregnant.

Pour 3 cups spring or filtered water into a small saucepan. Add 1 tablespoon dried and chopped echinacea root, 1 tablespoon dried sarsaparilla root (this is the good stuff you find in root beer; it's also anti-inflammatory, antibacterial, and antiviral), 1 teaspoon dried gingerroot or 2 teaspoons grated fresh, and 1 stick of cinnamon. Place on the stove and simmer for 10 minutes. Remove from the heat and strain out the roots, pressing as much liquid out of the roots as you can (there won't be much). Add a little water back to your decoction until you again have 3 cups. Decant 1 cup into a mug, sweeten with honey, stevia, or maple syrup, and add nut or soy milk, if you like. Drink a cup a day when you feel ill or when those around you are ill.

Tea for treating candidiasis. Pour 3 cups water into a saucepan and add 1 tablespoon echinacea and 1 tablespoon burdock root. Simmer for 10 minutes, then turn off the heat. Add 2 teaspoons thyme and steep, covered, for another 10 minutes. Strain the decoction and pour 1 cup into a mug (feel free to add a little water to dilute this a bit). Add 3 drops black walnut tincture (an antiparasitic herb). Add stevia and an unsweetened nut milk (*Candida loves* sugar and dairy). Drink a cup every day on an empty stomach, and wait 20 minutes to eat so that the herbs are maximally digested and absorbed. ***Note:*** If you are pregnant or have an ulcer or thyroid issues, leave out the thyme. All of the other herbs are completely safe.

Tea for internal healing. Pour 3 cups water into a small saucepan and add 2 tablespoons echinacea and 2 tablespoons dandelion roots. Simmer for 10 minutes. Strain out the roots, then add honey to taste. When the brew is cool, pour it into a clean quart jar. Add enough water so that you have 3 cups. Add 2 tablespoons marshmallow root.

Cap the jar and stick it in the fridge overnight (this is called a cold brew; it's the best way to extract the soothing medicinals and mucilage of the marshmallow root). The next day, strain out the marshmallow. Pour 1 cup into a mug, add unsweetened nut milk, if you like, and drink at least three times a day on an empty stomach. You can drink this cold or at room temperature. The liquid should be thick and syrupy; just think of that coating all the irritated parts of the throat, stomach, and intestines. ***Note:*** Marshmallow root likes to soak up everything around it and hustle it through the body, so don't take any medicines or supplements 30 minutes before or after you drink this tea.

recipes

BODY CARE

Salve for Healing Bites, Stings, and Wounds

The worst part about stings, bites, and wounds is the radiating pain and/or itchiness they cause. Enter echinacea, plantain, and beeswax for relief.

You can make this salve the slow way (if you're prepping a good, strong salve to last you all summer) or the quick way, which is fine, but perhaps not quite as effective.

- **2 tablespoons plantain leaf**
- **2 tablespoons echinacea root**
- **1 tablespoon yarrow flowers**
- **8 ounces olive, almond, apricot, or coconut oil**
- **1 ounce grated beeswax**
- **16 ½-ounce tins**

Slow Way

1. To a clean pint jar, add the plantain, echinacea, and yarrow, and cover with the oil (add more oil if the herbs aren't covered). Keep the jar in a nice, sunny window, and shake it every day for 2 weeks or until the oil takes on the color and aroma of the herb. At the end of the incubation period, strain into a double boiler or a heat-proof glass bowl sitting above simmering water. Add the beeswax and heat gently over low heat until the wax melts.
2. Test the hardness of your salve by dipping a spoon into the mixture and placing it in the freezer for a few minutes. Is the salve too hard? Heat the salve and add more oil (a teaspoon at a time). Too soft? Add more beeswax (again, a teaspoon at a time). Once you're happy, decant into little lip balm tins and place these conveniently in your purse, medicine cabinet, glove compartment, or first-aid kit.

Fast Way

1. Add the oil to a double boiler or heat-proof glass bowl sitting atop simmering water. Gently heat the oil, and then add the plantain, echinacea, and yarrow and remove from the heat. Let steep for at least 30 minutes.
2. Strain out the herbs and return the oil to the double boiler or heat-proof bowl. Add the beeswax and heat gently until it melts.
3. Test the hardness of the salve as outlined above, then decant into lip balm tins.

Makes 8 ounces

Echinacea-Lemon-Honey Throat Spray

I love combining honey, lemon, and brandy anytime I'm sick. There's something so soothing about it. It reminds me of staying home sick and getting to go over to my grandmother's house (minus the brandy, of course).

You can also use this concoction as a tea. Just omit the apple cider vinegar and drink a cup whenever needed.

- **3 tablespoons echinacea root**
- **2 tablespoons slippery elm bark**
- **1 tablespoon lemon juice (or more, depending on taste)**
- **1 tablespoon apple cider vinegar**
- **1 tablespoon raw honey (or more, depending on taste)**
- **Brandy to taste (optional)**

1. In a medium saucepan, combine the echinacea root and slippery elm bark with 4 cups water. Simmer over medium-low heat for 10 minutes. Strain the herbs, and add the lemon juice, apple cider vinegar, honey, and brandy, if using.
2. Decant the liquid into a spray bottle (you can find these in the travel section of the drugstore). Shake before using and use as often as needed. It should keep for a few months at room temperature, but when you're not actively using it, it's best to store it in the fridge. You can also gargle with this brew.

Makes 16 ounces

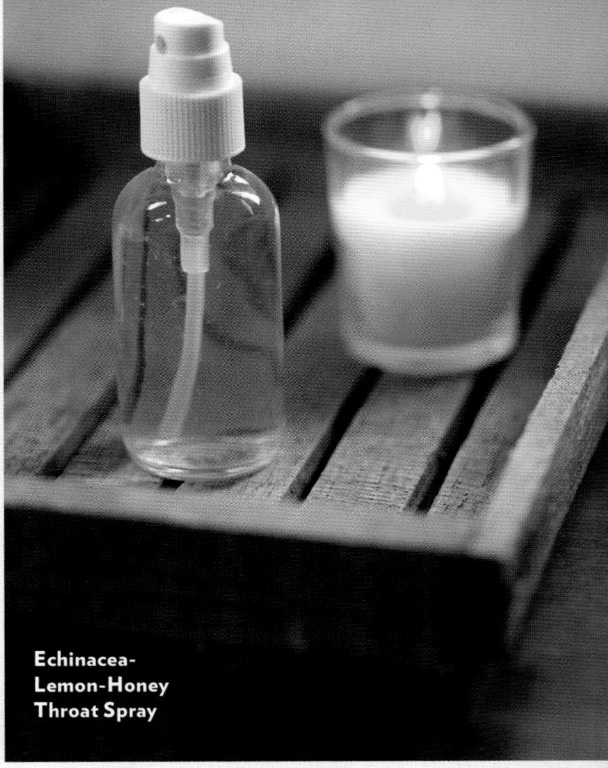

Echinacea-Lemon-Honey Throat Spray

Echinacea Wash for Yeast Infections or *Candida* Overgrowth

When you marry the immune-enhancing effects of echinacea with the yeast-destroying powers of good unpasteurized, unfiltered apple cider vinegar, plus the antifungal, antiviral, and antibacterial tea tree oil, you've got some amazing herbal juju right there at your fingertips. You can use this wherever the yeast infection appears, be it in the form of athlete's foot (use it as a foot soak), skin fungus (apply externally and bandage), or in the genital area (use as a douche or in the bath).

Recipe continues on next page

- 3 tablespoons apple cider vinegar
- 4 cups cool echinacea decoction (see page 180); use 1 tablespoon of dried root per cup of water)
- ½ teaspoon tea tree oil

In a medium bowl, mix together the vinegar, echinacea decoction, and tea tree oil. Stir well. Test a small area first for sensitivity. If this wash stings, dilute with more water and apply gently. Use this daily until the condition lessens and disappears.

Makes 16 ounces

Echinacea Vapor Rub

Vapor rub is a really good thing; it opens up the sinuses, warms and loosens the chest, and relieves coughing. The main problem with the store-bought variety is that it has a petroleum jelly base, and you don't really want those chemicals soaking into your vulnerable skin. So, instead, we turn to the magnificent, versatile oil-and-beeswax combo.

Note: Avoid thyme if you're pregnant, and peppermint (which may decrease breast milk) toward the end of your pregnancy and while nursing. Definitely don't use this rub on broken or irritated skin.

- ½ cup echinacea oil (see Appendix II)
- 2 tablespoons beeswax, grated
- 20 drops eucalyptus essential oil
- 10 drops sage essential oil
- 10 drops peppermint or thyme essential oil (depending on preference)
- 10 drops clove oil

1. Put the echinacea oil and beeswax into a double boiler or heat-proof glass bowl set over simmering water. Heat gently until the beeswax is melted. Remove from the heat and let cool 5 minutes.
2. Add the eucalyptus, sage, peppermint or thyme, and clove essential oils (if you're making this for kiddos, you can halve all the essential oils while keeping the echinacea oil and wax amounts the same).
3. Pour the mixture into a jar and use when hardened. If you need it now, apply it to the chest once it's cool enough not to burn. Once applied, place an old towel or T-shirt over your chest and keep the area warm with a heating pad or warm blanket. You can also rub some of this on the sufferer's feet. Trust me; it works and it feels amazing.

Makes 4 ounces

FOOD

Echinacea Popsicles

It's hard enough to get kids to take icky-tasting herbs like echinacea normally. But when they're sick? Yeah, you know how it is. Try these frozen treats and no one will ever be the wiser that there is a ton of immune-boosting herb power crammed in there. They are also particularly nice when the sufferer, child or adult, has a fever or a sore throat that needs soothing.

- **2 cups echinacea tea (1½ tablespoons dried herb per 2 cups water), cooled**
- **1 cup frozen berries of choice**
- **1 tablespoon lemon juice**
- **Honey, maple syrup, or stevia to taste**

Pour the tea, berries, lemon juice, and sweetener into a food processor or blender and blend until well mixed. Pour into popsicle molds or small paper cups with popsicle sticks in the center. Freeze until set (3 to 4 hours) and enjoy.

Makes six 3-ounce popsicles

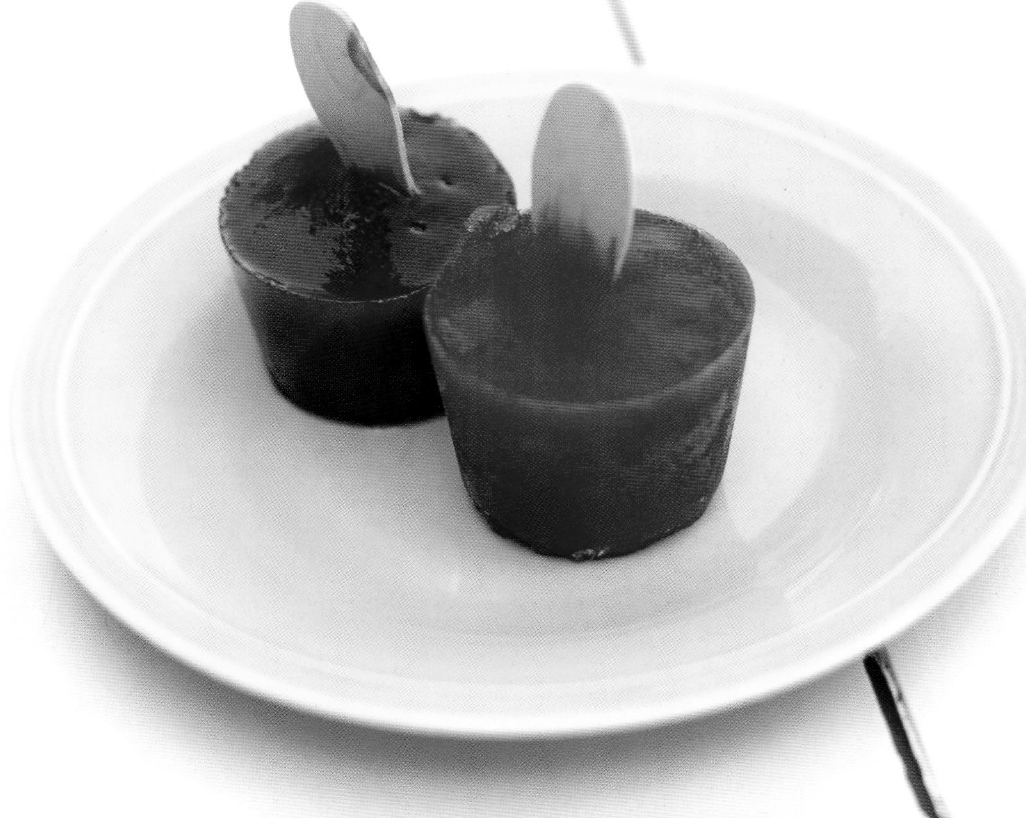

Echinacea-Lemon-Honey Jelly

As an herbalist, you need to be creative with the bitter herbs. Here's another "quick — hide the herbs in this sweet-tasting thing" recipe.

- **2 cups honey**
- **1 cup corn syrup or maple syrup**
- **1 cup echinacea tea (1 teaspoon herb per cup of recently boiled water steeped for 10 minutes and strained)**
- **3 tablespoons lemon juice**
- **1 pouch pectin**

1. Sterilize six 4-ounce jelly jars either by running them through your dishwasher or by boiling the jars for 10 minutes, adding the lids during the last minute. In a large saucepan, combine the honey, corn syrup, tea, and lemon juice. Stir and bring to a hard boil over medium-high heat. Add the pectin. As soon as the mixture comes to a rolling boil that can't be stirred down, start your timer; after 1 minute, remove the pan from the heat.
2. Skim off any film and pour the hot jelly in hot jars. Leave 1⁄8 inch headspace and screw on lids. Cool on a wire rack. Check the lids for a good seal, and store in a dark place for up to 1 year (any jars that don't seal can be stored in the refrigerator and used within a month).

Makes 24 ounces

Echinacea Maple Syrup

Here's another way to get some stellar immune-boosting power into kids or adults. As a bonus, you'll also receive all those good-for-you minerals found in real maple syrup. You can drizzle this syrup on your breakfast pancakes, stir it into tea, or take it by the spoonful to keep illness at bay.

- **2 cups grade B maple syrup (it has more minerals than grade A)**
- **2 tablespoons echinacea root**
- **1 tablespoon lemon juice**

1. Heat the syrup in a small saucepan over low heat for 5 minutes, or until just hot but not simmering. Add the echinacea and turn off the heat. Cover and let steep for 10 minutes.
2. Strain the syrup and stir in the lemon juice.

Makes 2 cups

ECHINACEA YOGA

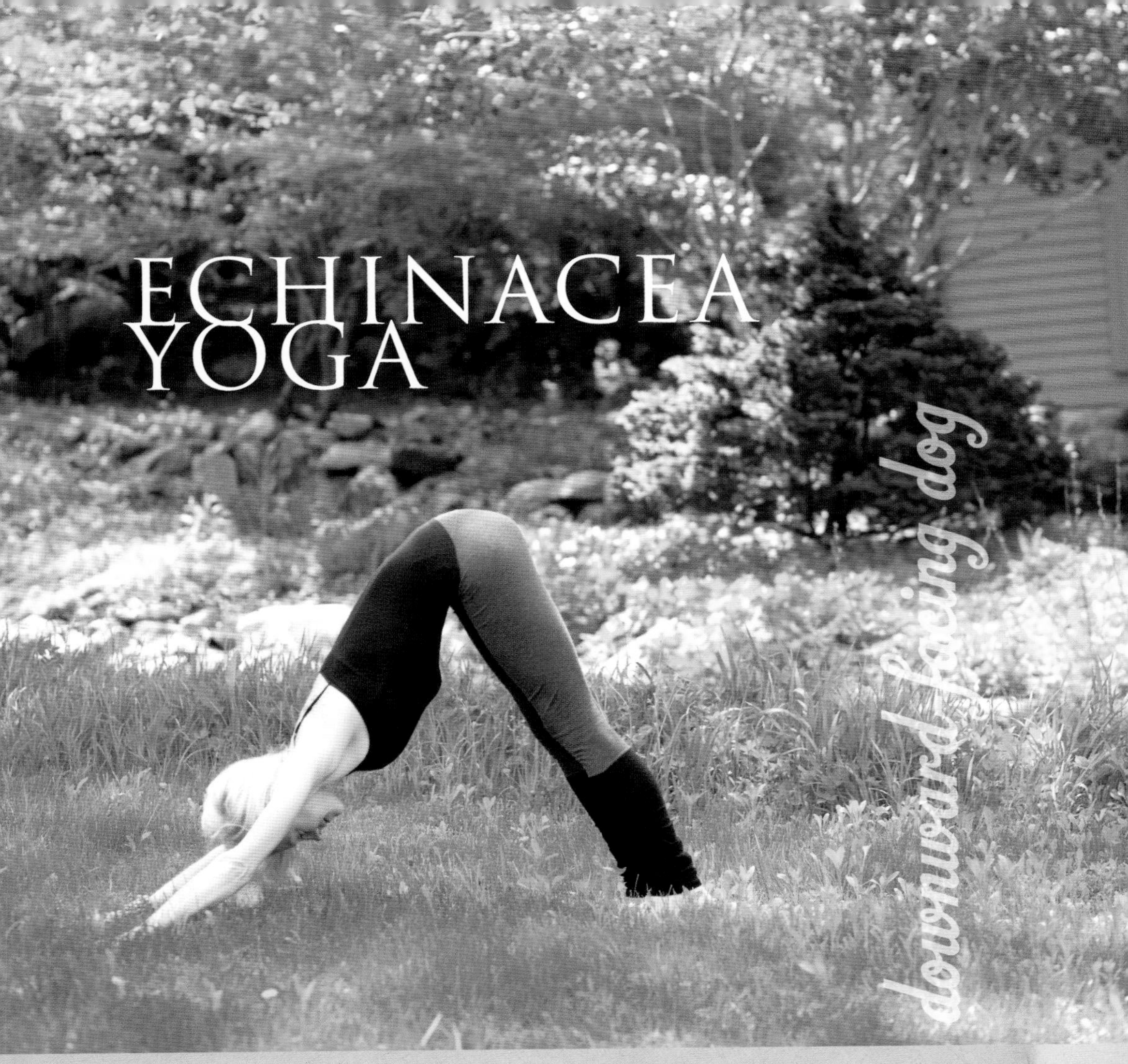

Since we've learned how well echinacea strengthens the immune system, we're going to do a strengthening and immune-boosting yoga pose. It's a little pose we like to call Downward-Facing Dog, Down-Dog for short (or *Adho Mukha Svanasana*).

Now, before we get into this, let your preconceived notions (read: hatred) of this pose drain right out of your head and stream away in little rivulets out your feet. I say this because if you've done yoga before, then you've probably learned this pose. And you probably hated it. I know most of my students do, and I did, too, when I first learned it.

Partly this is because the pose lengthens and stretches the sciatic nerve and hamstrings, which, in our culture of chairs and driving and desk jobs, tend to be tight and a bit shriveled. The sciatic nerve really, *really* dislikes being stretched, and it will let you know it in no uncertain terms. The other challenge inherent in this pose is the whole downward-facing bit. Your head is hanging between your arms, so the blood is rushing to your head and sinuses, making you feel uncomfortable.

Note: If you're *already* sick, skip this pose. Trust me, your congested head will thank you for waiting a day or two. But if you tend to suffer from chronic sinusitis, then Downward-Facing Dog will become your best friend. It opens up channels you never knew could be opened. This pose will also relieve chronic headaches, ease depression, and just give you an all-over good stretch and strengthening.

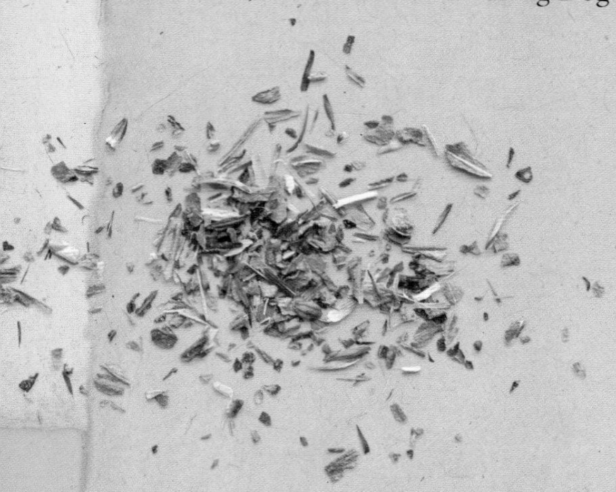

Starting position. Get down on all fours on your mat. Line up your knees under your hips and your hands a bit in front of your shoulders. Widen your fingers and really press those knuckles into the mat, especially your first finger and thumb. Ground here with your hands, making sure you're not slipping (a good mat will do wonders in this department; don't skimp on your mat purchase!).

Moving into Downward-Facing Dog. Inhale. As you exhale, start to straighten your knees — but don't go all the way just yet. Keep a slight (read: comfortable) bend. If you haven't warmed up yet, those hamstrings will be chattering away at you. You can do a few pedal pushes with the heels, just to get the blood flowing. Now, take a gander at your feet. We want them to be parallel to each other, so that means you'll probably have to push your heels apart a bit. Ah, feel that stretch down the outside of your calves? That's the stuff.

Draw your navel in toward your spine to lengthen your back while you tilt your sit bones toward the ceiling. This will stretch your hammies even more, so if it's too much, ease off. We don't want to stress your back here, so if you feel a pinch in your low spine, bend your knees more so you can stretch those sit bones, tilting them up.

Fine-tuning. Now try to lengthen your heels toward the mat (they may not make it, and that's totally fine — they may never make it, depending on how your bones are shaped; just do your best) and gently straighten your knees, but don't lock them. You may also find that you *just don't want* to straighten your knees. That's okay. Again, do your best.

From here, you want to rotate your thighs slightly inward. This just means that you're changing the shape of your pelvis slightly, making more room for your low back.

Finishing. Spend 30 seconds to 1 minute in Down-Dog. Let your head and neck relax. Breathe. You'll want to hold your breath, but don't. Breathe through the desire to stop breathing. When done, rest in Child's Pose (see page 55).

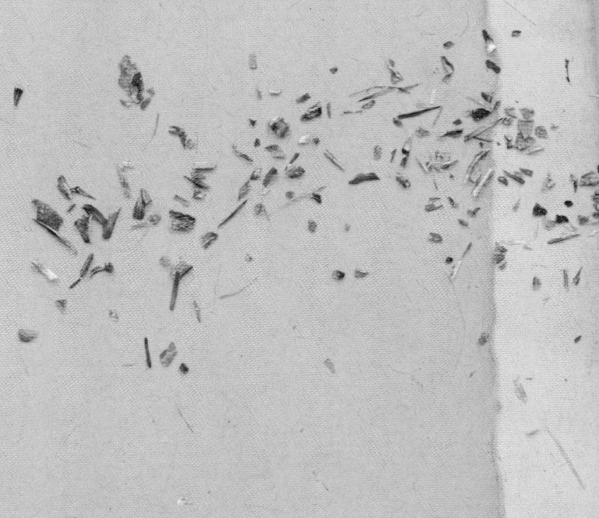

INWARD THIGH ROTATION

If you're not sure how to rotate your thighs inward, take a break for a moment and sit down on your mat or lie on your back. Stick your legs out straight in front of you. Now, from your *hip* (this is important, hence the carefully chosen italics), roll your legs outward. Your feet will look like duck feet, and your knees should point away from each other. That's outward rotation.

Now, bring your legs back to neutral. Next, do the opposite. Roll your legs in toward each other so that your feet are pigeon-toed. If you lie on your back and do this, you'll notice that during this *inward rotation*, your low back and upper pelvis open just slightly. If you *can't* feel that, there's nothing wrong with you, I promise. It takes time to become sensitive to these minor changes in the body.

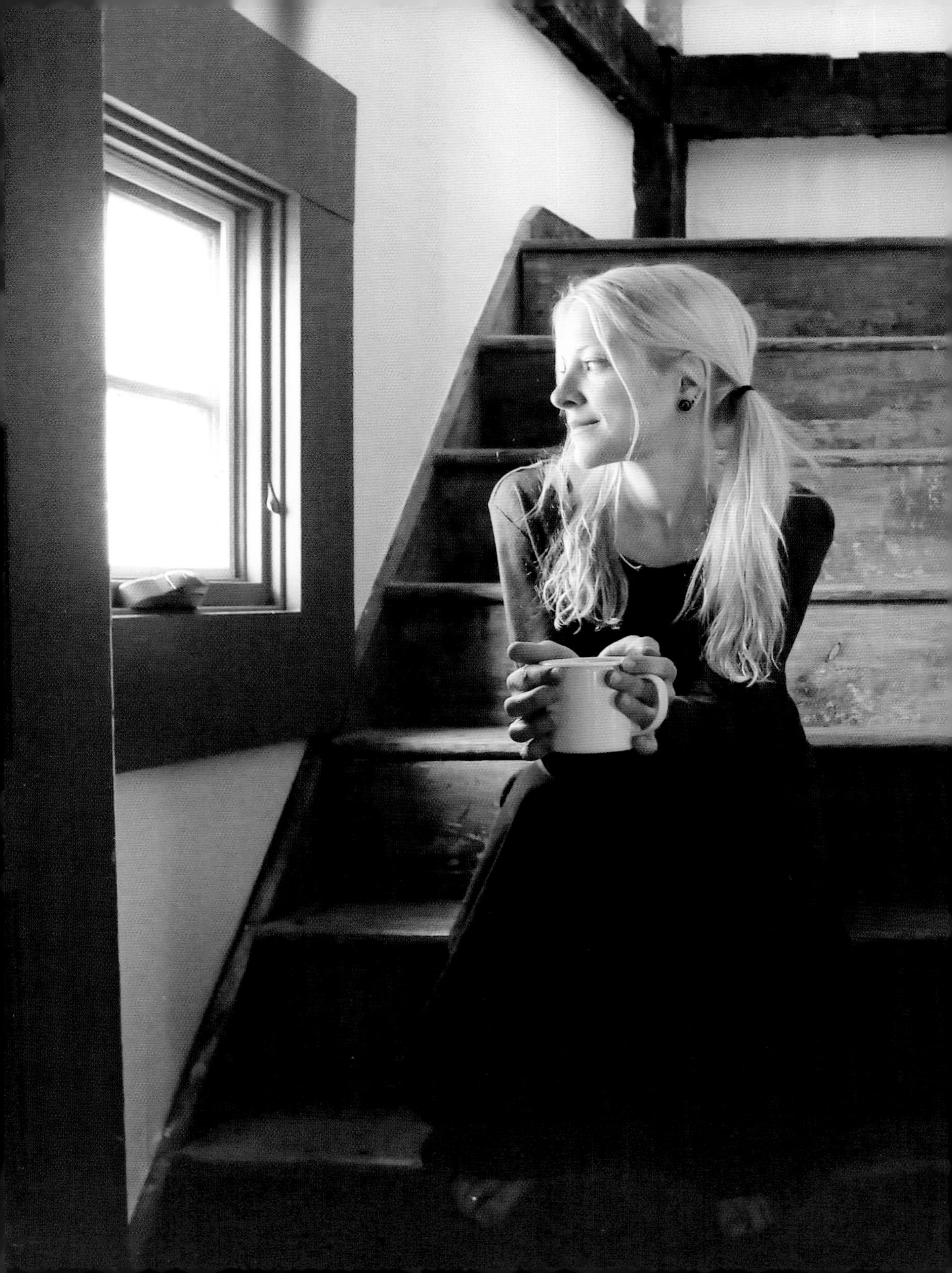

10

The Many Wonders of the ELDER PLANT

We have come to my absolute favorite herb: elder (*Sambucus nigra* and *Canadensis*). (Have I said that before about a different herb? Oh, probably. I think herbs are kind of like children: you love them all equally, but there are just some you sometimes like better than others.)

Not only is this herb insanely diverse; it's also just plain beautiful (ripe elderberries make the most fabulous blue-purple dye). There's also a ton of folklore associated with the elder tree, including faeries and underworlds. And I haven't even mentioned elderberry wine.

You can use the flowers, berries, and bark of this shrub, though I don't recommend using the bark unless you're working with an experienced herbalist. The bark has exactly the same qualities as the flowers and berries, but it's much, much stronger; in other words, all your systems need to be in good working order before using the super-strong medicine found in the flesh of the shrub. The berries and flowers are gentle and safe.

Most people think elder plants are trees, but technically they are shrubs. They tend to grow wild all along the East Coast, and even as far inland as the Central Plains. At my home in Maine, I would just scavenge the surrounding woodlands for elder. If you know what you're doing, you'll find elder everywhere. In June and July, look for fragrant white flowers growing in flat, star-like clusters. The deep purple-black, blue, or dark red berries arrive in late summer. The stems are greenish brown and, when broken, reveal a white pith. Leaves grow opposite one another and have an uneven number of leaflets (usually 5 to 11). I'm sure you don't need me to remind you to be sure you're confident identifying elder before you go picking berries!

For medicinal purposes, you want black or Canadian elder. Avoid red elder, as it tends to be a little too toxic for the human body (resulting in some uncomfortable digestion issues and poor assimilation). The flowers are the best-tasting and easiest part of the plant to harvest for herbal preparations; harvest these after they bloom, but before they wilt away. Pick in midday, after the dew has dried. Harvest the berries when they're ripe and pluck easily from the stalk. Never eat raw berries; they'll make you sick unless you cook or dry them — then they're perfectly safe.

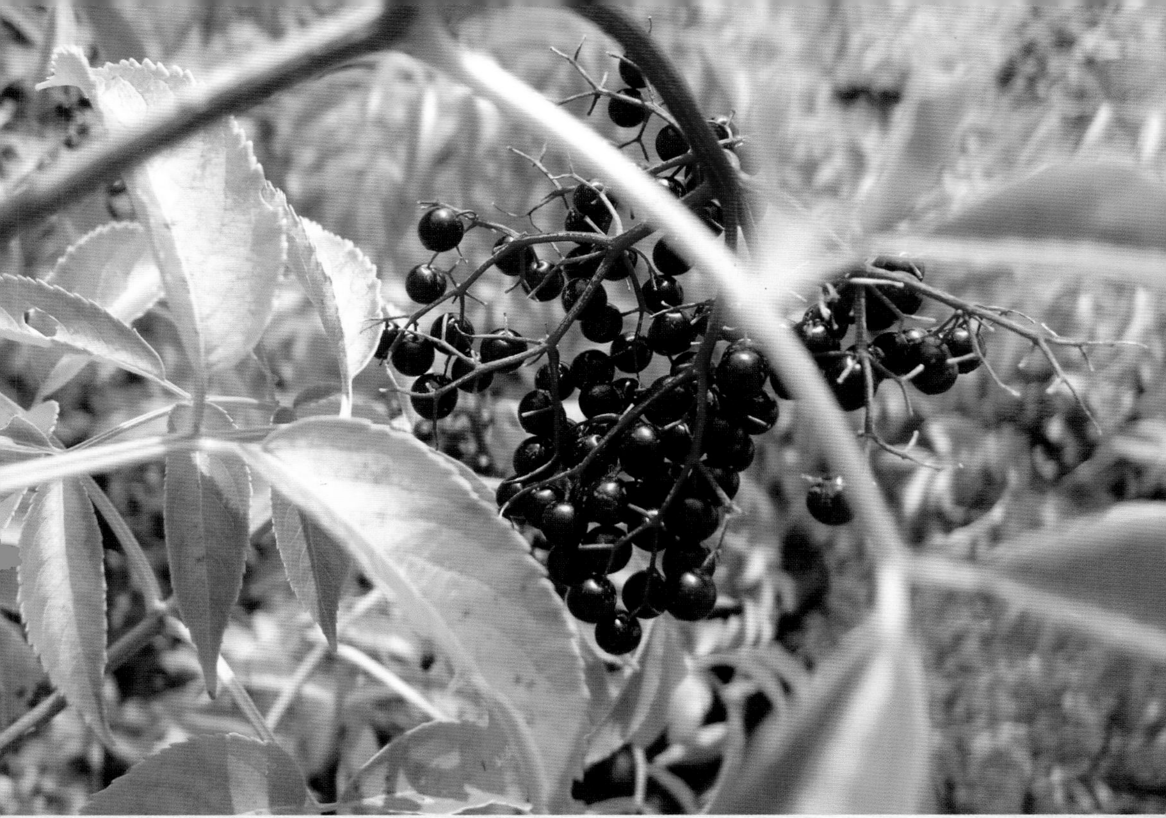

for the Body

Elder is what we herb nerds call a diaphoretic, which means that it brings blood to the surface of the body, causing the body to sweat. Why on earth would you want to induce a sweat? For one, if you're cold-blooded like me and you're constantly chilly, elder is a really good method of staying warm. You won't really sweat, but you'll be able to make better use of the heat your body produces. ***Just a note:*** You'll want to use fresh-flower tea to heat the body.

If you're a hot-blooded type of person, elder can help you cool down. As it brings blood to the surface of the skin and induces sweating, your body releases heat. This is really useful if you have what's known in Traditional Chinese Medicine (TCM) as a "hot condition." Use dried flowers for this benefit.

But elder isn't just for opening up the pores and vessels of and near the skin; it also opens up every channel of the body. These channels include blood vessels, bronchioles (those bits that, when closed, make it difficult to breathe), colon, and kidneys — basically anything that pumps or transports anything. This opening up allows fresh oxygen to move more swiftly and easily through the body, bringing energy and health to stagnant organs. It also allows waste to be removed more quickly and easily. This action is relaxing and good for things like spasmodic coughs.

Finally, elder is also an astringent, which means that it tightens tissues. This makes it good for cleansing and toning the skin as well as soothing sore throats, drying mucus, and easing such conditions as bleeding gums, ulcers, and sores in the mouth.

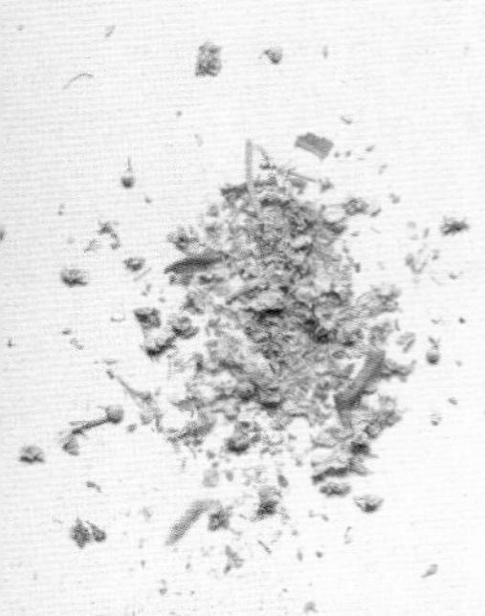

All that I've described are benefits of the fresh or dried flowers, as well as the berries. But the burgundy-colored berries also help build the blood. All that color indicates a rich supply of nutrients vital to healthy blood and organs, especially vitamins A and C. And all that vitamin C makes elder a fantastic virus (read: cold and flu) fighter. Brew up a cough syrup or flu-fighting tea (see page 197) as soon as the sniffles show up. Of course, a nightcap of elder cordial or wine (see page 203) isn't such a bad idea, either.

ELDER

Sambucus nigra and *Canadensis*

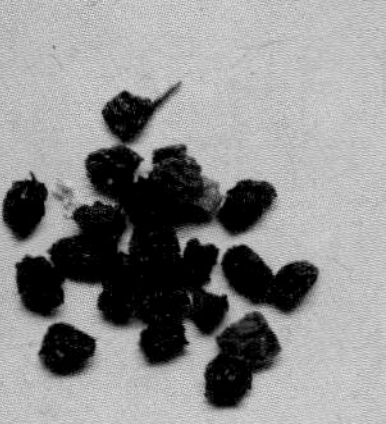

Parts used: Berries, flowers

How to harvest: Elder grows wild, so if you're foraging, choose a spot far from a roadside and well away from any potential pesticide/chemical fertilizer use

Effects on body: Immune-boosting, astringent, nutritive

Effects on mind and spirit: Opens channels, moves stuck energy, inspires joy and resolve

Safety first: Always, always cook or dry your berries. Though raw elderberries aren't life-threatening, they might make you ill. Never, ever ingest the bark.

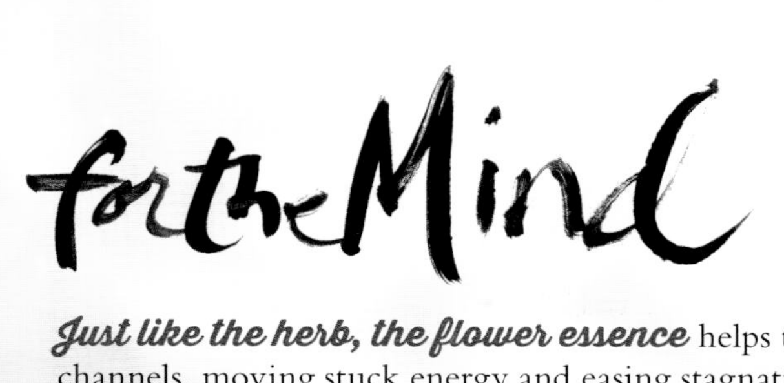

for the Mind

Just like the herb, the flower essence helps to open channels, moving stuck energy and easing stagnation. Use the elder essence when you feel helpless, hopeless, overwhelmed, or stuck in one place or pattern. Or, use it to gently redefine and ground yourself if you feel as though you're constantly drawn into other people's orbits, unable to disentangle your own energy from theirs.

Elder helps you send down your own roots, inspiring your own sense of joy and resolve. When you feel grounded, protected, and safe, you are able to explore your own personality, and your own wants and needs, without undue influence of those around you. That same deep, nutrition-laden quality of the elder plant reintroduces itself in the flower essence, giving you a new sense of vigor, strength, and (inner and outer) beauty.

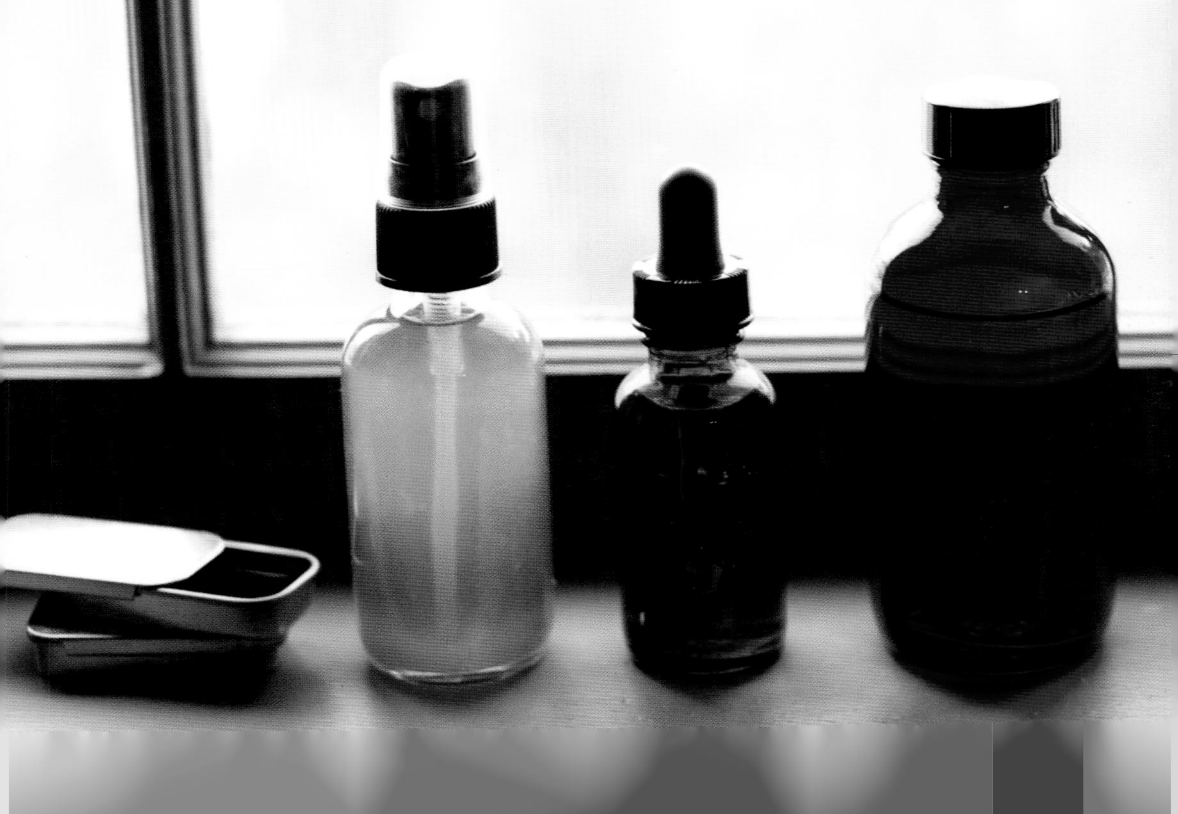

for the Spirit

Elder, perhaps even more so than any other herb we've explored thus far, has a long, long folk and spiritual history. The folklore goes as far back as pre-Christian Britain, Ireland, and Scotland (the Celtic trifecta). There, elder was called "Hylde Moer" ("Elder Mother"), in part because elder was so versatile and could heal (or at least help) pretty much any condition.

"Little Elder Mother" was said to dwell in the tree, and it was through this place that one could enter the dominion of Faerie. When the plant was in flower, it allowed anyone sitting beneath it on Midsummer (the summer solstice) to see the troops of faeries marching past. So, you definitely wanted to take care around the elder plant, and you certainly didn't want to fall asleep beneath it, lest you awoke in that foggy between-time known as Faerie.

Not only could elder heal the body, but it was also believed that pleasing (or at least thanking) the Elder Mother would help bless and protect the land as well. Native Americans, for instance, placed offerings beneath elder shrubs before harvesting from them, thanking the seemingly powerful plant spirit for her offering. Elder was thought to ward off malevolent forces and spirits, keep away storms and plague, and protect livestock and homesteads.

Elder is associated with the planet Venus, the female gender (the crone, to be specific — she is Elder Mother after all), and the element water. It is used in spells for protection, banishment, health, prosperity, and wisdom, and for gaining sight and direction. Because elder marks the entrance to the underworld, it's also associated with the darkest time of the year — Yule or midwinter. Because the underworld is, well, kind of dark and scary, elder is a protection against this dark time of the year, reminding us that it is a necessary phase before the inevitable rebirth in spring. Taken a bit deeper, elder is also a reminder that no energy is destroyed; it only changes form, which means that there is, in reality, no true death, just transformation.

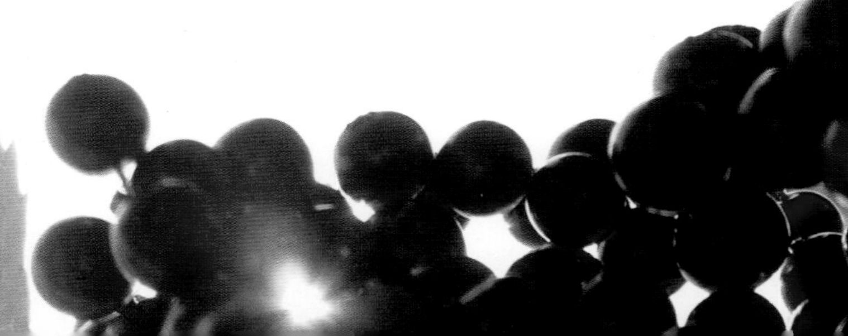

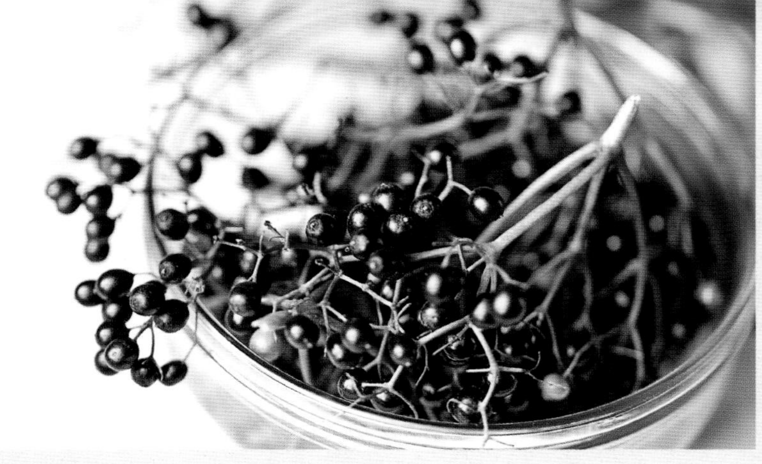

TEAS

Flu-fighting tea. Elderberries make an incredibly flavorful and comforting beverage for the cold and flu season. Simply simmer 1 tablespoon dried elderberries and 1 teaspoon elder flowers (if you have them) in 1 cup water for 10 minutes. Strain, then add honey or sweetener of choice, a dash of lemon, and a touch of brandy (optional but especially good if you're trying to get to sleep). Feel free to drink three cups a day. You probably won't have any discomfort from this tea, but a few individuals can experience intestinal discomfort. If you do, just scale back the frequency of the dose, or cut the quantity of elderberries in your brew.

Tea for breaking a fever. Elder and yarrow flowers are ideal for breaking a fever. Now, remember: Most fevers are perfectly normal and you can let them run their course; all a fever is doing is raising the body's temperature enough to make it an inhospitable environment for the current unwanted tenant. Nonetheless, fevers are uncomfortable and it's nice to get them over with as quickly as possible.

Put ½ tablespoon elderflowers, 2 teaspoons yarrow flowers, and 1 tablespoon chamomile flowers in a preheated mug (if making it for kids, use 1 teaspoon of each herb). Pour a cup of boiled water on top, cover, and steep for 10 minutes. Strain, then add honey and lemon juice to taste. Adults can drink a cup four times daily (and it's safe for women who are pregnant or breastfeeding).

ELDERBERRY MAGIC

FOR PROTECTION

When you have a plant called "the queen of herbs," you can be pretty secure in its innate power to protect. The shrub itself has long been planted on properties, not just because it can help treat almost anything, but because the plant itself has such protective properties.

Carry some leaves, flowers, or berries with you when you travel. Place windfall branches over doors or windowsills (you can cut branches, but never burn elder — it's considered bad luck). Alternatively, you can drink a strong elder tea or sprinkle elder infusion around the perimeter of your house for extra protection.

TO CULTIVATE STRENGTH AND SOFTNESS

Drinking and/or bathing in an herb is a great way to bring the strength of the plant into your body. Use elder when you're trying to be persuasive. Similarly, use elder before making big purchases, signing contracts, or doing any other scary thing that needs strength of will but softness and openness of spirit. Elderberry wine is a fantastic way to erase anxiety while keeping presence of mind and strength of will. (Just don't drink *too* much and lose presence of mind along with the anxious thoughts!)

FOR PROSPERITY

The easiest, and arguably most effective, way of keeping prosperity close is to grow the shrub in your garden. The growing plant has some powerful juju. You can also gather a few leaves and slip them into your wallet or purse, allowing the natural attraction of the plant to draw prosperity to you.

Drink the tea or bathe in elderflower-infused bathwater before a big interview or a possibly lucrative meeting. Carry a few flowers in your pocket when you go to the interview (or even gift your interviewer with a bouquet from your garden or a bit of elderberry wine). Remember: All that really matters is intention. The right herb just helps transmit your intention to the universe.

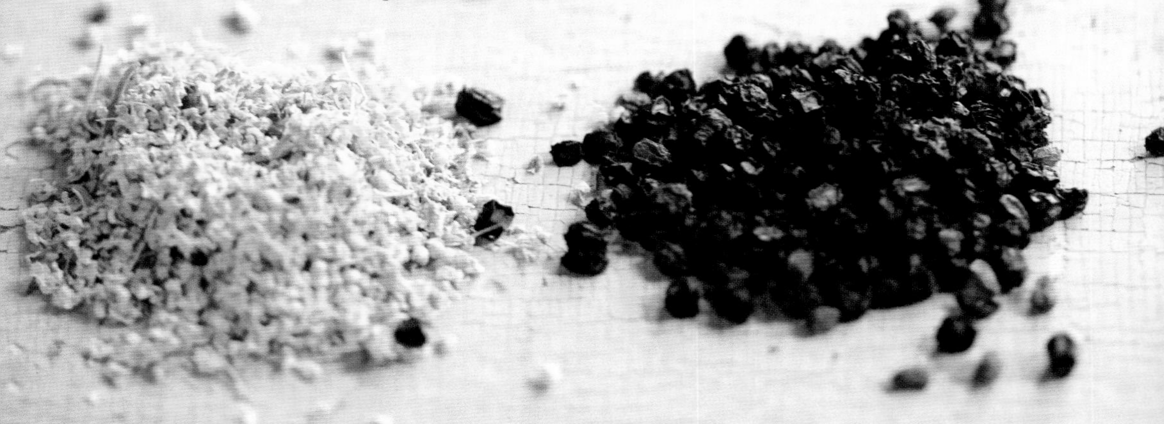

Note: If your fever persists longer than a few days or is higher than 103°F/39°C, seek medical advice.

For kids under 1 year old, drink 1 teaspoon of tea every 3 hours (minus the honey), up to four doses per day. For kids ages 1 to 2, drink 2 teaspoons every 3 hours, up to four doses per day. For kids over 2 years old, drink ½ cup every 3 hours, up to four doses per day. Keep hydrated, everyone.

Tea for internal inflammation. For every cup of water, use 2 teaspoons elderberries, 1 teaspoon dried ginger (or 2 teaspoons fresh), and 1 teaspoon marshmallow root. Put the berries and gingerroot in a small saucepan, add water, and simmer, covered, for 10 minutes. Strain into a clean jar and let cool to room temperature. Add the marshmallow root, cover, and refrigerate overnight. The next day, strain and drink a cup, hot or cold, adding sweetener and nondairy milk to your taste. You can drink up to three cups a day. **_Note:_** Don't take any medicines or supplements 30 minutes before or after you drink this tea, since marshmallow tends to hustle them through the body.

Elderflower tea for detox. For every cup of water, use 1 teaspoon elder flowers. If you tend to be a cold person (I'm talking temperature, not temperament), or you're in the dead of winter, throw in a cinnamon stick — it's good for warming the body and moving the blood. If you're a hot person (again, temperature, not

HOW TO FIND THE RIGHT HERB

Often, there are many herbs you could use to treat one condition (a virus like the cold or flu, for instance). How do you know the right one to use, when, and on whom?

Partly, that intuition comes with trial and error, your own experience, and your own journals, but I think part of it can also come by learning the history of a plant and its spirit (its essence, aura, or energy). For example, since elder is associated with the crone, perhaps this would be a better remedy than echinacea for building health in an older individual.

Whatever you do, follow your interests. When you let go of your expectations, you'll find that you instinctively design your own journey, educating yourself in a way that honors your curiosity and deepens your awareness of the world around you.

catwalk material), try adding 1 teaspoon sage. Pour boiling water over the herbs, steep 10 minutes, and strain. If using cinnamon, drink hot; if using sage, drink cold or at room temperature. Drink one cup at a time and feel free to sweeten and/or add non-dairy milk to your taste.

Tea for insomnia. Here, we're talking about the type of insomnia that occurs in the middle of the night, after you've already been sleeping for a bit. It's usually accompanied by sweaty, agitated, and annoyed discomfort. Depending on what time you're waking up, this kind of insomnia is usually caused by blood sugar (high or low) or an organ detoxing (such as liver, kidneys, or lungs, each of which has its own accompanying emotion of fear, anger, or anxiety). (This all comes from Traditional Chinese Medicine or TCM; see the Resources section for more information.) Elderberries lower the temperature of the body and steady the blood sugar while lemon balm calms anxiety, cools the body, and relaxes the mind.

Bring 4 cups water to a boil. Put 2 tablespoons elderberries and 2 tablespoons lemon balm in the bottom of a quart jar, and add the boiling water. Let steep 10 minutes, strain, and drink right away or bottle and stick in the fridge. You could also pour the cooled tea into ice cube trays, freeze, and then pop the cubes into a plastic bag in the freezer. Whenever you need a dose of tea, gently warm the cubes until just melted or heated through. Four large cubes equals about 1 cup.

BODY CARE

Elder Chest Rub for Easing Asthma

Remember our vapor rub from the previous chapter (page 184)? We're going to use the same basic recipe, but with different herbs. This is the beautiful thing about these recipes — once you know them, you can just change up the herbs, depending on what's going on in the body.

Note: All of these essential oils are safe for kiddos, adults, and pregnant or breastfeeding women.

- **½ cup elderflower oil (see Appendix II)**
- **2 tablespoons beeswax, grated**
- **10 drops ginger essential oil**
- **10 drops lavender essential oil**
- **10 drops chamomile essential oil**
- **10 drops rose essential oil**

1. Add the elderflower oil and beeswax to a double boiler or a heat-proof glass bowl set over simmering water. Heat the wax until it melts, then remove from the heat and let cool for 5 minutes. Add the ginger, lavender, chamomile, and rose essential oils.
2. You can pour this salve into a jar and use it once hardened or, if you need it now, apply once the salve is cool enough not to burn. Once applied, place an old towel or T-shirt over the chest and keep warm with a heating pad or warm blanket. You can also rub some of this on the sufferer's feet.

Makes 4 ounces

Elderflower-and-Carrot Anti-aging Mask

I love it when the stuff I put on my face is like food. This one, I guess, *could* actually be food. It will keep in the fridge for a day or so, but there are no preservatives in this particular recipe, so it's best to use it immediately after you make it.

Carrots contain vitamin A (also known as retinol, which should be a familiar word if you ever read antiwrinkle-cream ads). Vitamin A helps keep the skin toned and youthful. Add to that the antioxidant power of elder and the moisture-drawing qualities of honey, and you have seriously good food for your face.

Recipe continues on next page

2 tablespoons dried elder flowers
1 medium carrot, grated
1 teaspoon honey
1 tablespoon oat flour

1. In a small bowl, combine the elder flowers and enough warm water to cover. Soak just long enough to rehydrate the flowers (about 5 minutes). Strain, reserving the liquid.
2. In a medium bowl, combine the grated carrot and elder flowers. Mash together, then add the honey and oat flour. Mix until the paste is sticky enough to hold together. If it's too dry, add some of the reserved elderflower water; if it's too wet, add a little more flour.
3. Here's the fun part: Put on an old T-shirt, stick your clean hands in the bowl, and coat your face with this foodie goodness. Relax 10 minutes or so, then rinse with warm water.

Makes 1 treatment

Elderberry-and-Milk Cleanser

This is a super-gentle cleanser you can use daily. Milk adds vitamin D to your skin, honey moisturizes, oats exfoliate, and elderberries add antioxidants (another one of those cosmetics you could actually eat). Honey is a good preservative, so feel free to make enough for a week at a time; you can store it right in your bathroom (no need to refrigerate).

1 tablespoon powdered milk (goat's milk, cow's milk, or buttermilk)
1 tablespoon oatmeal flour (or grind your own in a food processor or coffee grinder)
3 teaspoons honey
Brewed elderberry tea (you won't need much, but brew some with 1 cup water and 1 teaspoon berries)

1. In a small bowl, combine the powdered milk and oat flour. Add honey and dribble in enough water to make a thin paste. Mix well.
2. Wet your face and apply the cleanser with your fingers, massaging in small circles. Rinse with warm water.

Makes enough for 3 applications

FOOD

recipes

Elderberry Wine

It is just wicked fun to gather friends together to go elderberry picking, go back to someone's house (the one with the biggest kitchen) and make big batches of wine, and then get together a year later to celebrate opening that first bottle.

- **4 quarts loosely packed ripe elderberries (you really have to use fresh ripe berries for this, not dried)**
- **6 cups cane sugar (I like evaporated cane juice)**
- **1 cup organic raisins, chopped**
- **1 ½-inch piece of ginger, chopped**
- **2 cinnamon sticks**
- **2 teaspoons whole cloves (optional)**
- **5 wine bottles and corks**
- **5 balloons**
- **Sealing wax (optional)**

1. De-stem your elderberries. To do this, you can use a fork or a wide-toothed comb, or simply freeze the stems for a couple of hours and just shake off the berries.
2. Preheat a gallon-size mason jar by filling it with really hot water from the tap and dumping out the water. Add the de-stemmed berries, ginger, cinnamon, and cloves.
3. Bring 2 quarts of water to a boil, and pour over the jarred elderberries, leaving 1 inch of headspace at the top of the jar for the fermenting berries to expand.
4. Drape plastic wrap over the mouth of the jar, secure it with a rubber band, and loosely put on the lid (you want some venting space). Place the covered jar in a sunny place — either in a window or outside if it's warm enough — for 3 days.
5. Bring in your jar and strain the liquid through cheesecloth, a wine bag, or a jelly bag. Squeeze the life (i.e., the juice) out of those berries and return the juice to your jar. Stir in the sugar. You want the sugar to dissolve, so if your fermenting juice isn't warm enough, heat just enough water to dissolve the sugar and then pour this into the juice.
6. Add the raisins (these are the magic fermenting ingredient), and cover loosely (I use a clean tea towel and rubber band). Keep in a warm, indoor place for 3 weeks. Here's where we really begin bubbling. The raisins, with their yeast-growing ability, should do the trick, but if you don't see bubbles within a couple of days, add a commercial wine yeast so your wine doesn't become moldy.

Recipe continues on next page

7. Strain the liquid again, squeeze out the raisins, and decant into sterile, narrow-necked glass bottles (such as old wine bottles or mineral water bottles). Okay, the fun part: Slap a balloon over the mouth of the bottle (the gases from the yeast will expand the balloon; it's very cool). Once the balloon stops expanding, then cork the bottle tightly and store it on its side. You can go ahead and seal this with wax, if you like. Age for 1 year before you pop the cork.

Makes approximately 1 gallon

Elderberry Syrup

This is one of my favorite ways to take elderberries. Since I'm not a fan of honey, I usually replace it with good, grade B maple syrup (local, if possible). This is also a good option if you're making this for kiddos under 1 year old.

To take this sweet remedy, try a tablespoon either on its own or dissolved in some warm water. This is especially fabulous first thing in the morning during the cold and flu season.

- **1 cup fresh or ½ cup dried organic elderberries**
- **½ teaspoon clove powder**
- **1 teaspoon ginger powder**
- **1 teaspoon cinnamon**
- **1 cup raw honey or grade B maple syrup**

1. In a medium saucepan, combine the berries, clove, ginger, cinnamon, and 3 cups water. Bring everything to a boil, then reduce the heat and simmer for 30 minutes (the water will boil off a bit; that's okay).
2. Using a potato masher or the back of a ladle, smush all the berries into the liquid, then strain the whole business. Let cool for 10 minutes.
3. Add the honey or maple syrup and blend well. Bottle and store in the refrigerator. It should keep for about 3 months.

Makes 8 ounces

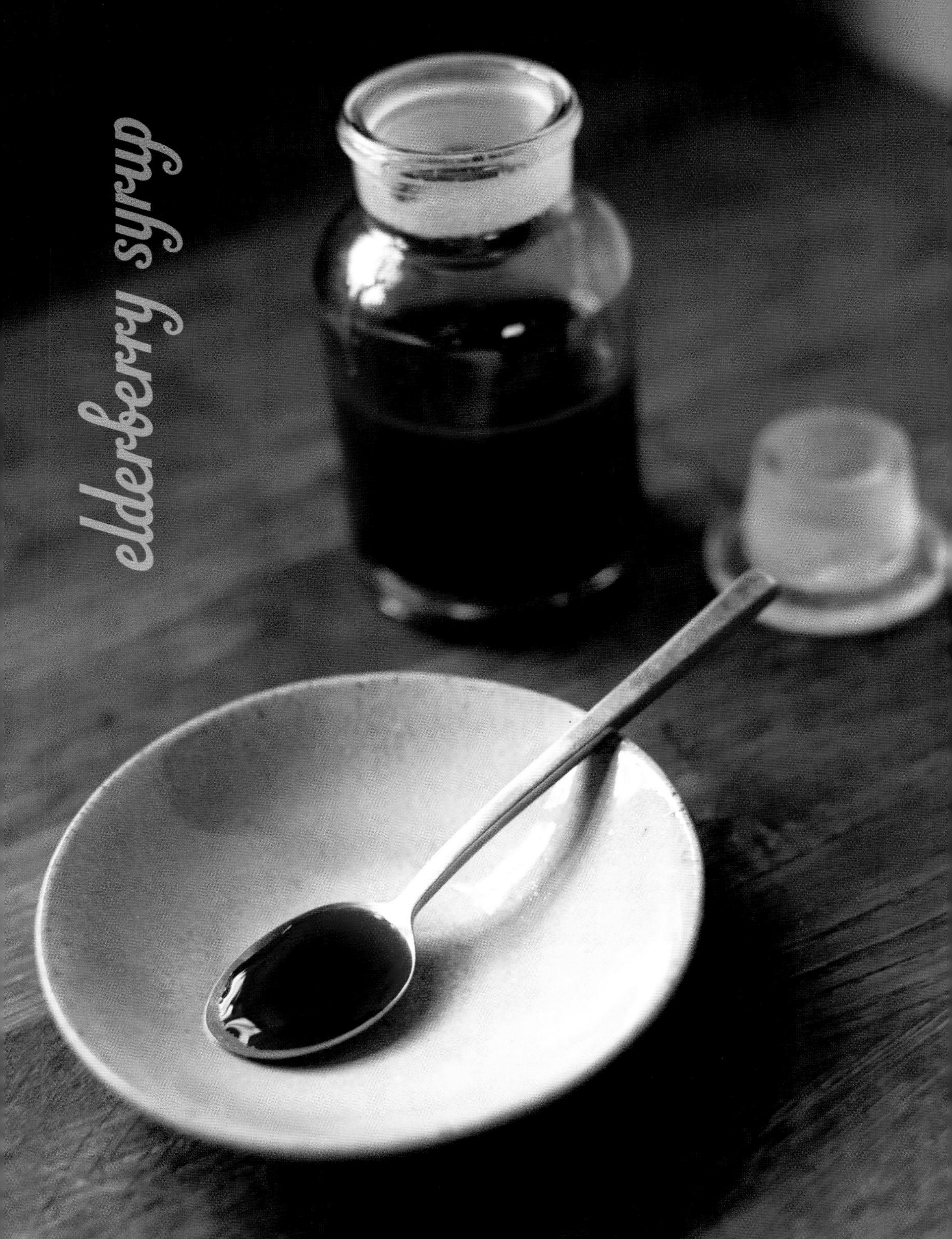
elderberry syrup

Elderberry Toffee Cookies

Um, look at the title. Do I need to say anything else?

- 1 cup butter (vegan or dairy)
- 1 cup brown sugar
- 1 egg or vegan substitute
- 2 cups flour
- ½ teaspoon salt
- 1 teaspoon vanilla
- 1 8-ounce package milk chocolate chips or 8-ounce bar
- 2 tablespoons dried elderberries
- ¼ cup nuts of choice, chopped (optional)

1. Preheat the oven to 350°F/180°C and line a baking sheet with parchment paper.
2. Cream together the butter and brown sugar. Add the egg and mix well. Add the flour, salt, and vanilla and mix together. This makes a super-stiff dough.
3. Using a butter knife, spread the dough very thinly over the baking sheet until it's about ¼-inch thick. Place another piece of parchment on top and another cookie sheet on top of that, and press down on the top cookie sheet. You're making a cookie crust, basically. Remove the top sheet and parchment, then place the dough in the oven and bake for 15 to 20 minutes.
4. While the dough is baking, simmer water in a small saucepan. Once it simmers, turn off the heat and place a heat-proof glass bowl over the water (it's okay if it touches the water). Pour the chocolate and elderberries into the bowl and stir until the chocolate melts.
5. Remove your cookie crust from the oven and let it cool a few minutes. While it's still warm, spread the chocolate mixture over the crust. Sprinkle nuts, if using, on top of the chocolate (or sprinkle whatever the heck catches your fancy). Let the chocolate harden, then cut into squares. The cookie crust is crunchy and gets better after it sits for a day or two in an airtight container, if you can make it last that long.

Makes 3–4 dozen cookies

ELDER YOGA

Because elder magic (and medicine) is all about opening channels and transitioning, I thought it would be good to do a little transitioning on the mat. In general, we spend so much time focused on the beginning of a journey and the end result that we rarely notice the transitions. The same holds true in our yoga practice. We focus on a certain pose in a sequence, hoping to get it as "right" as possible, then move on to the next pose, not realizing that the transition *between* poses is as much a pose as any other. You're still breathing, you're still aware, so it must be important. If you're taking the time to move from place to place, pose to pose, then the journey must be as important as the destination.

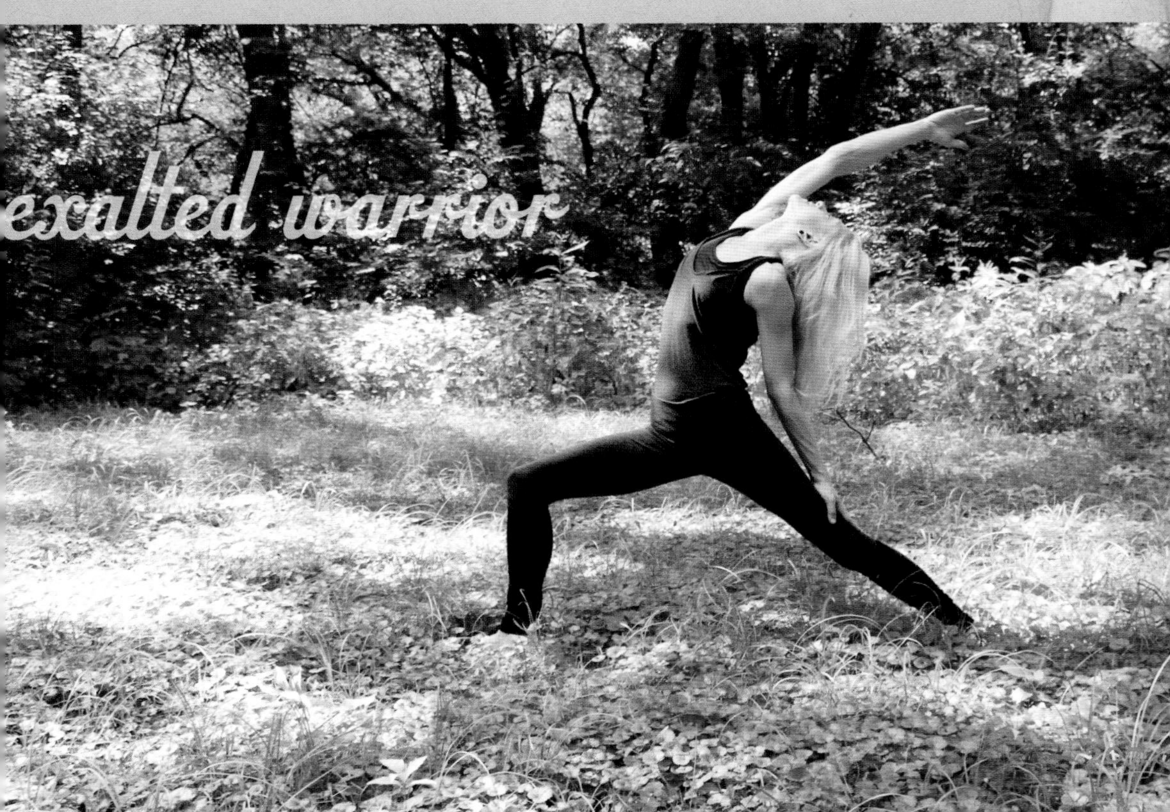

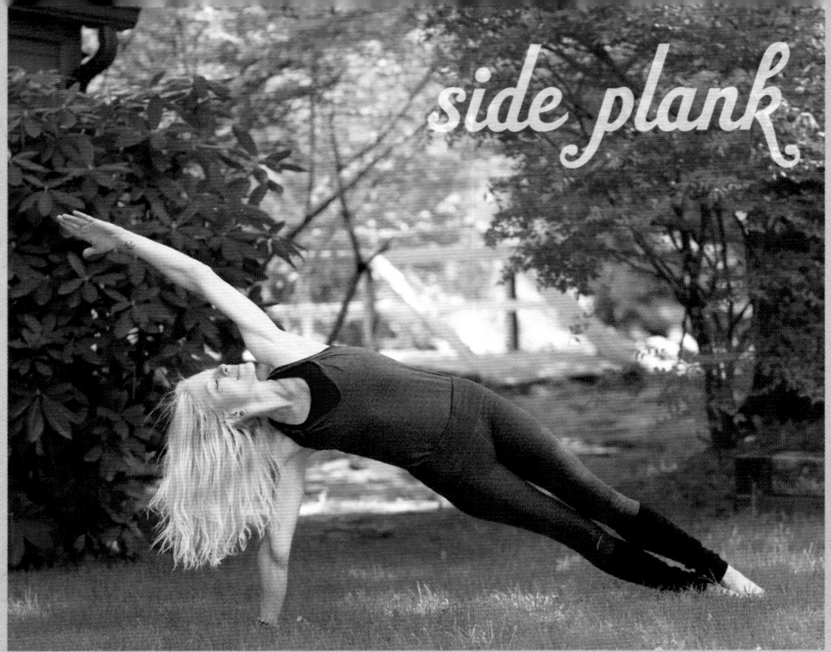

To appreciate and become fully aware of the transition between poses, we're going to move carefully and slowly so that we feel every muscle do its part to get us from A to B. We're going to start in turmeric's pose, Warrior II (*Virabhadrasana II;* see page 168), and transition into Exalted Warrior and then into the Side Plank (*Vasisthasana*).

Beginning in Warrior II. Move yourself into a nice, steady Warrior II pose. Let's start on the right side (meaning your right leg will be the bent one and you'll be looking out over your right hand). Breathe here for a few moments.

Transitioning into Exalted Warrior. Now we're going to add a little flair to our transition (we're healers, herbalists, and heralds of the earth spirit; we like flair). Inhale and flip that right hand over so that your palm faces the ceiling (or the sky, if you're lucky enough to be outdoors). As you inhale, keep lifting your arm up and back, allowing your left hand to lower until it reaches (or reaches toward) your back left leg. Your torso, chest, and head will all follow this movement as well.

Your movement is kind of like a big seesaw; your right hand is the kid on the seat going up, hoping your left hand (the kid on the seat going down) won't suddenly step off the darned thing. This pose is called Exalted Warrior, and trust me, you'll feel that whole exalted thing as you stretch your right arm up toward the sky.

Transitioning into Side Plank. Now, exhale and come back down through to Warrior. Keep going until you can rest your right hand on the floor. Now, begin to place your weight in that right hand, especially through your first finger knuckles and your thumb. Then bring your right knee down and step your left foot out so that it rests in line with your hips behind you, instep to the floor (you'll be in one long line, supported by the lowered knee).

Reach your left arm up to the sky, straight out of your left shoulder. Engage your core and pull up through the sides of your waist. This will keep you stable and keep you from dropping into that right hip. If you're feeling the stability here, feel free to step your right foot out to meet your left. That right foot can either come in front of the left for the sake of balance, or you can stack them, left on right. Keep reaching your left arm toward the ceiling, looking out into the distance or, maybe, even up at that extended hand.

Keep your right, supporting, arm engaged. Hug it into your shoulder socket and keep pressing through your knee (if it's on the ground) and the sides of your feet, continuing to lift through your waist and hugging your thighs toward each other. Hold there for a few breaths.

Transitioning back into Warrior II. If you're completely stacked in the pose, then return your right knee to the mat. Placing both hands on the ground, use them to support you as you get that right foot beneath you. See if you can — by engaging and coordinating the breath, your core, and your right quadriceps — draw back and up with your left hand, bringing yourself back into Warrior II.

Finishing. You can switch sides here, or keep this sequence going a few times. I only ask this: that you move slowly through these transitions (as if you're moving through the richest maple syrup you can imagine or, if you're feeling feisty, elderberry syrup). Each moment of the transition is its own pose; it takes up its own space, its own varied muscles, and its own emotional and physical response. All of those aspects of the pose are important. Feel them. Be in them. Use the spirit of elder to ground those feet; that will give you the freedom and confidence to let the rest of you soar.

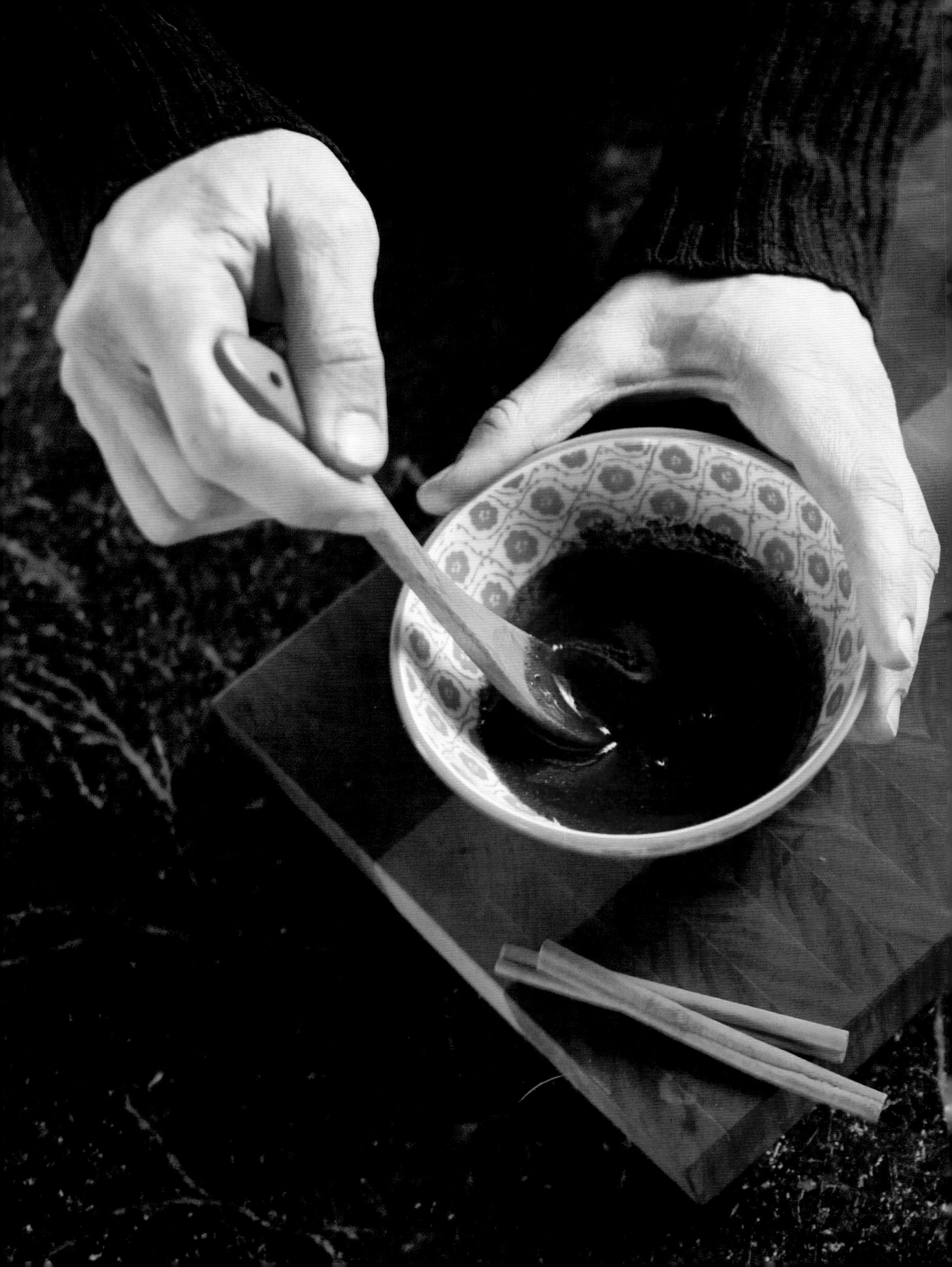

11

Versatile and Singular CINNAMON

For me, no other scent induces a bout of nostalgia more so than cinnamon (*Cinnamomum cassia*). Whether I'm doing a little holiday baking, steeping cinnamon tea, or simmering a few sticks on the stovetop to instill a warm atmosphere on a damp winter day, I'm instantly brought back to childhood and all that cheery, warm holiday fuzziness.

Think about your own memories and associations with cinnamon for a moment. What comes to mind? Warmth? Ease? Excitement? Optimism? Happiness? Comfort? Well, there's a reason for that.

Cinnamon is warming and flavorful, associated with cold winter days and festive holidays. It helps you digest heavy foods while keeping your blood sugar steady. It's not really a surprise that it shows up in indulgent holiday baking.

Most likely, you haven't considered cinnamon to be a medicinal plant; most people are surprised to learn that it functions as anything other than a kitchen spice. Most spices, however, are herbs (as we'll see in the next chapter as well), and it's no coincidence that we find them in particular foods and during particular times of the year.

CINNAMON

Cinnamomum cassia

Parts used: Inner bark of the tree

How to harvest: Strip the bark from smaller branches; never take cuttings from the trunk (for the sake of the health of the tree)

Effects on body: Warming, stimulating, astringent; promotes and enhances digestion

Effects on mind and spirit: Joy-inducing, freeing, inspiring

Safety first: Avoid medicinal doses (in other words, large doses — anything other than amounts used for flavoring) while pregnant or breastfeeding; though rare, some people have a cinnamon allergy, so go slowly if you have allergic tendencies

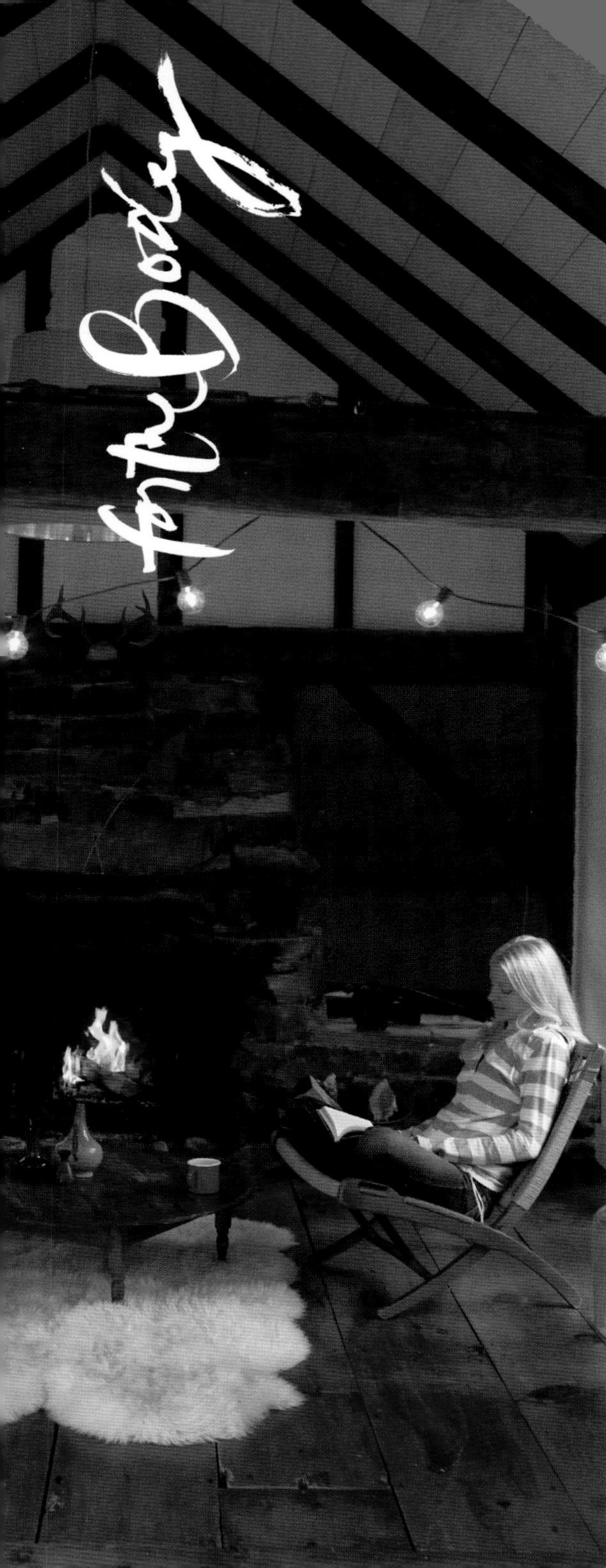

We've already touched on cinnamon's ability to warm the body, making it perfect for winter consumption. It's stimulating as well, so the next time the sun begins to set at 4 P.M. and you still have hours to go before you sleep, brew up a warm and energizing pot of cinnamon tea (which will also get the digestive system primed and ready and in peak shape).

Cinnamon is also an astringent. Astringents tone tissues, which is why you use them on your face to prevent sagging and tighten pores. When taken internally, cinnamon can help halt bleeding (especially good postpartum) and stem diarrhea, especially when there's been a lot of fluid lost. In this case, cinnamon eases chills brought on by those nasty digestive upsets, while also stabilizing blood sugar if there's a loss of appetite.

Speaking of appetite, cinnamon helps digestion and prevents flatulence, bloating, heartburn, and nausea. Since it helps stabilize blood sugar and appetite, warming and stimulating the whole system, it's a great herb for supporting weight loss and a powerful ally when one is dealing with type II diabetes.

Cinnamon's antibacterial, antimicrobial, and antifungal qualities make it a wonderful addition to cold and flu remedies, with the added bonus of masking the flavor of less appetizing herbs. The essential oil of cinnamon (when mixed with a carrier oil) is warming and healing for strained muscles, fungal infections, and cuts and scrapes.

for the Mind

The cinnamon tree has incredibly spicy-sweet and fragrant flowers, which bees and birds find irresistible. They're small and creamy white to yellow in color, and the scent itself is uplifting, reminding us (there's that nostalgia factor again) of the burden-less joy of ideal childhood. So it's not really all that surprising that the cinnamon flower essence would connect us with that inner child, bringing to the fore that bubbling fountain of extroverted joy and ease and the effortless ability to be thoroughly in the moment.

Think about childhood for a moment. Expression and invention were at your fingertips; you didn't need to sit and find time to create, did you? You were by nature a creative, and creating, being. Ideas flowed so readily that they were your reality, not a fantasy that you had to drum up in brainstorming meetings, think-tanks, or stream-of-consciousness painting or drawing.

Cinnamon flower essence will help you express yourself creatively and with ease by bringing those latent expressive abilities, so often lost with childhood, to the forefront of your daily life. The added bonus? By feeling and expressing your emotions, you are "unpacking" your emotional baggage and leaving the bags behind. I mean, think about it — how many two-year-olds hold a grudge? They feel it, they express it, and they move on. How freeing is that? Once these latent emotions can be loosened and expressed, joy comes more readily to us.

You can take cinnamon flower essence over a period of time, as you slowly begin to let go of old patterns and states of emotional disease. Or take it before making a big presentation, walking on stage, speaking in public, or showing up at a family gathering or party (especially if you're an introvert like me).

for the spirit

Cinnamon's element, unsurprisingly, is fire, and the fiery heavenly bodies it's associated with should also come as no surprise: the sun, Mars, and Mercury. Cinnamon also carries a masculine-gendered energy. Long used as incense, cinnamon is a wonderful aid in cleansing, clearing, and purifying sacred spaces, such as temples, altars, and hallowed land. It raises energy — both the surrounding energy as well as your own — and is helpful in boosting success and protection, honing your intent, and aiding and clarifying psychic visions. It energizes the nervous system and sharpens instinct, thought, and impressions. Just don't bathe in it or anoint yourself with its undiluted essential oil — it's pretty strong stuff and can hurt sensitive skin.

Cinnamon is also pretty versatile in magical workings. You can ingest it, burn it, or carry cinnamon sticks or chips in a pouch on your person. No matter how you choose to use it, it will help draw positive energy to you (whether that's in the form of luck, money, love, or success — whatever you're working toward).

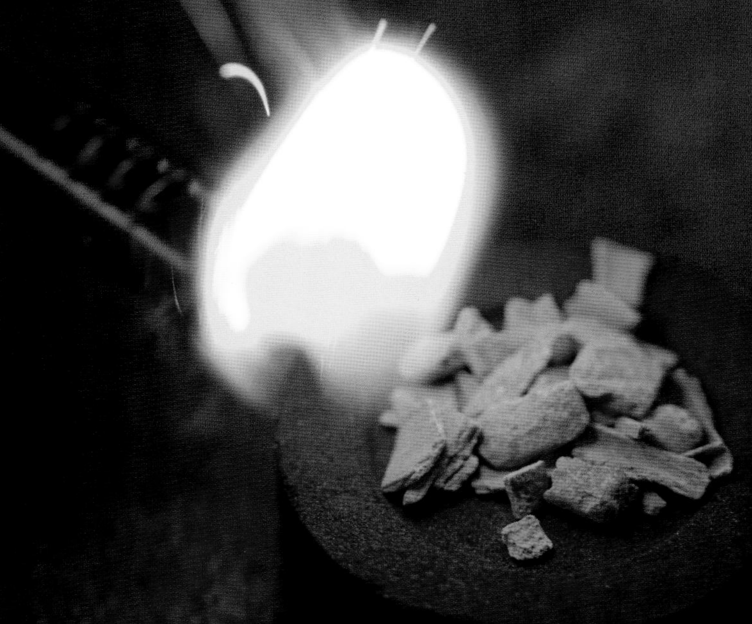

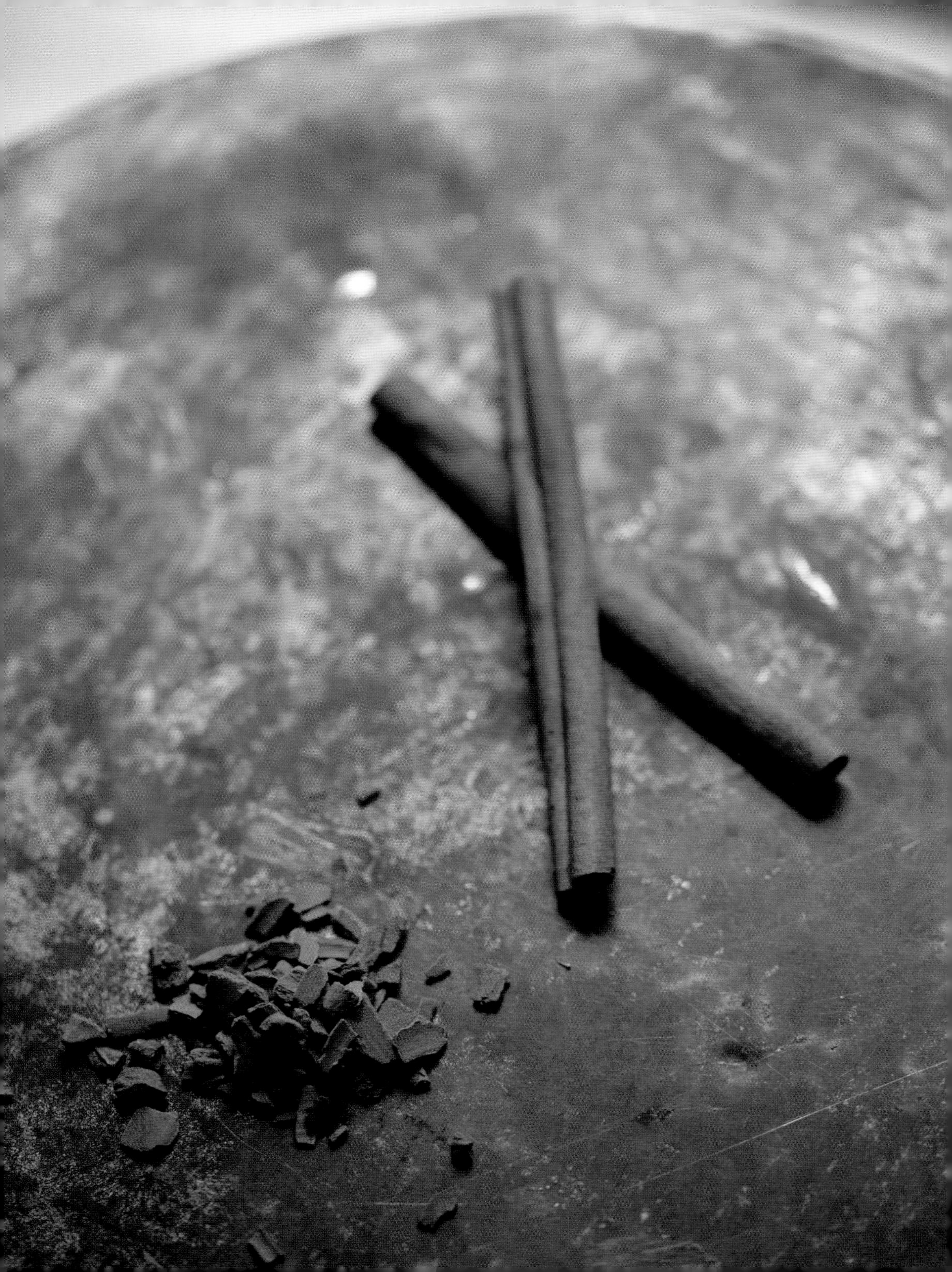

CINNAMON MAGIC

TO INSPIRE SUCCESS

I'm a big believer in the power of scent, and, as we've discovered, cinnamon's scent carries a lot of nostalgia and power. When I need a little boost of courage or confidence, I pour a few drops of cinnamon essential oil into a teaspoon of carrier oil (such as almond) and anoint my pulse points. Not only does the scent make me feel powerful, potent, and secure, but it also fires me up, warms my blood, and raises my awareness of the environment around me.

Don't want to smell like a cookie? That's okay. Just carry a vial of cinnamon essential oil (or even cinnamon gum or candy will do in a pinch). Take a sniff before a big moment, after a minor setback (real or imagined), or when confronting a person with whom you're uncomfortable. Cinnamon may not be able to speak for you, but it allows you to do something even better — confidently speak for yourself.

FOR HAPPINESS AND HARMONY

Here's another olfactory spell, redolent of the first day of winter, cozy fires, wool socks, and homemade cookies. After a terrible, dreary, hard day, I like to simmer a bit of water on the stove and toss in a few cinnamon sticks (you'll notice these have a different scent from the essential oil; while the oil is pungent, fiery, and powerful, the simmering sticks are warm, subtle, homey, and welcoming). I turn the heat way down and just keep this cooking all day long (be sure to keep an eye on the water level, though — don't let it all evaporate). Sometimes, after a seriously horrible day, I just stand over the stove and inhale the steam (from a safe distance), releasing my troubles into the steam and letting the resulting space fill with warmth, comfort, and security. Cinnamon helps you remember that there is good in the world, even when things seem darkest.

FOR MANIFESTATION

Cinnamon oil and simmering cinnamon are definitely powerful juju. But what about burning the cinnamon as incense, using the smoke to heighten and strengthen your intent? Now that is some kind of power right there.

When I'm working with intention, manifestation, or wish fulfillment, I always feel like I need an extra boost. In these cases, I turn to incense. I usually light a small charcoal disk and either sprinkle some cinnamon powder (for short-lived incense) or cinnamon chips (for a longer, slower smolder) on it. I close my eyes and meditate, focusing first only on the scent of the smoke, then second on my intention. I marry my intention to the scent and the smoke and let it rise, making my wishes known and, at the same time, offering this smoke as a gift of thanks to whoever is listening.

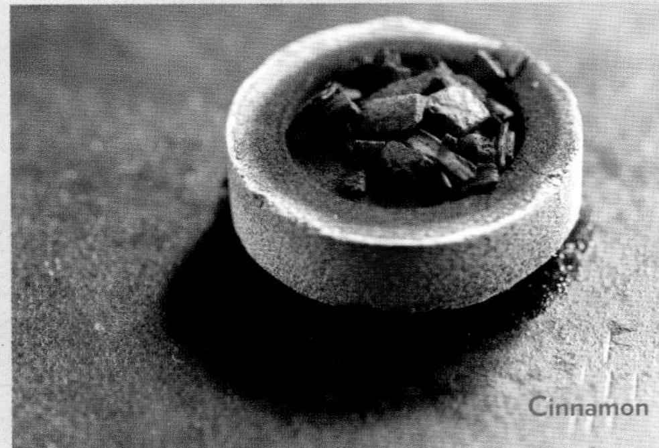

TEAS

Cinnamon tea for blood sugar. I like to simmer up a big quart jar of cinnamon tea and keep it in the fridge, just for ease of access. Pour 4 cups water into a small saucepan and add 4 good-quality (organic) cinnamon sticks. Cover and simmer for 10 minutes, then doctor with stevia (a sweetener that won't affect your blood sugar), unsweetened nut or soy milk, and a dash of vanilla. If you battle high blood sugar (hyperglycemia), drink this tea 20 minutes after your meal, and if you battle low blood sugar (hypoglycemia), drink it throughout the day on an empty stomach.

Cinnamon tea for digestive complaints. Pour 3 cups water into a small saucepan, and add 1 tablespoon each of fennel, licorice root, and cinnamon chips (or one stick cinnamon). Simmer, covered, for 10 minutes. Strain and sip 20 minutes before or 30 minutes after a meal. You can doctor this tea up, but try to keep some of the pungent flavor of these potent aromatic herbs (in other words, don't make a frappe-type sweet drink this time around). Drink daily, if needed. ***Note:*** If you have low blood pressure, substitute anise for the licorice.

Cinnamon tea to instill warmth in the body. In a small saucepan, combine 3 cups water, 1 tablespoon cinnamon chips (or one stick), 1 tablespoon gingerroot (fresh or dried), ½ teaspoon rosemary, and ¼ teaspoon sage. Cover and simmer for 10 minutes. Doctor to your taste.

Holiday cinnamon tea. Boil 4 cups water in a medium saucepan. Remove from the heat and add 3 cinnamon sticks, 1 tablespoon grated fresh gingerroot (1 teaspoon powder), ¼–½ teaspoon nutmeg, 1 tablespoon cardamom pods (1 teaspoon powder), ½ teaspoon allspice, and 1 tablespoon fennel seeds. Simmer for 10 minutes or longer, depending on how strong you like this stuff. Strain and pour into preheated mugs. Add a few drops of vanilla extract, sweetener, and a bit of milk. Sip hot or iced, as often as you'd like.

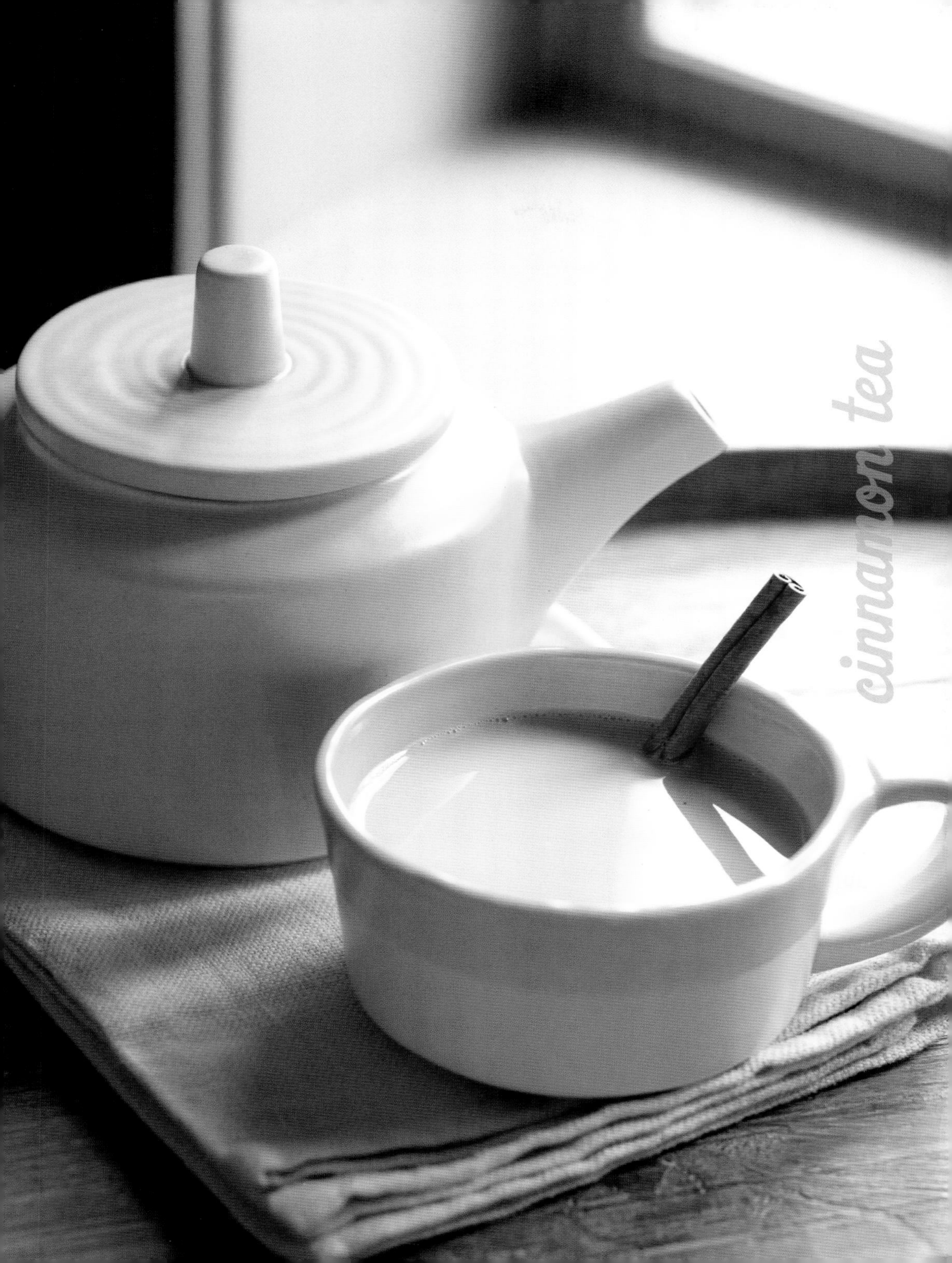
cinnamon tea

recipes

BODY CARE

Cinnamon-Coffee Skin Scrub

This little invention is probably the best holiday gift I've ever concocted. I think it was inspired by a much-needed cup of coffee one early winter morning that I happened to lace with cinnamon. I sat in my pj's, watched the snow, and thought "Man, it would be awesome to bathe in this brew." Thus, this scrub was born.

If you're a coffee drinker, you can use your brewed grounds in this recipe (recycling!), or you can buy a small package of coffee, brew it, and use the grounds.

- ½ **cup brewed coffee grounds**
- 1 **tablespoon ground cinnamon**
- ¼ **cup sugar (any granulated kind you have on hand will work)**
- ¼ **cup almond oil (a bit more or less as needed to make a paste)**

1. Place your coffee grounds in a small bowl and add a little water to moisten, if necessary. Add the cinnamon, sugar, and enough almond oil to make a nice, spreadable paste.
2. Get into the tub (because this stuff is messy), and scrub all over, rubbing the exfoliating scrub into rough patches — knees, elbows, heels. Then run a nice warm bath and soak up the warmth and moisture. Shower off the scrub and follow with a dab of almond oil to seal in moisture. Make sure you scrub the tub before the next bather. This stuff is pretty slippery.

Makes approximately 6–8 ounces

Cinnamon Clay for Acne Treatment

Cinnamon, with its heating and antibacterial properties, makes a great spot treatment for acne and troubled skin. I like to mix up a little of this paste and apply it to outbreaks before I go to bed, rinsing it off in the morning. The combination of cosmetic clay and cinnamon helps dry out the skin, draw out toxins, and heal inflammation and redness.

- 1 **tablespoon French green clay, bentonite clay, or white cosmetic clay**
- ½ **teaspoon cinnamon powder**

In a small bowl, mix together the clay and cinnamon. Add just enough water to make a paste. Apply the paste to affected areas, and leave it on for 10 minutes or overnight, washing the face as usual in the morning.

Makes 1 treatment

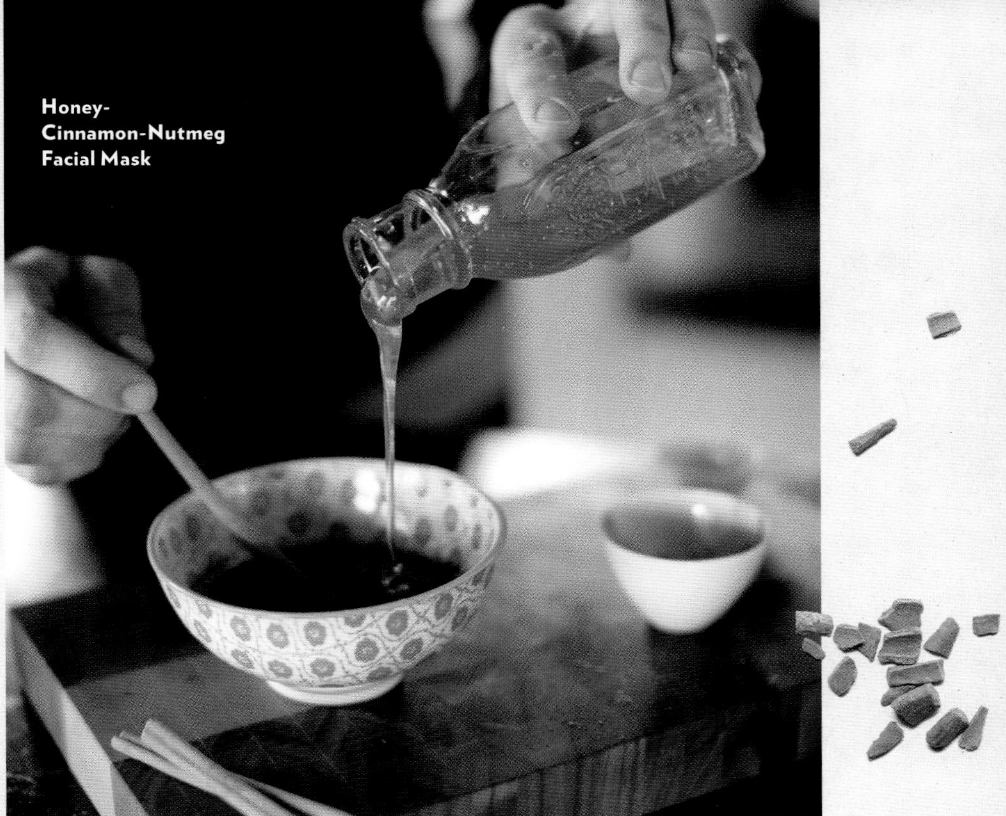
Honey-Cinnamon-Nutmeg Facial Mask

Honey-Cinnamon-Nutmeg Facial Mask

Let the holiday-inspired cosmetic scrub making continue! I think the idea for this one came in the midst of the maiden voyage of the above scrub. As we've learned, honey draws moisture to the skin and nutmeg gently exfoliates while also drawing blood to the surface of the skin. What does that mean? You end up with a glowing, healthy, radiant complexion void of pore-clogging oils and environmental toxins.

This makes enough for one (maybe two) treatments. Since honey is a wonderful preservative and since this cleanser is gentle enough for daily use, feel free to mix up a week's worth (or more) and keep it right in your bathroom.

1 tablespoon raw honey

1 teaspoon cinnamon powder

½ teaspoon nutmeg powder

1. In a small bowl, combine the honey, cinnamon, and nutmeg. Add just enough warm water (or almond oil if you have very dry skin) to make a spreadable, cleansing milk–like consistency.
2. Wet your face, and, using small circles, massage the cleanser into your skin. Rinse with warm water and moisturize, if needed.

Makes 1 treatment

recipes

FOOD & DRINK

Chai Tea Latte

Mmmm . . . a chai latte that's just like the one at your favorite coffeehouse (but maybe a tad healthier).

- ¼ teaspoon cardamom seeds
- 6 whole cloves
- 1 3-inch-long cinnamon stick
- 6 black peppercorns
- 2 ¼-inch-thick slices fresh ginger
- 4 black tea bags
- 2 cups soy milk
- Sweetener of choice (optional)

1. In a small saucepan, combine the cardamom, cloves, cinnamon, peppercorn, ginger, tea, and 2 cups water. Bring to a boil, then reduce the heat and simmer for 20 minutes. Strain and return to the pan.
2. Add the soy milk and reheat over low until hot.

Serves 4

Cinnamon–Coconut Milk Ice Cream

This stuff is amazing. My brother loves to make ice cream, so this recipe is courtesy of his mad skills.

- 3 quarts coconut milk
- 2–3 cups white sugar
- 3 tablespoons vanilla extract
- 2 teaspoons cinnamon
- 3 eggs or vegan alternative, slightly beaten

1. In a large pot or double boiler, mix together the coconut milk, sugar, vanilla, cinnamon, and eggs. Cook, stirring, over low heat until the mixture is just about to boil. Remove from heat and cool.
2. If you have an ice cream maker (highly recommended), go ahead and use it, following the directions for your device. Alternatively, you can put this into a freeze-proof tub and stick it in the freezer for a few hours or

until just set. Then use a stick blender or food processor to blend until smooth and creamy.

3. Serve immediately, refreeze any leftovers, and blend again before serving.

Serves 4 (or 1 if you're like me)

Cinnamon Granola

I LOVE granola. It's a really good thing I have some self-control.

- 3 cups rolled oats
- 1 cup shredded coconut
- ¾ teaspoon sea salt
- 1½ cups raw nuts and/or seeds of choice, whole or chopped
- ½ cups coconut or safflower oil
- 1 teaspoon vanilla extract
- ¾ cup honey, maple syrup, or other liquid sweetener
- 1 teaspoon cinnamon
- 1 cup raisins or other dried fruit (optional)

1. Preheat the oven to 300°F/150°C and line two baking sheets with parchment paper.
2. In a large mixing bowl, combine the oats, coconut, salt, and nuts, and mix together.
3. In a medium bowl, combine the oil, vanilla, sweetener, and cinnamon. Whip or beat until thoroughly combined. (If you're using honey and it's super-solid, just heat it gently in a small saucepan over low heat until it flows easily).
4. Pour the honey mixture over the dry ingredients, and mix with your hands (I like to oil my hands first), making sure everything is coated. Spread the mixture on the parchment-lined cookie sheets. It should be about ½ inch thick — any thicker and it doesn't get crunchy; any thinner and it tends to burn.
5. Place in the oven and cook for 30 to 40 minutes or until the granola is light brown. ***Note:*** Your granola may not be super crunchy by the end of 40 minutes; it hardens as it cools. Stir after the first 15 minutes and every 15 minutes after that.
6. Remove from the oven and mix again. Let it cool, then place in a large bowl and add raisins or dried fruit of your choice, if using. Store in an airtight container up to 2 weeks.

Makes 6 cups

CINNAMON YOGA

We're going to have a little fun on the mat (well, don't we always?) with a pose called Wild Thing (or *Camatkarasana,* which translates as "the ecstatic unfolding of the enraptured heart" — gorgeous, right?). Since cinnamon is all about invoking childlike joy and cultivating creativity while also warming the body, Wild Thing is the perfect pose. It's a backbend, which is, in itself, inherently warming to the body. But backbends also open the heart area, which, as we've learned, is essential for opening up the path of creativity by loosening old emotions and allowing new experiences to enter into our lives.

When you see the pose (and, indeed, when you do it yourself, no matter how "accomplished" you are in the pose), you immediately sense the joy and happiness it inspires. So let's get started.

Starting position. Assume the Downward-Facing Dog position (see page 187 if you need to reacquaint yourself). From here you're going to inhale and bring yourself onto your right side, rolling onto the outside of that right foot and keeping your right hand on the mat. Your torso will face the left side. If you need to bring your left knee down here, go right ahead.

Moving into Wild Thing. Keep that right hand firmly on the mat (you can even increase your grip by making a scrunching motion on the mat). Inhale and lift your hips, stepping your left foot behind you. Place your toes on the floor and keep that left knee bent just a bit.

Now sweep back with your ribcage (think back to when you were a kid and one of your parents picked you up when you refused to go somewhere; perhaps you let your head and ribcage drop back to spite them, while they kept hold of your hips . . . yeah . . . it's kind of like that), extending your heart and letting your left arm stretch into space, aiming it toward the floor.

Finishing. Keep lifting your heart and hips with the inhale and let that right foot be solid on the mat. Hold for 5 to 10 breaths, then slowly and carefully make your way back to Downward-Facing Dog. Repeat on the other side, first taking a break in Child's Pose (see page 55) if you want.

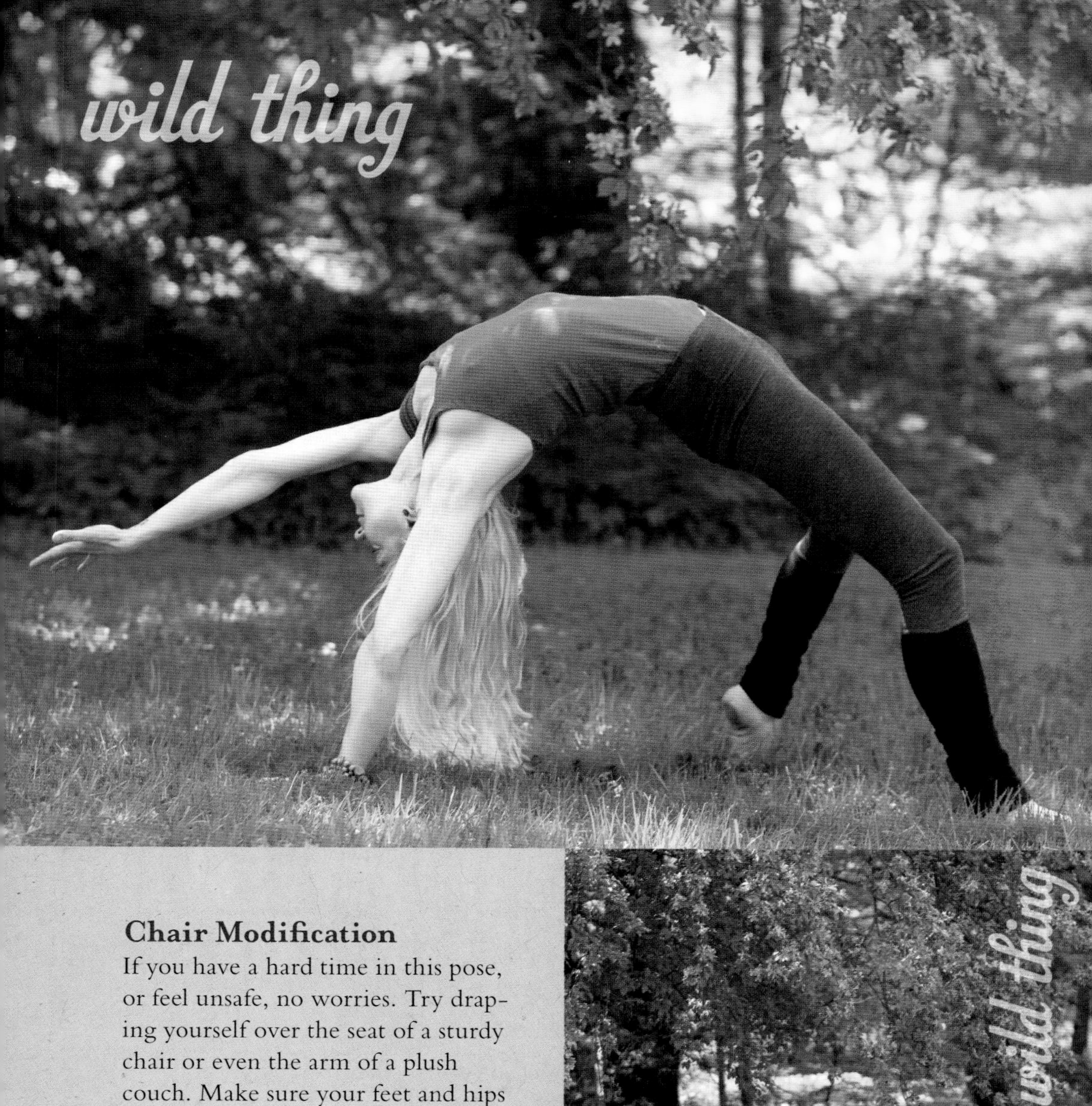

Chair Modification

If you have a hard time in this pose, or feel unsafe, no worries. Try draping yourself over the seat of a sturdy chair or even the arm of a plush couch. Make sure your feet and hips are stable, and let your arms stretch down into space. You'll get the same feeling of lift, exultation, and joy, while feeling safe and supported (and isn't *that* just the ultimate expression of an ideal childhood?!).

modified wild thing

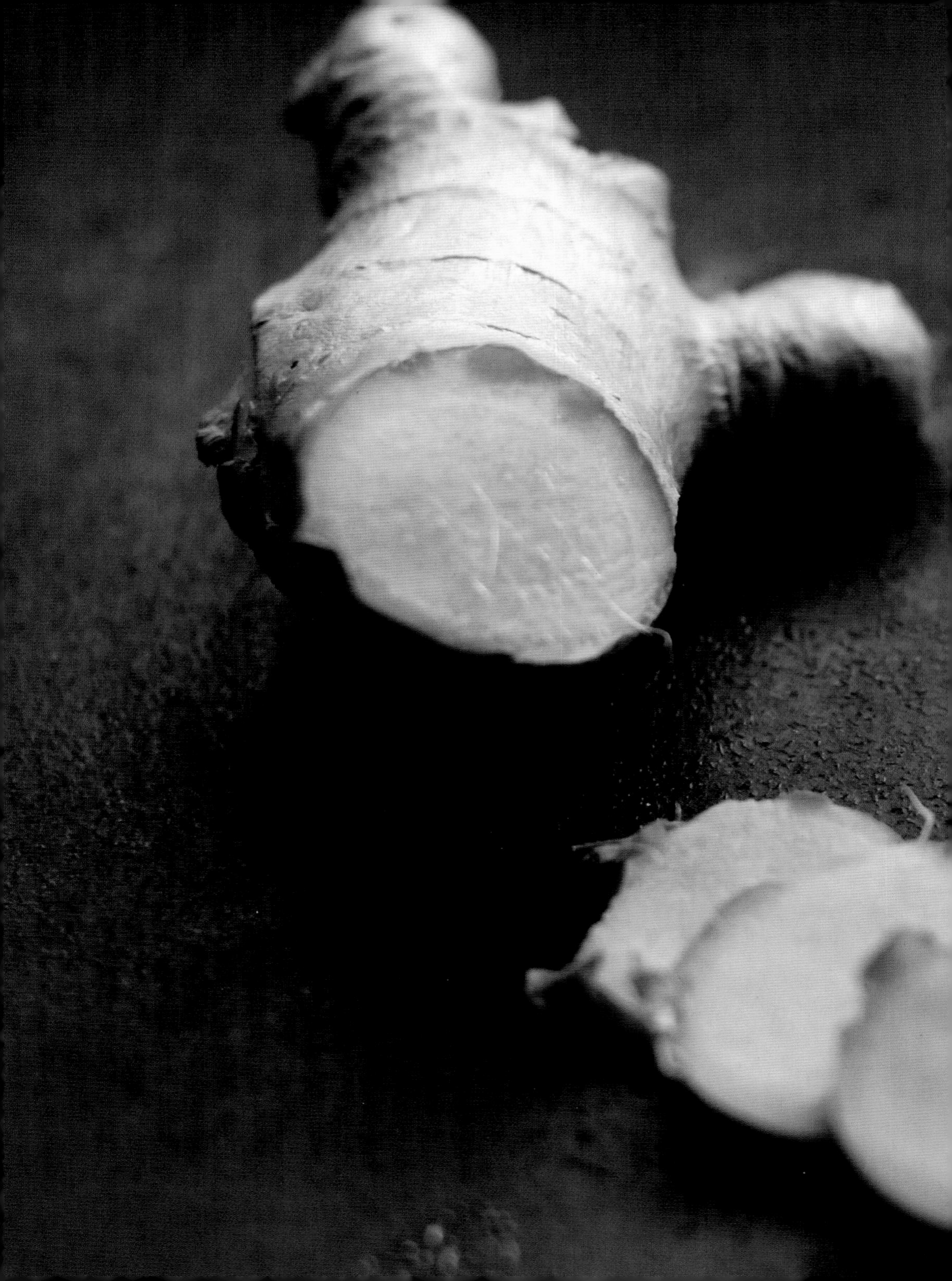

12 Jiving It Up with GINGER

Much like cinnamon, ginger (*Zingiber officinale*) is another kitchen spice-turned-medicinal (or more accurately, medicinal-turned-spice). Also like cinnamon, ginger is one of those warming herbs we associate with winter and its myriad holidays. The scent of ginger baking, sautéing, or steeping may transport you back to a family meal or holiday.

If you've ever accidentally (or on purpose) bitten into a piece of ginger, you know how warming it is. The intense, spicy burn of the root is immediate. The herb does the same to the body as it does to the tongue — it stokes the inner fire — which means better digestion and circulation.

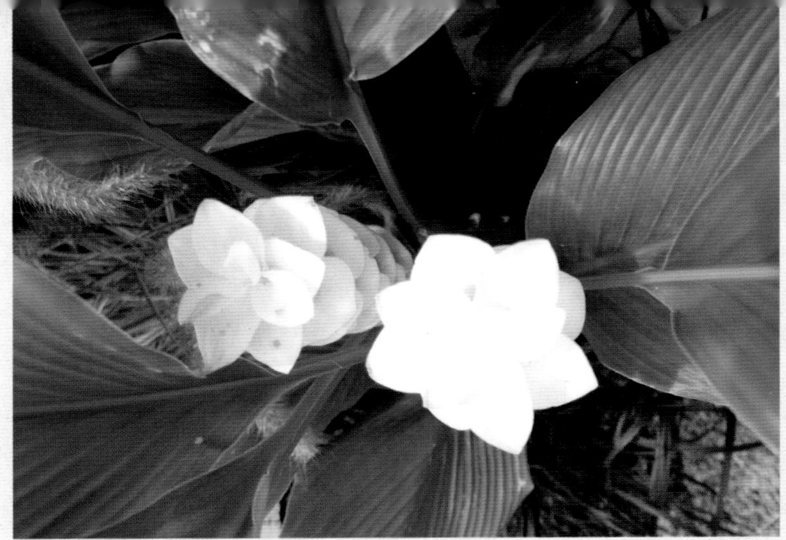

Growing ginger in pots indoors at home (unless you live in a very warm region; then you can plant it outside) is remarkably easy. In fact, you may have accidentally started a ginger plant somewhere along the way. Oh, and even though we say "gingerroot," we're not actually eating the root of the plant. We eat and use the rhizome, which has roots of its own. But, meh. Semantics. For our purposes, we'll talk about the root.

GINGER

Zingiber officinale

Parts used: Rhizome

How to harvest: After the plant has died back for winter (its dormant season), carefully dig up the root and cut a few fleshy rhizomes; return the rest of the root if you'd like new growth in the spring

Effects on body: Warming, stimulates digestion, eases pain, eases nausea, regulates blood sugar, and fights viruses

Effects on mind and spirit: Enhances and strengthens familial bonds and opens you up to creating new, lasting bonds with others

Safety first: Avoid large (medicinal) quantities if you're already prone to being overly warm or are prone to chronic heartburn; it is considered safe for pregnant women when used moderately (up to 3/4 teaspoon of the herb three times per day)

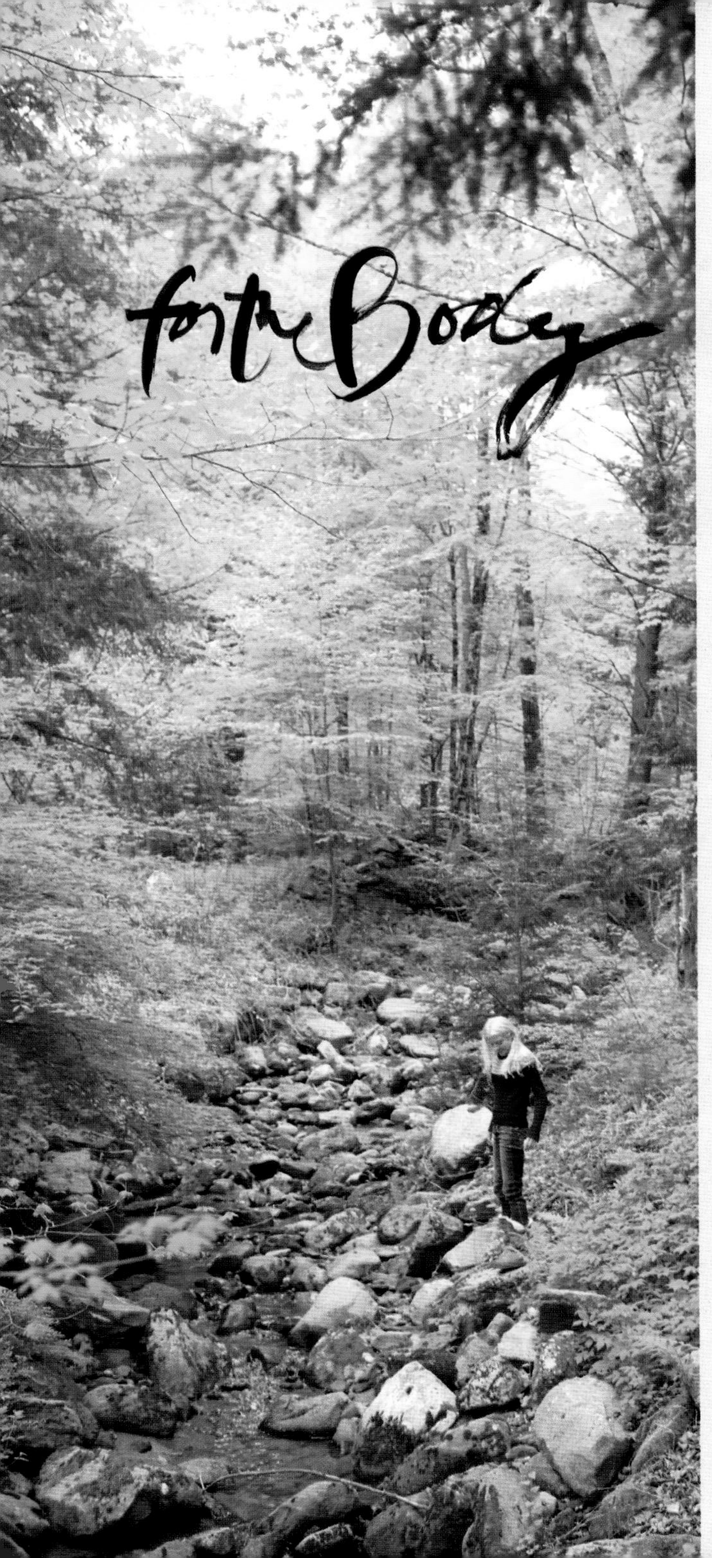

for the Body

It's kind of cool the way that plants are made. A plant's chemistry is what gives it its medicinal qualities, taste, and scent. For example, ginger has two oleoresins, called gingerol and shogaol (an oleoresin is a substance that is both oil and resin and occurs naturally in a plant), and volatile oils that cause the root to be warm and stimulating when ingested. The oleoresins and oils open up capillaries to release heat (and warm you up at the same time), warm the stomach (and improve digestion — especially fat digestion), and stimulate the intestines (relieving gas and helping things just move along, in general). Ginger's special affinity for the stomach and digestion is also what eases nausea and both motion and morning sickness.

On top of those active constituents, ginger also has an enzyme called zingibain in its arsenal. Zingibain helps break down protein, making ginger an excellent digestive aid. But, further, zingibain is also an anti-inflammatory, helps regulate blood sugar, and helps to relieve autoimmune conditions.

Ginger's also pretty spectacular when applied topically. Just as ginger warms and loosens stagnation internally, it does the same when applied externally. Ginger essential oil, when rubbed on the chest (for coughs), the belly (for indigestion and bloating), the intestines (for constipation or gas), or any muscles (for cramps), is flipping amazing. Seriously, it begins to work within minutes and you don't even need a carrier oil. (Although, do please do a skin patch test if you're the keeper of sensitive skin.)

You know how a fresh ginger rhizome kind of looks like an arthritic hand, with its gnarled root and finger-like protrusions? Well, here's the crazy bit: ginger is actually really good for arthritis. Not only is it an anti-inflammatory, which eases pain all on its own, but it also opens blood vessels and thins the blood, bringing more fluid and lubrication to the cartilage and the joints and allowing much more movement to happen.

Since ginger is so warming, if you're already a warm-blooded person (both in constitution and in temper), it's probably best to avoid large quantities of this herb. Skip the ginger tea, but feel free to eat the gingerbread (sparingly, of course).

Finally (just because we can and because it's impressive), here's a short list of conditions relieved in part or in total by dosing yourself with ginger: arthritis, athlete's foot, body odor, bunions, colds, coughs, cramps, dandruff, depression, dizziness, fever, heart disease, high cholesterol, indigestion, morning sickness, motion sickness, nausea, pain, and viral infections. Whew!

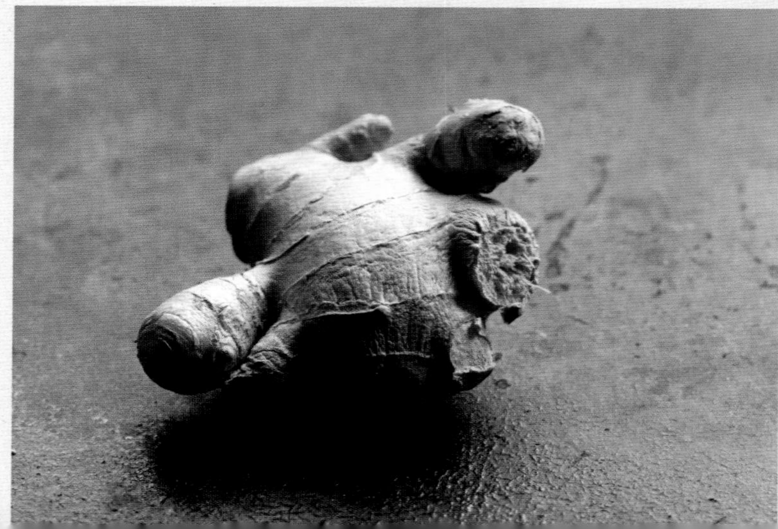

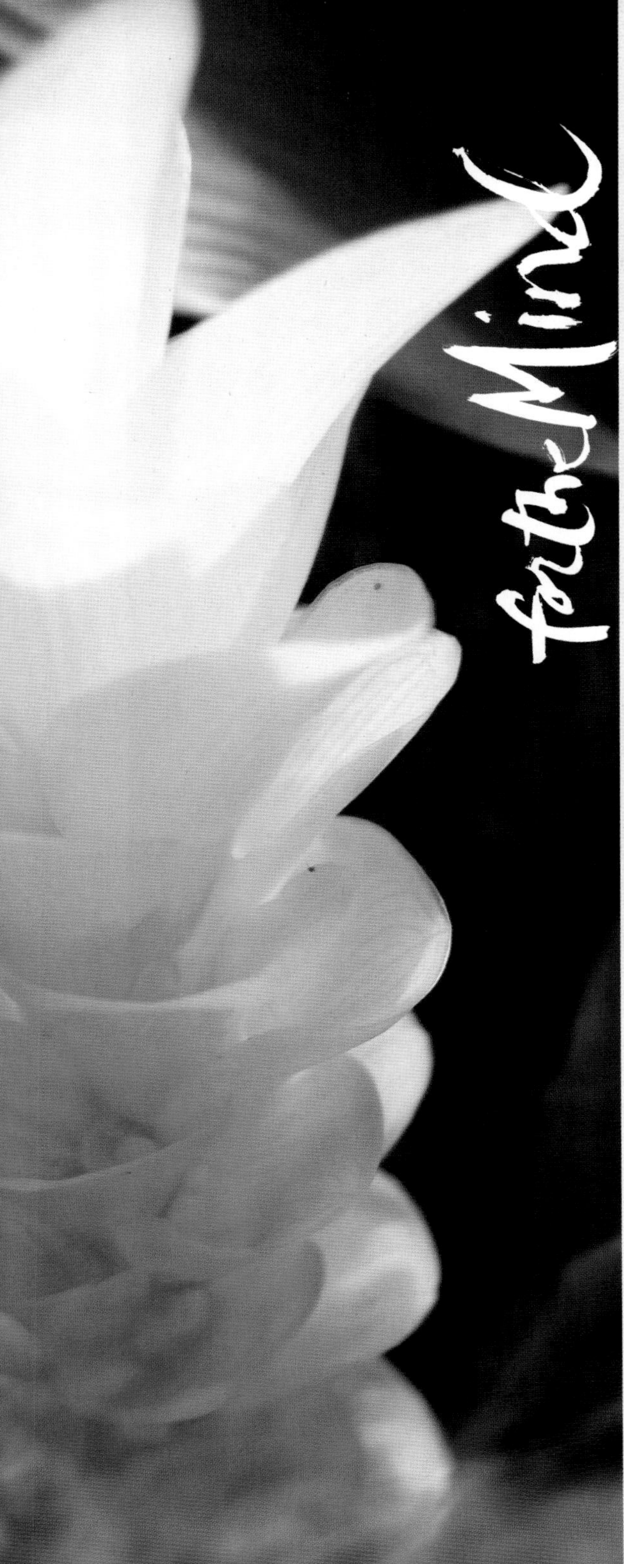

Part of the folklore around ginger, as an herb, is that it creates strong bonds between family members (and I'd go so far as to say natural families as well as urban and adopted families). In fact, in some cultures where the entire family is present for the birth of a new member, everyone shares one cup of ginger tea in order to heighten the warmth of connection and to strengthen the bond in the room.

Given this, it shouldn't be a surprise that the ginger flower essence is used exactly for that kind of bond. Take this where estrangement is or has been present, where families (or friends) are reunited after a long absence, or after a long emotional rift has done its damage.

The flower essence will also attract sweet, healthy relationships into your life, easing any bitterness that might keep you (knowingly or subconsciously) from creating bonds with others. This is especially effective if you tend to attract (or be attracted to) needy, one-sided, or unhealthy relationships.

Just like the herb, the flower essence helps to spread warmth, both between as well as within individuals. For example, if you're the type of person who fears rejection or new situations, ginger essence will help you tap into the welcome feeling and warmth that exists right alongside the scary newness. Or, if you tend not to be comfortable sharing yourself, your feelings, and your life with others (and you would like to), ginger can help cultivate that level of comfort, especially if that hesitancy is caused by past trauma.

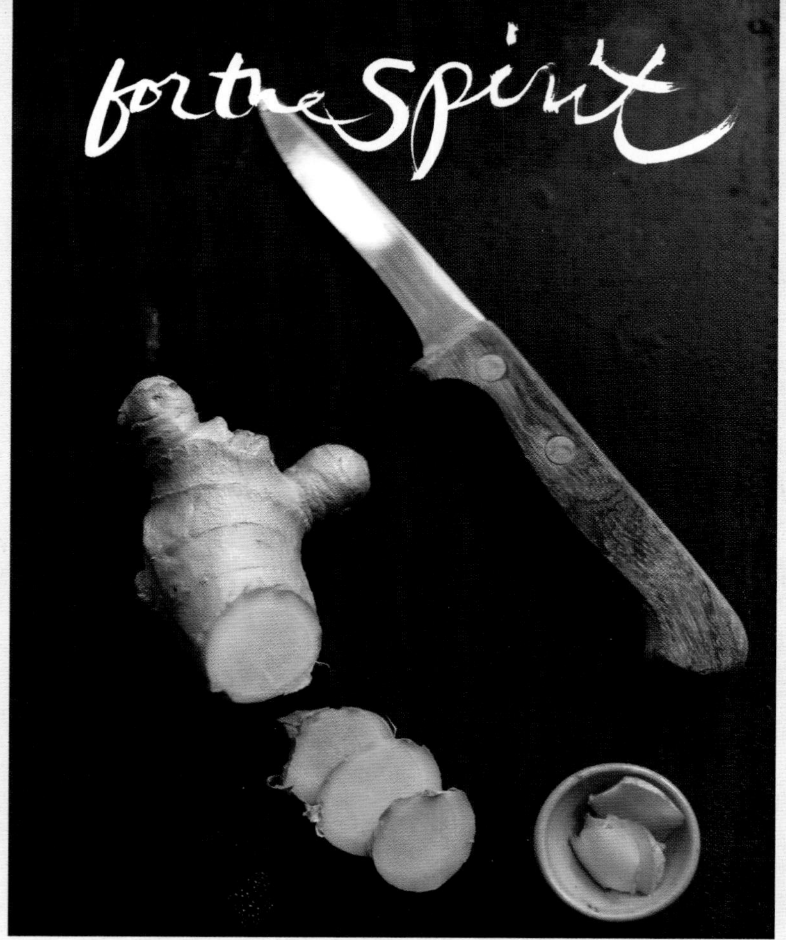

Ginger is associated with the planet Mars and carries masculine energy; its element is fire (not really surprising). Ginger is known for its attraction powers — whether it be to attract love, prosperity, success, strength, courage, or health. Ginger tea or the candied root is often eaten or drunk before casting spells in order to strengthen the spell itself or the practitioner, or to sweeten resolve or the effects of the casting. The fire of the herb will act to stoke your own power and internal fire (especially helpful in love spells, I would imagine).

Ginger is often planted in the home for harvest, yes, but also to attract money, success, and prosperity. You might want to have several pots going. Fill up the house with the warmth, power, and prosperity of this wild, warm, and humble plant.

GINGER MAGIC

FOR SUCCESS

Ginger essential oil is a must in the magical apothecary. I like to rub a few drops between my palms before meeting and greeting a new group, client, or student. I don't use enough to be noticeable, but enough to transmit confidence — both in myself and so that the people I'm meeting have confidence in me as well.

You can also use ginger when drafting or signing legal documents, making art, or completing a writing assignment — anything you feel needs a little extra boost. You can either put a little smoke from ginger incense on the pen, paper, computer, or paintbrush in question, or dress your hands in a little ginger oil and hold the object. Sip ginger tea for extra inspiration.

FOR INVOKING COURAGE

When it's a question of courage, I love using olfactory magic — whether it's steam, incense, or essential oil. There's something so empowering about scent; it uplifts, grounds, and encourages. Plus, carrying a little vial of essential oil in my hand is comforting when I feel especially vulnerable. If I have time to meditate before the event in question, I'll burn a little dry ginger on a charcoal disk and just inhale the scent, imagining that fiery courage taking root in my solar plexus — the center of all of our bravery and will.

If I don't have time for that, I'll brew a strong tea and inhale the steam. You can put it in a travel mug so that it's mobile, and you don't even need to drink it. Or carry the essential oil and either dress your pulse points or take a surreptitious sniff when needed. You can also do the ginger-oil-in-the palm trick or carry a bit of root in a sachet tucked into your purse or pocket.

FOR LOVE

There's something instantly sensual about the mellow sweetness and heat of ginger. Add some essential oil to a carrier oil, and dress your pulse points (wrists, neck, and behind the knees). Burn ginger candles, or cook a gingery curry for your date night. Candied ginger is a wonderful, sweet heat-builder. If things get even more intimate, there's nothing wrong (and, actually, everything right) about spiking some massage oil with a little ginger essential oil. Just add 10 drops essential oil per 2 cups almond oil. Heat gently and apply.

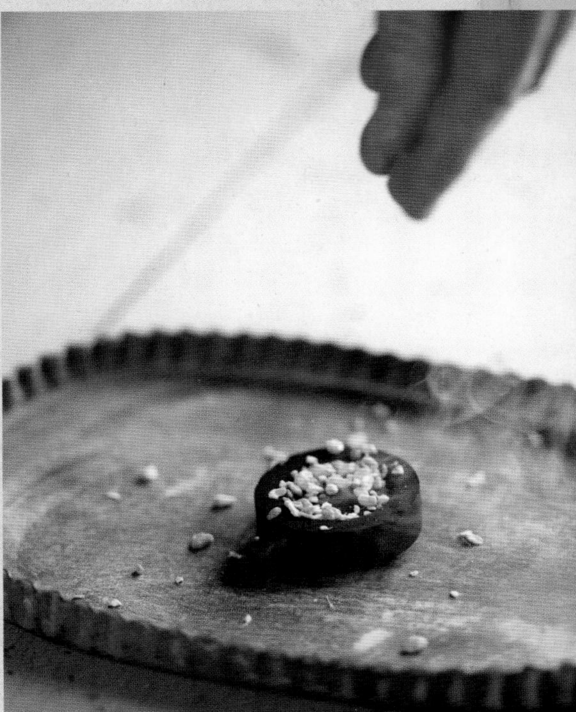

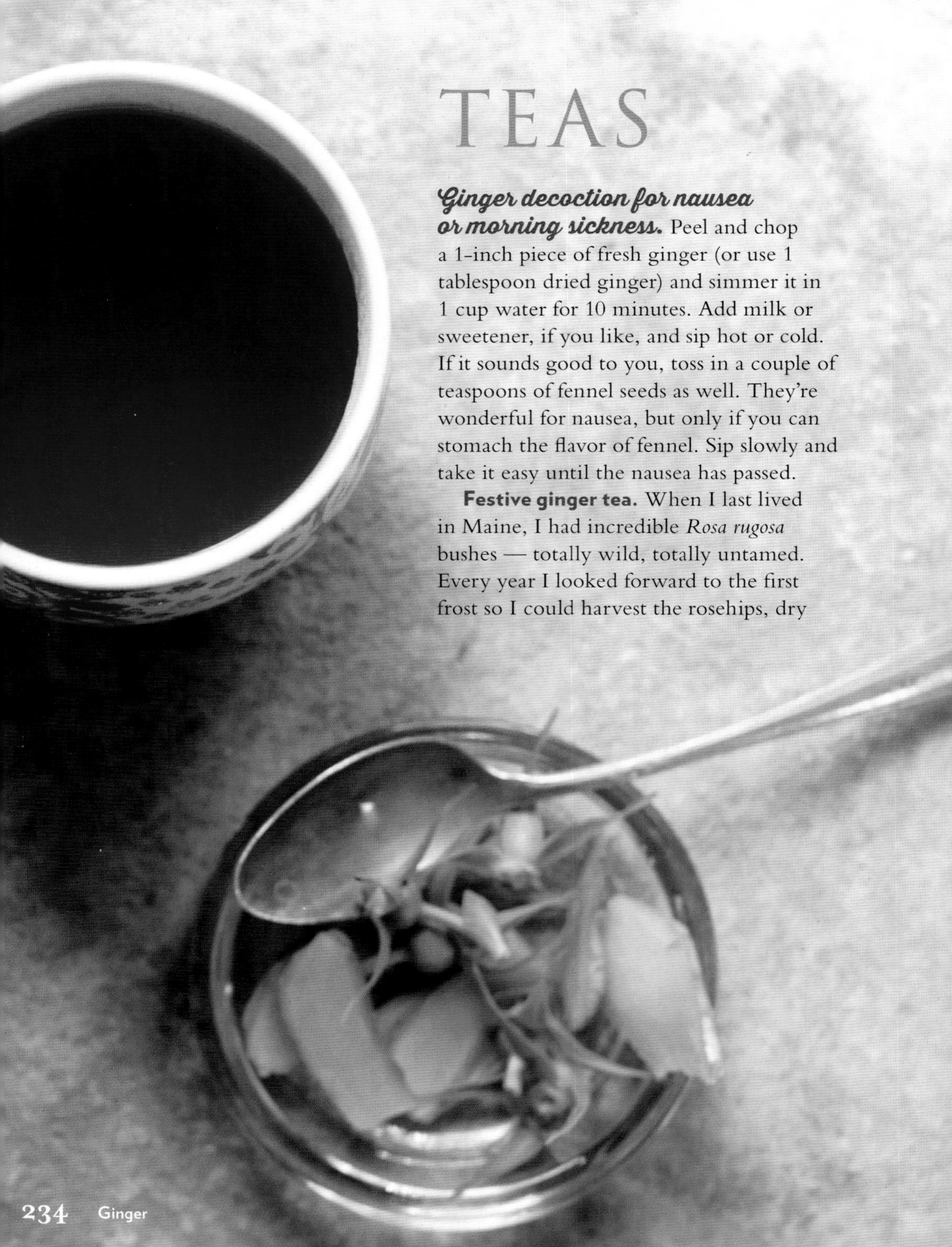

TEAS

Ginger decoction for nausea or morning sickness. Peel and chop a 1-inch piece of fresh ginger (or use 1 tablespoon dried ginger) and simmer it in 1 cup water for 10 minutes. Add milk or sweetener, if you like, and sip hot or cold. If it sounds good to you, toss in a couple of teaspoons of fennel seeds as well. They're wonderful for nausea, but only if you can stomach the flavor of fennel. Sip slowly and take it easy until the nausea has passed.

Festive ginger tea. When I last lived in Maine, I had incredible *Rosa rugosa* bushes — totally wild, totally untamed. Every year I looked forward to the first frost so I could harvest the rosehips, dry

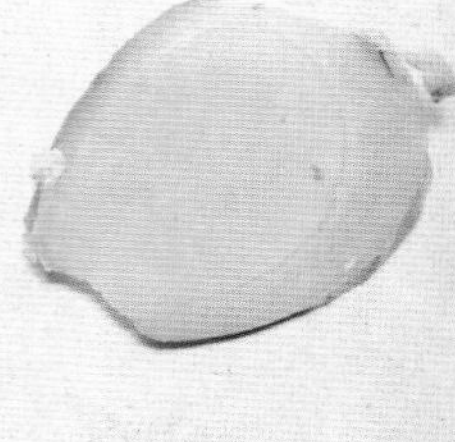

them, and use them all winter. Thus my absolute favorite middle-of-January blizzard tea was born — with only three (or four) ingredients!

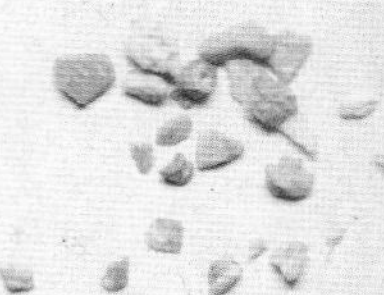

Place 1 tablespoon dried ginger and 1 tablespoon dried rosehips in a preheated mug or teapot. Pour 2 cups recently boiled water (or 2 cups gently heated milk) on top, cover, and steep for 10 to 15 minutes. Strain and sweeten the tea, and then watch the snow-drifts gather without a care in the world.

Ginger tea for digestion. Combine 1 tablespoon dried ginger, 2 teaspoons fennel seeds, and 2 teaspoons dandelion root in a small saucepan. Pour 3 cups water into the pan and simmer for 10 minutes. Strain 1 cup into a mug and enjoy. You can drink this hot or cold, either 20 minutes before or 30 minutes after a meal. Just don't sweeten or doctor it — you want the pungent flavors to stimulate the digestive system. Drink one cup at a time as needed throughout the day. ***Note:*** Ginger and heartburn aren't such good friends, so don't use this tea if that's your current complaint.

Flu-fighting ginger tea. The fiery nature of ginger is perfect for opening up sinuses, clearing the chest, and moving colds and the flu out of the system. I like to combine 1 tablespoon ginger, a pinch of cayenne powder, 1 teaspoon peppermint (sinus-opening goodness), and 2 teaspoons dried rosehips (for that vitamin C action) in a small saucepan. Pour in 3 cups water and simmer for 10 minutes. Strain and doctor with lemon, honey, brandy, or non-dairy milk. Drink as often as needed, one cup at a time, throughout the day.

BODY CARE

Invigorating Ginger Toner

If you have troubled, tired skin, ginger can jolt the life and health right back into those pores. Combining apple cider vinegar, ginger tea, ginger essential oil, and peppermint essential oil with a touch of witch hazel will have you looking forward to getting up in the morning and splashing some of this blend on your face.

- **1 cup strong, cool, ginger tea (1 tablespoon ginger steeped for 10 minutes in 1 cup water)**
- **1 tablespoon apple cider vinegar**
- **1 tablespoon witch hazel**
- **5 drops ginger essential oil**
- **1–2 drops peppermint essential oil (test before adding more)**

Combine the ginger tea, apple cider vinegar, witch hazel, ginger essential oil, and peppermint essential oil in a clean jar and shake it up. Feel free to add more of either essential oil, but make sure you test it first — essential oils can be too strong for some skin types. With a cotton pad, smooth a bit of this toner over your face whenever needed to awaken, revive, and refresh.

Makes 8 ounces

Warming and Invigorating Ginger-Lemon Scrub

I love, love, love ginger and lemon together. The scent itself is magical, and the acidity of the citrus helps slough off dead skin and correct discoloration, leaving behind a bright and glowing complexion.

- **1 cup granulated sugar**
- **1 tablespoon grated lemon rind**
- **2 teaspoons powdered ginger**
- **10 drops lemon essential oil**
- **5 drops ginger essential oil**
- **Enough almond or apricot oil to make a spreadable paste**

Combine the sugar, lemon rind, powdered ginger, lemon and ginger essential oils, and almond or apricot oil in a small bowl, and mix them together. Climb into the tub and scrub the mixture into your skin, paying special attention to your knees, elbows, and heels. Rinse with warm water. Clean out the tub when you're finished — this stuff is slippery.

Makes 8 ounces

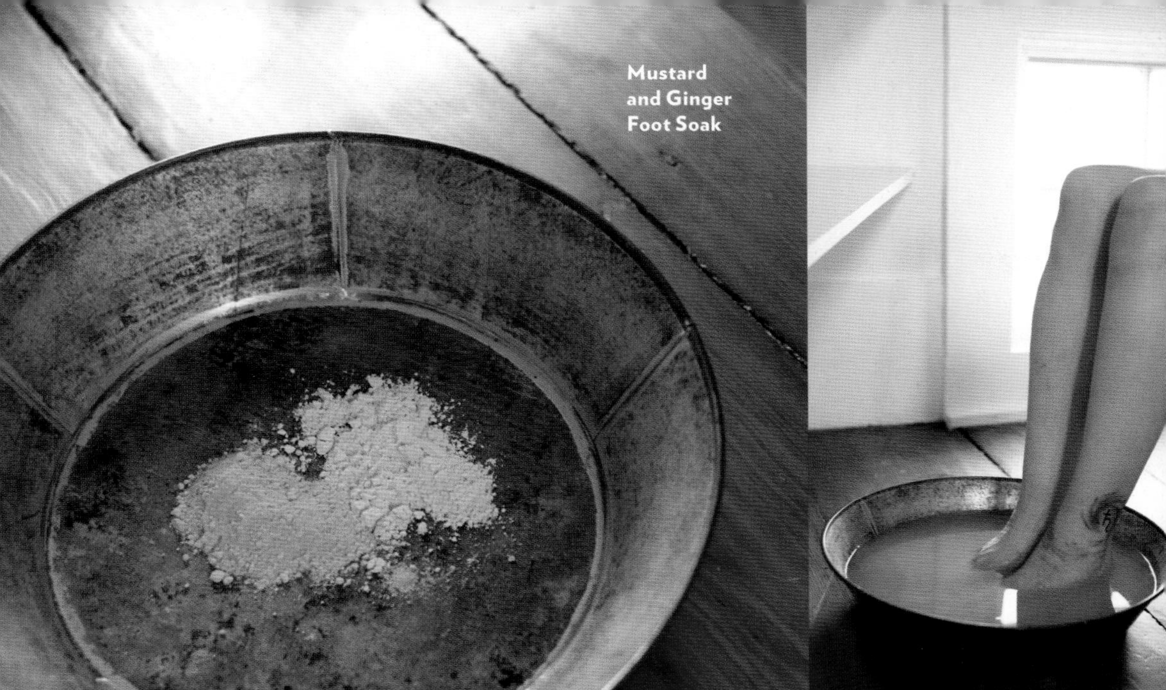
Mustard and Ginger Foot Soak

Cinnamon and Ginger Bath Salts

Bath salts are one of my favorite projects because they are just so, so easy. And when put in a pretty jar, they make a great gift.

- **1 cup Epsom salt**
- **2 tablespoons cinnamon**
- **2 tablespoons ginger**
- **10 drops ginger essential oil**
- **5 drops cinnamon essential oil**

In a medium bowl, combine the Epsom salt, cinnamon, ginger, and essential oils (add more essential oils if you like, but first test your skin's sensitivity). Mix and decant into the jar of your choice. Use 1⁄4 to 1⁄2 cup per bath.

Makes 8 ounces

Mustard and Ginger Foot Soak

Wake up tired feet and heal athlete's foot with mustard and ginger powders.

- **3 tablespoons ginger powder**
- **6 teaspoons mustard powder**

In a container big enough for you to soak your feet, combine the ginger powder and mustard powder with 3 cups water. Soak your feet daily for 15 minutes until the problem has passed. For especially tired feet, add a few drops of peppermint essential oil.

Makes 1 treatment

recipes

FOOD

Quintessential Gingerbread

What's a chapter on ginger without gingerbread? I had to include this recipe, especially since it was passed down to me by my grandmother and reminds me of cold, snowy days in their Rhode Island home. The sauce recipe that follows is optional but awesome.

- **2 eggs, beaten or vegan alternative**
- **1 cup brown sugar**
- **1 cup molasses**
- **½ cup shortening or butter**
- **1 cup boiling water**
- **2½ cups flour (add more if batter is too soupy)**
- **2 teaspoons baking powder**
- **½ teaspoon baking soda**
- **1½ teaspoons powdered ginger**
- **2 teaspoons cinnamon**
- **½ teaspoon salt**
- **1 cup raisins or chopped, candied ginger (optional)**

1. Preheat the oven to 350°F/180°C and grease a 9×12-inch pan or 2 muffin tins (that hold 12 muffins each). Put the kettle on to boil water.
2. In a large bowl, mix together the eggs, brown sugar, molasses, shortening or butter, and boiling water. In a medium bowl, mix together the flour, baking powder, baking soda, ginger, cinnamon, and salt. Add the dry mixture to the sugar mixture and stir until well combined.
3. Pour the batter into the pan or muffin tins. Add the raisins or dried ginger, if using, and use a fork to lightly press them into the batter. Place in the oven and bake for about 30 minutes for the pan and 20 minutes for the muffin tins, or until a toothpick inserted into the center comes out clean.

Sauce

- **1 cup water**
- **½ cup confectioner's sugar**
- **2 tablespoons arrowroot powder or cornstarch**
- **1 teaspoon vanilla extract**
- **1 teaspoon butter (vegan or dairy)**

In a medium saucepan, combine the water with the sugar and arrowroot powder or cornstarch. Cook over medium-low heat until clear. Remove from the heat and stir in the vanilla and butter. Pour (while hot) over the cake or muffins when ready to serve.

Makes 2 loaves or approximately 18 muffins

Pickled Ginger

Pickled ginger is my favorite part about sushi. Try eating a bit of this with your meal to aid digestion.

- **3 ounces fresh gingerroot, peeled and sliced thin**
- **½ cup water**
- **½ cup raw apple cider vinegar**
- **½ cup sugar**

1. In a small saucepan, combine the ginger with the water. Bring to a boil over high heat, and boil for 1 or 2 minutes, depending on thickness of your ginger slices. Remove from the heat and strain off the water. Add sugar and stir.
2. Fill a clean glass jar with the vinegar. Add the strained ginger, cover, and store on the counter for 24 to 48 hours (check it after 24 hours; if you like the taste, stop there). Store your pickles in the refrigerator. This stuff will keep for several weeks.

Makes 3 ounces

Pear-Ginger-Squash Soup

This is one of my favorite meals for a dark winter evening.

- **1 medium-size butternut squash, peeled and chopped**
- **4 cups vegetable broth (more for a thinner soup, less for a thicker one)**
- **1 ripe pear, cubed (leave the peel on)**
- **1 orange, zested and juiced**
- **1 teaspoon minced gingerroot**
- **Salt and pepper to taste**
- **Allspice to taste**
- **Dried cranberries for garnish (optional)**

1. In a medium saucepan, combine the squash and vegetable broth. Boil over medium-high heat for 20 minutes or until tender (just keep checking).
2. Using a stick blender (or food processor), puree the squash. Return this to the stove and add the pear, orange zest and juice, ginger, salt and pepper, and allspice. Simmer for about 15 minutes. Serve hot with a sprinkling of dried cranberries, if you like.

Serves 4

GINGER YOGA

Because ginger focuses on the digestive system, stokes the body's fire, and provides for all-around toning of the circulatory system, we're going to gear our yoga toward the same end: the abdominals, but also toning and heating the entire body. The pose? Upward Plank (or *Purvottanasana*).

If you have tight shoulders (and who doesn't, really?), you're going to have a love/hate relationship with this pose. No worries. Just go as far as you can, and build from there.

Warming up. Do a few arm circles and forward bends, just to warm up a bit. There's no need to do a whole yoga practice first.

Starting position. Sit on your mat with your legs straight out in front of you (this is called Staff Pose, or *Dandasana*, by the way). Walk your hands a few inches behind your hips, trying to keep them in line with your shoulders as much as possible. If comfortable, point your fingers toward your feet. (If you have serious wrist issues, feel free to come down onto your elbows.)

Moving into Reverse Tabletop. Bend your knees and plant your feet on the mat. On an exhale, push your body up into a Reverse Tabletop by pressing into the mat with your hands and feet, drawing your belly in, and using as much core strength as possible in order to keep nice and flat. Your knees may want to splay out; try to keep them parallel to each other and coming right out from your hips, knees stacked over ankles. *Only* if it's comfortable in your neck, let your head drop back. Otherwise, just keep looking forward.

Good? Okay, on an exhale come on down. If you found that challenging, stay here for a while, building strength in your core, arms, shoulders, and thighs (quadriceps).

Moving into Upward Plank. Stretch your legs out in front of you. You're going to push up again, but this time with straight legs into Upward Plank.

As you are doing this, rotate your legs in toward each other; your feet will stay touching and you will really feel this in your inner thighs. Ideally, you also want to keep the soles of your feet on the mat. You'll really use your core here and lift as much as you can with your hips. Think of your hips moving forward, rather than up. Again, drop your head back only if it's comfortable.

If you feel any strain or pinching in your low back, draw that belly in tighter and lift more with your hips. If that doesn't help, lower back down and stick to Tabletop for a while.

Finishing. Hold the pose for 30 seconds or so, then lower on an exhale. You may find that folding forward here feels really good on your back, but do whatever counter-pose your body is asking for.

Chair Modification

Take a seat. Grasp the sides of the seat and walk your feet out. Press them into the floor, internally rotate your thighs, and lift your pelvis. Hold as long as you can, then sit back down. Fold forward.

Practice this until you feel confident doing the full pose.

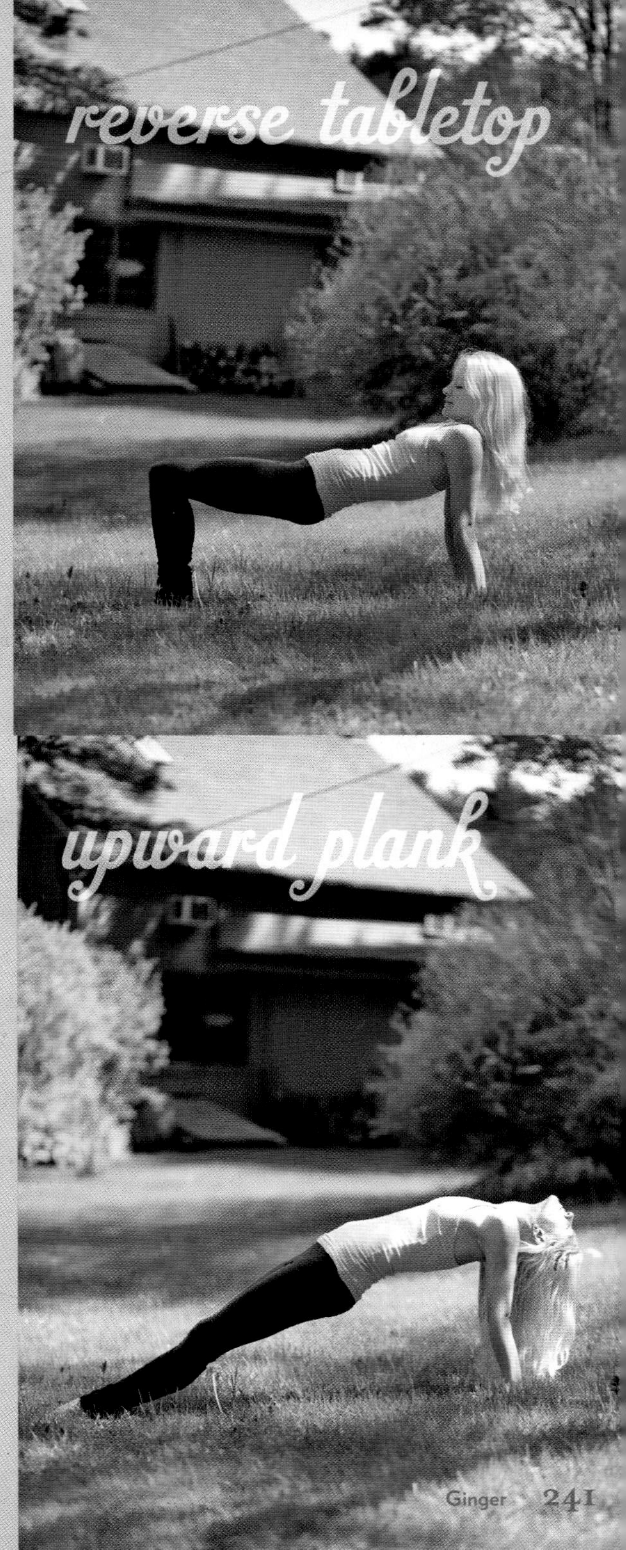

Appendix I: Flower Essences

To make your own flower essence, choose a dry, sunny day to visit your flowers (you'll have to grow a patch indoors or plan this project for the summer months). Bring a clear glass bowl with room-temperature spring water. Set it aside and sit with the flowers for a while, just meditating on the sight, smell, and healing qualities of the plant; thank the flowers for their contribution to your mental and physical well-being. When you're ready to begin, follow these instructions.

Clear glass bowl
Spring water
Sterile scissors
Cheesecloth
Dark glass bottle
Small, dark dropper bottle
Brandy or glycerin (for preservation)

1. Fill the bowl with water, then use sterilized scissors to snip enough flowers to cover the surface of the water (don't touch the flowers; just let them fall into the bowl). Leave the bowl on the ground, in the sun (preferably near the patch you harvested from) and allow the water to infuse for a few hours.

2. Strain the water through cheesecloth, and add the used flowers to your compost pile (karma-wise, you may want to offer the plot of flowers a little of the infused spring water as well, in gratitude).

3. Fill a sterilized dark glass bottle halfway with the infused water. Top off the jar with brandy; this will keep bacteria from growing in your bottle (alternatively, if you'd prefer not to use alcohol, you can use glycerin as a preservative). This is your Mother Bottle; you'll make your own flower essence from this bottle.

4. To make a stock remedy that you'll take when needed, fill a small, dark dropper bottle halfway with water. Add 7 drops infused water from the Mother. Shake the bottle against the palm of your hand for 2 minutes, sending your own vibrations of wellness into the remedy. Top the bottle with brandy (or glycerin) for preservation.

5. Take a few drops of flower essence under the tongue as needed throughout the day. (Bonus: once you're familiar with all of the herbs in this book, you'll be able to expertly blend several flowers into one essence, depending on your needs.)

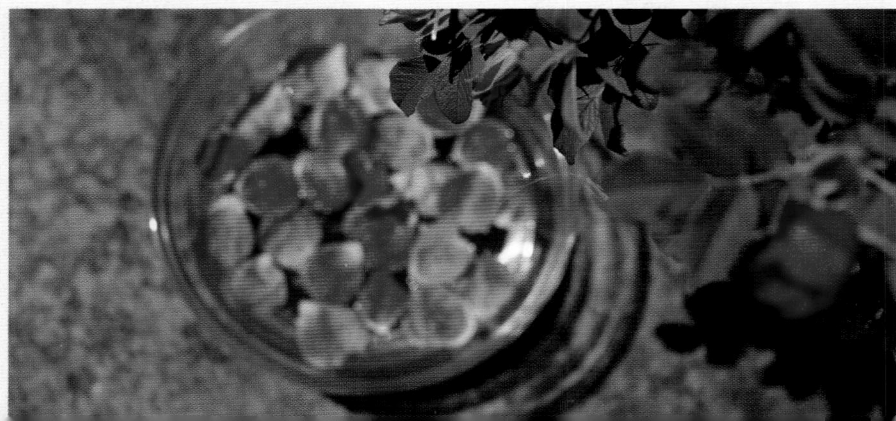

Appendix II: Herbal Oils

Making herbal oils is really no different than making a salad dressing with savory herbs; it's just a way to get the fat-soluble constituents out of the herb and into the oil. I have two ways here: the fast way and the leisurely way. For a stronger oil, use 2 parts herbs to 5 parts oil and if using the solar method, let it infuse for 4 weeks. If you notice mold, cloudiness, signs of fermentation, or anything else that looks unusual, discard immediately.

1 part dried herb(s) of choice (measure by volume)

5 parts oil of choice (measure by volume)

Sterile glass container

Cheesecloth

The Fast Way

1. In a double boiler, heat your herbs and oil and cover with a tightly fitting lid. Bring the water to a simmer and slowly, slowly (yes, even in the fast method you want to keep that heat on low) heat the oil for 30 minutes. Keep checking the oil — you don't want to cook the herbs! (Brown, crunchy herbs don't have much to contribute here.) Remove from the heat and let cool enough to handle.
2. Decant your oil into a (super) dry, sterilized jar. Using cheesecloth, squeeze as much oil as you can out of the herbs. You can store your oil in the fridge for a longer life.

The Slow (or Solar) Way

1. Place the herbs and oil in a glass mason jar and cover tightly. Place in a sunny window (with no drafts!), and let infuse for 2 weeks or so, shaking daily.
2. Using cheesecloth, strain the oil into a sterilized jar. Squeeze as much oil as you can out of the herbs. Cap tightly.

Appendix III: Herbal Salves

Salves are just basically solid herbal oils. We make them solid by adding beeswax (or candelilla wax, as a vegan alternative) to our herbal oil. See also the recipes for Calendula Salve for Injured and Infected Skin on page 124 and Salve for Healing Bites, Stings, and Wounds, page 182.

- 4 parts herbal oil of choice (measure by volume)
- 1 part wax of choice (measure by volume; this is much easier if the wax is grated first)
- Essential oils (how much you use will depend on your personal preference; for your basic salve, begin with 10 to 20 drops per cup oil and go from there)
- Clean, sterile containers of choice (such as tins or glass jars)

1. For a firm salve, heat 4 parts herbal oil (see Appendix II) and 1 part wax in a double boiler until the wax melts (for a softer salve, use 6 parts oil to 1 part wax). If you want to check the consistency of the salve, dip a spoon in the blend and put it in the freezer for a few minutes. Add more oil if the salve is too hard, or more wax if it's too soft.
2. Let the salve base cool a bit (5 minutes or so) before adding any essential oils (if you're using them), then package in clean, sterile containers. This stuff keeps pretty much forever.

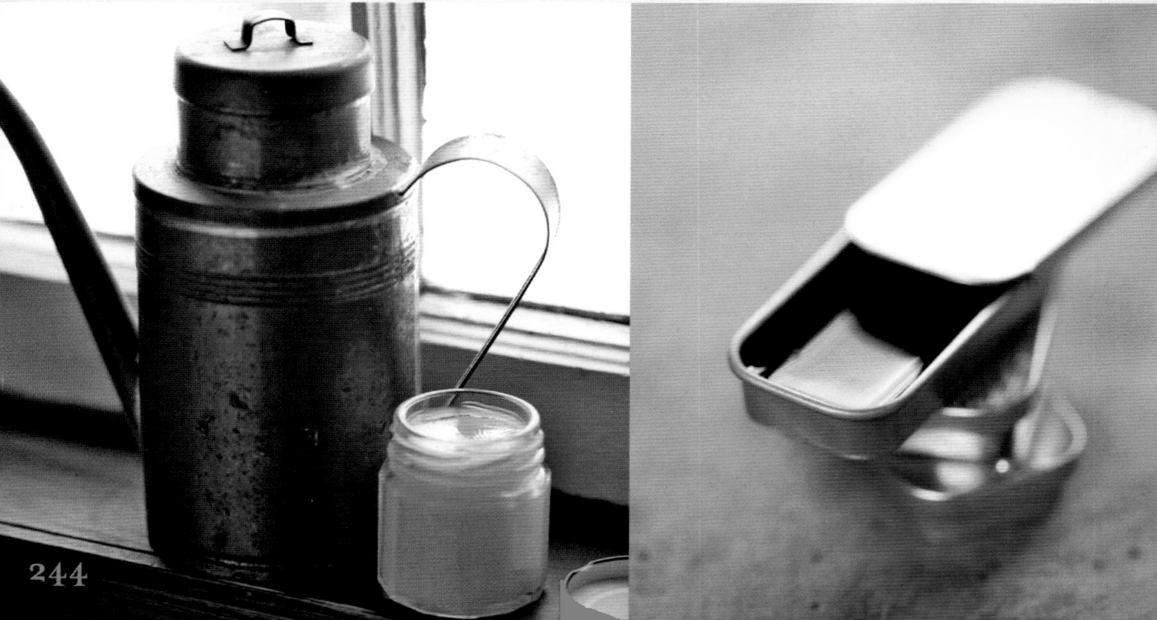

Appendix IV: Herbal Tinctures

Tinctures are just another extraction method for herbs. I vastly prefer taking tinctures over capsules, as they are much stronger. You can use alcohol (the higher the proof, the better, such as brandy, vodka, or Everclear), or apple cider vinegar or glycerin.

- 1 part dried or fresh herb of choice, chopped or ground as finely as possible (measure by volume)
- 5 parts liquid of choice, such as alcohol, vinegar, or glycerin if using dried herbs (measure by volume) or 2 parts liquids of choice if using fresh herbs
- Clean, sterile glass jars for the brewing portion
- Small amber or blue glass dropper bottles for decanting tinctures into once they've finished brewing

1. Chop, grind, or crush your herb as much as possible — we want lots of surface area. Combine 1 part dried herb to 5 parts liquid (or 1 part fresh herb to 2 parts liquid) in a sterile jar.
2. Stir the mixture, cap your jar, and label it with the date you made it. Store it in a dark, cool place for 2 weeks, shaking daily. Check the liquid level — if your herb swells past the top of the liquid, add more liquid (move it into a larger jar, if necessary).
3. Strain your tincture, squeezing out as much of the liquid as possible. Label and store in amber or blue glass bottles. If you don't use alcohol, keep it in the fridge for a longer shelf life. Most tinctures should be replaced after a year, just for potency's sake.

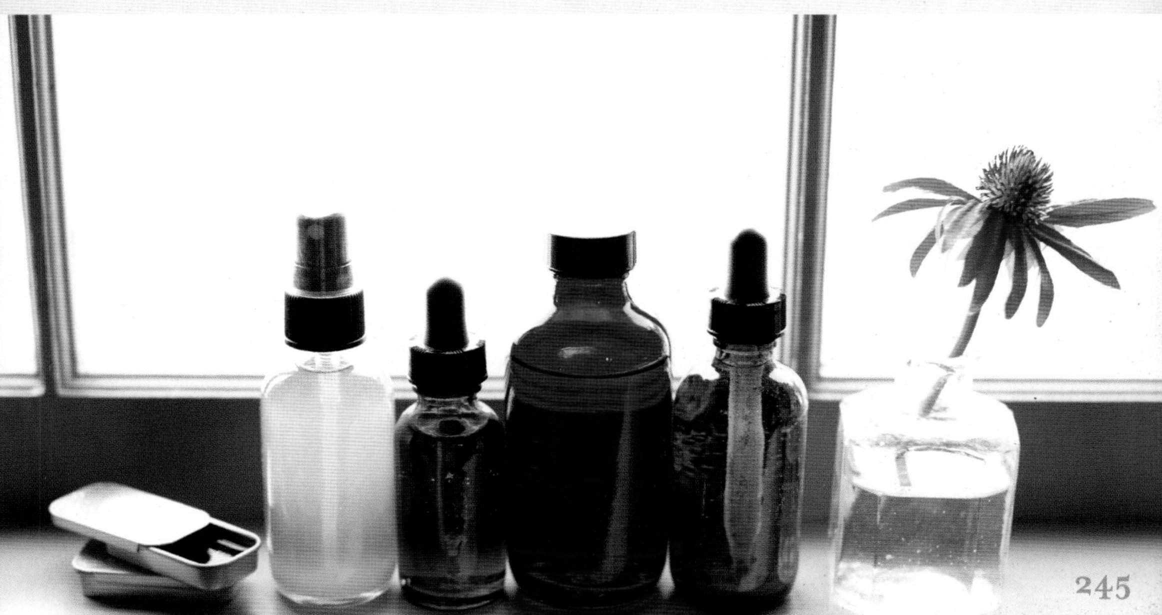

Appendix V: Herbal Vinegars

While not your typical culinary herbal vinegar, this recipe will make a lovely vinegar for the kitchen. My favorite is an herbal infusion of rose petals and rice wine vinegar.

Materials

- 1 part dried or fresh flowers or leaves of herb of choice (measure by volume)
- 5 parts vinegar of choice (measure by volume)
- Clean, sterile jar for brewing
- Pretty upcycled glass bottle or jar for storing (optional)
- Fresh or dried herb sprigs (optional)

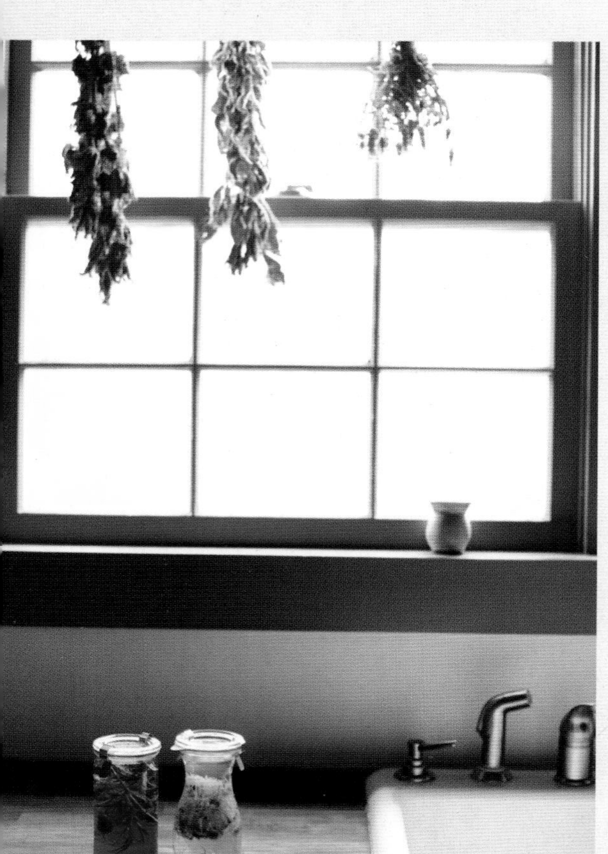

1. Sterilize the jar by boiling it for 10 minutes or running it through the hottest cycle in your dishwasher.
2. If using fresh herbs, wash and pat dry and chop roughly. Place the herbs (fresh or dried) in the sterilized jar and fill with vinegar. Cover the container tightly and place in a dark, cool place to steep. Allow the vinegar to infuse for 2 to 4 weeks, or until the desired flavor has developed.
3. Strain out the herbs, and pour the infused vinegar into sterilized bottles or jars. You can add fresh sprigs or dried herbs before sealing to make the bottle more attractive and to further enhance the flavor.
4. Label with the ingredients and date. That's it! To retain the flavor, it's best to store vinegars in a cool, dark place and use within 4 to 6 months, or keep the vinegar refrigerated. If you notice mold, cloudiness, signs of fermentation, or anything else that looks unusual, discard immediately.

Resources

Here are some of my favorite spots for products as well as further instruction and research.

Herbs and Supplies

Avena Botanicals

866-282-8362

www.avenabotanicals.com

I might be just a tad biased by saying that Avena has some of the best teas, tinctures, salves, and herbal formulas out there. They are, after all, in my home state of Maine, and I've taken many a class there. Deb Soule, owner of Avena, is an incredible, intuitive, kind, talented, and generous herbalist.

Bramble Berry

360-734-8278

www.brambleberry.com

Soap-making supplies including kits, exfoliants, essential oils, herbs, botanicals, containers, and packaging

Bulk Apothecary

888-968-7220

www.bulkapothecary.com

Herbs, spices, soap and candle making supplies, essential oils, raw ingredients, fragrance and flavor, supplements, unscented bases, containers, and more

Bulk Herb Store

877-278-4257

www.bulkherbstore.com

Organic, wild-crafted, and conventional bulk herbs

Cultures for Health

800-962-1959

www.culturesforhealth.com

Culture supplies, including kefir, kombucha, yogurt, sourdough, cheese, and soy starters

Dr.ChristophersHerbs.com

www.drchristophersherbs.com

My go-to resource for black drawing salve

Frontier Natural Products Co-op

800-669-3275

www.frontiercoop.com

Don't have a natural grocery store or co-op nearby? Never fear! This is a fantastic go-to site for all kinds of organic foods, spices, teas, and cosmetic craft supplies.

Healing Spirits Herb Farm and Education Center

607-566-2701

www.healingspiritsherbfarm.com

Wide variety of herbal teas, tinctures, syrups, cosmetics, supplies, and unusual flower essences, not to mention all kinds of classes if you happen to be in the Finger Lakes Region of New York

Mountain Rose Herbs

800-879-3337

www.mountainroseherbs.com

Bulk herbs, aromatherapy, containers, supplies, bottles, candles, clays, and pretty much anything herb-crafty related

Pacific Botanicals

541-479-7777

www.pacificbotanicals.com

This is another great resource for bulk, organic, or wildcrafted herbs. You can even get fresh herbs for your preparations if you'd like! If you're a professional herbalist without access to enough land on which to grow your own medicinals, Pacific Botanicals can grow or source what you need.

Penn Herb Company

800-523-9971

www.pennherb.com

Herbs, spices, natural remedies, and essential oils

Starwest Botanicals

800-800-4372

www.starwest-botanicals.com

Bulk herbs and botanicals

Research/Education

The American College of Healthcare Sciences

800-487-8839

www.achs.edu

ACHS (my alma mater) was founded in New Zealand in 1978. Now located in Portland, Oregon, it has become a fully accredited college offering holistic health education. The faculty is incredibly diverse, with herbalists from both Eastern and Western traditions. ACHS encourages sustainable, safe, and responsible herbal practices.

Avena Botanicals

866-282-8362

www.avenabotanicals.com

Healing Spirits Herb Farm and Education Center

607-566-2701

www.healingspiritsherbfarm.com

The Medicine Woman's Roots

http://bearmedicineherbals.com

Want to make your own black drawing salve? Here you'll find an authentic recipe using pine pitch.

MindBodyGreen

www.mindbodygreen.com

Articles on natural health/herbs (to which I am a contributor)

Mother Nature Network

www.mnn.com

Natural soap-making tutorials

Quiet Earth Yoga

www.quietearthyoga.com

My website. It is chock-full of all kinds of fun stuff — from blog posts to art, herbal references, yoga fun, and DIY yoga, herbal, and lifestyle videos. Come visit!

Sacred Pregnancy

www.sacredpregnancy.com

This is a great educational resource for all of the green mamas and green mamas-to-be out there. Offerings include classes, an online community, books, magazines, and wellness retreats.

Traditional Chinese Medicine World Foundation

212-274-1079

www.tcmworld.org

Traditional Chinese Medicine originated thousands of years ago and has evolved ever since. TCM practitioners use herbal medicines, acupuncture, meditation, and tai chi to treat or prevent disease. It's a holistic form of medicine, focusing on food, herbs, and mind/body practices.

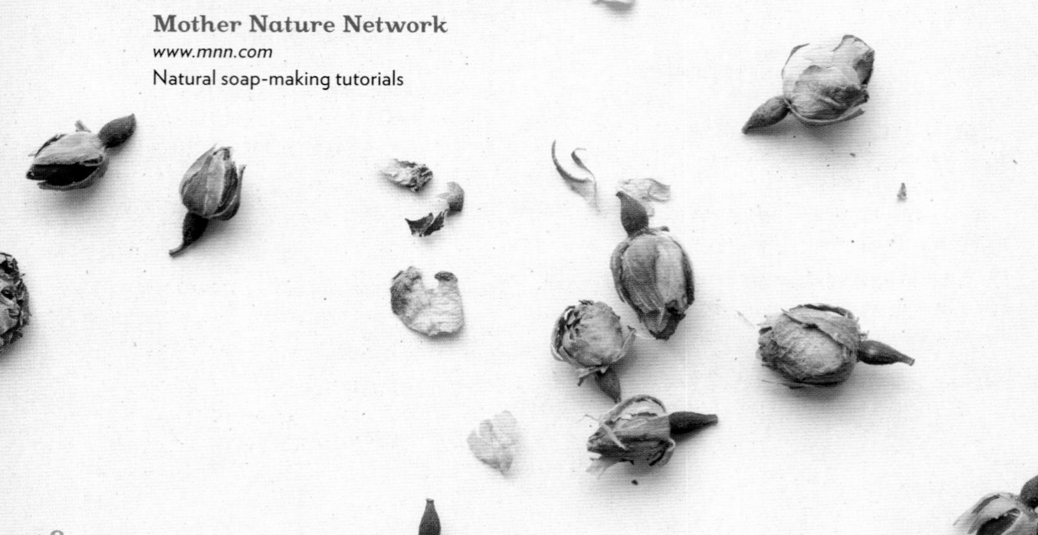

Suggested Reading

Collected here are the invaluable resources I used as I wrote this book. They have been my constant friends since I began this journey in 2002, and I reference them again and again. There is so much out there, so remember: this is by no means a complete list! Follow your own intuition, reading whatever suits your fancy. That's the beautiful thing about the herb world: It's practically boundless and inexhaustible in its applications for the mind, body, and spirit.

Alfs, Matthew. *300 Herbs: Their Indications & Contraindications*. Old Theology Book House, 2003.

Angier, Bradford, and David K. Foster. *Field Guide to Edible Wild Plants*, 2nd ed. Stackpole Books, 2008.

Breedlove, Greta. *The Herbal Home Spa: Naturally Refreshing Wraps, Rubs, Lotions, Masks, Oils, and Scrubs*. Storey Publishing, 1998.

Cech, Richo. *Making Plant Medicine*. Horizon Herbs, 2000.

Cunningham, Scott. *Cunningham's Encyclopedia of Magical Herbs*, rev. ed. Llewellyn Publications, 2012.

Dugan, Ellen. *Garden Witch's Herbal: Green Magick, Herbalism & Spirituality*. Llewellyn Publications, 2009.

Duke, James A. *The Green Pharmacy*. St. Martin's Press, 1997.

Foster, Steven, and James A. Duke. *A Field Guide to Medicinal Plants and Herbs of Eastern and Central North America*, 2nd ed. Houghton Mifflin, 2000.

Grieve, M. *A Modern Herbal, Volumes I & II*. Dover Publications, 1971. First published 1931 by Harcourt, Brace & Company.

Harrison, Karen. *The Herbal Alchemist's Handbook*. Weiser Books, 2011.

Hoffmann, David. *Holistic Herbal*, 3rd ed. Thorsons Publishing, 2002.

Mabey, Richard, ed. *The New Age Herbalist*. Simon & Schuster, 1988.

Scheffer, Mechthild. *Bach Flower Therapy: Theory and Practice*. Healing Arts Press, 1986.

———. *The Encyclopedia of Bach Flower Therapy*. Healing Arts Press, 2001.

Soule, Deb. *A Woman's Book of Herbs: The Healing Power of Natural Remedies*. Carol Publishing, 1998.

Tenney, Louise. *Today's Herbal Health: The Essential Reference Guide*, 6th ed. Woodland Publishing, 2007.

Tourles, Stephanie. *Organic Body Care Recipes: 175 Homemade Herbal Formulas for Glowing Skin & a Vibrant Self*. Storey Publishing, 2007.

Uliano, Sophie. *Do It Gorgeously: How to Make Less Toxic, Less Expensive, and More Beautiful Products*. Hyperion, 2010.

White, Linda B., and Steven Foster. *The Herbal Drugstore*. St. Martin's Press, 2000.

Wood, Matthew. *The Earthwise Herbal: A Complete Guide to Old World Medicinal Plants*. North Atlantic Books, 2008.

———. *The Earthwise Herbal: A Complete Guide to New World Medicinal Plants*. North Atlantic Books, 2009.

Glossary

adaptogen. An herb that helps the body, mind, and spirit adapt to stress. It modifies the response of the body to stressful situations so that peace and calm can prevail.

analgesic. An herb that lessens pain.

antibacterial. Combating bacterial infections in and on the body.

antifungal. Inhibiting fungal growth.

antihistamine. An herb that stops the histamine response to an allergen.

anti-inflammatory. An herb that soothes swelling and inflammation, internally or externally.

antioxidant. A substance in an herb (or any food) that helps the body rid itself of free radicals.

antiviral. Destroying viruses in the body.

astringent. A substance that tightens the tissues of the body — internally and/or externally.

bentonite clay. A powerful healing clay that, when mixed with water, becomes electrically charged and swells into a healing sponge of sorts. Because it carries a negative charge, it will pull impurities, such as heavy metals and toxins, out of the skin.

compress. A cloth that has been soaked in an herbal solution and applied externally to a painful, inflamed, or infected area of the body.

decoction. Basically, a tea that is made by simmering the hardy parts of plants (bark, roots, stems, and seeds) in water for 10 minutes or longer.

demulcent. An herb that soothes mucus membranes with its own brand of mucilaginous qualities.

diaphoretic. An herb that induces sweating (usually used to break a fever).

diuretic. An herb that increases the elimination of water from the body (increases urination).

drawing salve. An herbal salve made with pine tar and renowned for drawing out splinters, insect venom, and infection.

essential oil. The aromatic oil that is distilled from plants.

expectorant. An herb that helps expel mucus from the body, especially in the lungs.

flower essences. Liquid extracts made from the vibrant (and vibrational) energy of fresh flowers, used therapeutically to ease specific mental, emotional, spiritual, and physical issues.

French green clay. A cosmetic clay used in skin-healing and detoxifying preparations, French green clay is a powerful drawer of oil, toxins, and impurities from the skin. Because of this quality, it is best used on oily and troubled skin.

infusion. What we, in the herbal world, call a tea. It's made by steeping herbs in hot water for a period of time.

mucilage. The gelatinous substance found in some herbs that helps soothe mucus membranes of the body.

nervine. An herb that soothes the nervous system.

poultice. An external application of moistened herbs applied to an affected area of the body.

rhizome. Not a root itself, it is the often-fleshy stem that grows horizontally away from the root. It's found just under the surface and has nodes on it from which other stems can grow.

salve. An ointment made by combining an oil extraction of an herb with enough beeswax to make it solid yet malleable.

sedative. An herb that soothes and (often) induces sleep.

stimulant. An herb that acts, in general, to increase action in the body — from energy levels to circulation to eliminating waste.

tincture. A preparation of herbal matter that most often involves alcoholic extraction but can include vinegar, honey, and/or glycerin.

white cosmetic clay. A fine, light clay used in skin-healing and detoxifying preparations. This clay, while a good drawer of toxins, oils, and impurities, is gentle and best suited for dry, sensitive, or mature skin.

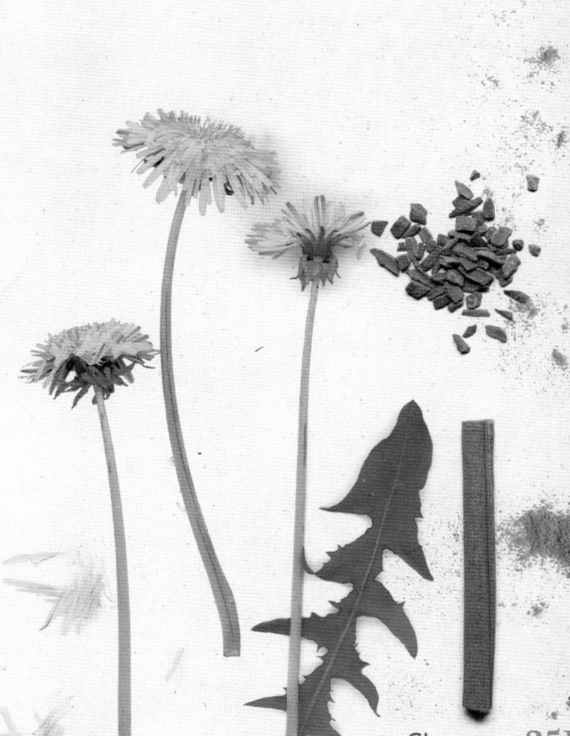

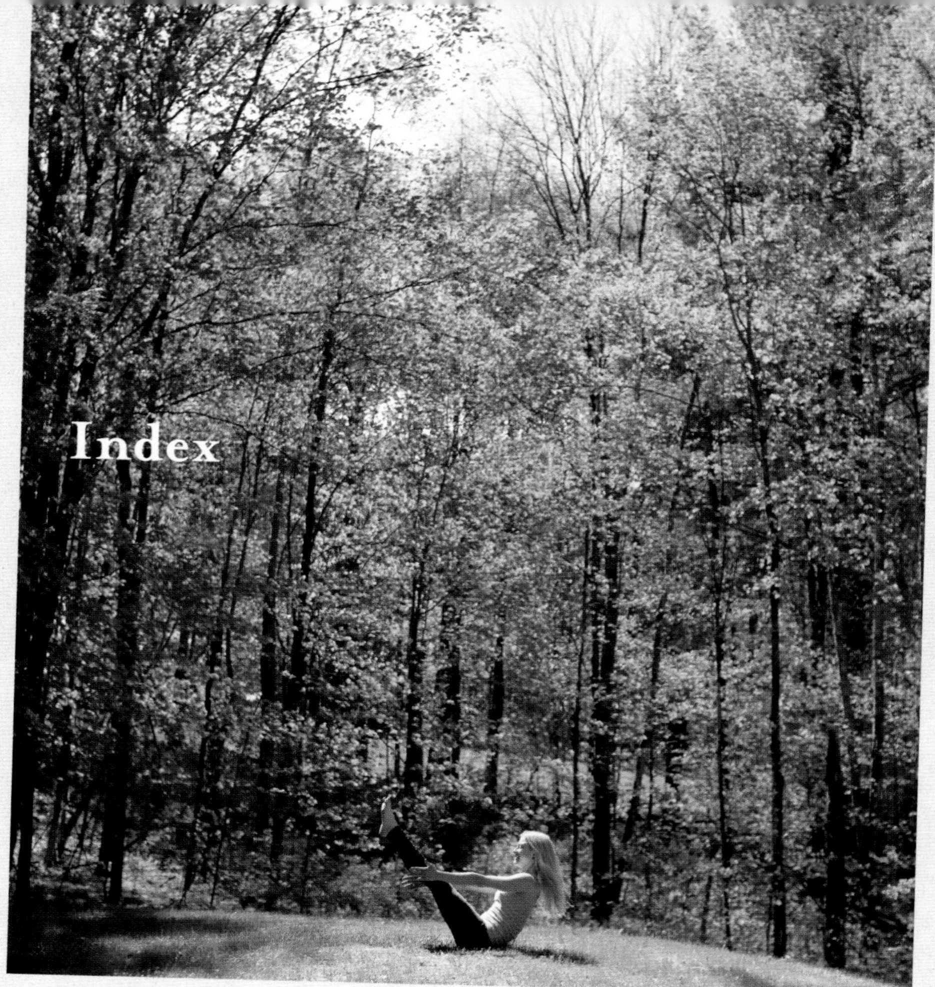

Index

Page numbers in *italic* indicate photos.

a

b

c

d

e

f

g

h

i

j

l

m

n

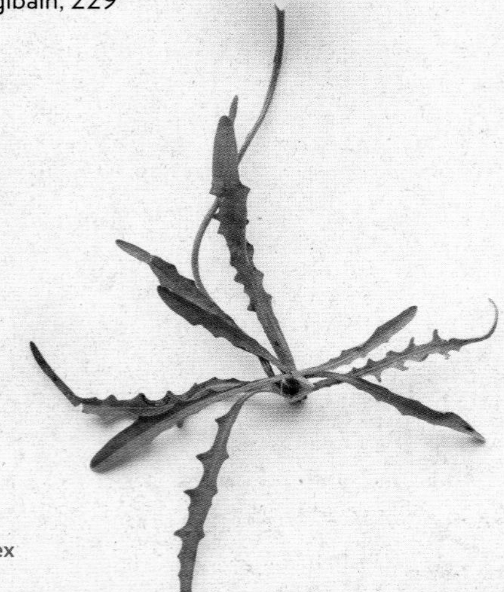

PHOTOGRAPHY CREDITS

© Adam 88xx/iStockphoto.com, 203; © Antonel/iStockphoto.com, 33; Carolyn Eckert, back cover (author photo), 1, 5, 13 (right), 21, 23, 38, 43, 52 (right), 57 (flower), 61, 70, 71, 72, 76 (top), 77 (left), 101, 114 (top), 115, 117, 133, 136, 151 (top), 173, 176–177, 190–191 (everything but herbs), 193, 196, 228 (top), 231; © Dmitris 66/ iStockphoto.com, 18; © If_VISAWAN/ iStockphoto.com, 152; © Joe Biafore/ iStockphoto.com, 238; © John Polak, 47, 134; Mars Vilaubi, 4, 14 (left), 17 (flower), 20, 25, 27, 46, 58, 63, 67, 74 (leaf), 76 (bottom), 77 (right), 80 (leaves), 83, 85, 87, 98, 104, 112 (flowers), 116, 124, 126, 137, 153, 154, 165, 171 (flower), 172 (top), 175, 180 (top), 188, 189, 200, 202, 212 (top), 218, 220, 222–223, 235 (bottom), 248; © Nailia Schwartz/iStockphoto.com, 197; © narinbg/iStockphoto.com, 214; © Patrick GUEDJ/Gamma-Rapho/Getty Images, 150; © Picture Partners/iStockphoto.com, 44, 192 (flower); © Sean Jirsa, 207; © stuartbur/ iStockphoto.com, 157; © Supersmario/ iStockphoto.com, 151 (bottom); © triocean/ iStockphoto.com, 22